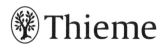

For all of you who continue to ask questions, search for answers, and follow diligently the pursuit of good research practice

Advanced Concepts in Surgical Research

Edited by

Mohit Bhandari, MD, PhD, FRCSC

Professor and Academic Chair
Division of Orthopaedic Surgery
McMaster University
Hamilton, Ontario, Canada

Bernd Robioneck, PhD

Research and Development Leader
Stryker Osteosynthesis
Schönkirchen/Kiel, Germany

Associate Editor:

Emil Schemitsch, MD, FRCSC

Department of Surgery
Division of Orthopaedics
St. Michael's Hospital
Toronto, Ontario, Canada

Managing Editor:

Sheila Sprague, MSc

Program Manager
Department of Clinical Epidemiology and Biostatistics
McMaster University
Hamilton, Ontario, Canada

With contributions by
Volker Alt, Laurent Audigé, Simrit Bains, Lauren A. Beaupre, S. Samuel Bederman, Mohit Bhandari, Dianne Bryant, Brett D. Crist, Monica Daigl, Ivan R. Diamond, Tania A. Ferguson, Rajiv Gandhi, Vanja Gavranic, Anthony Gibson, Charles H. Goldsmith, Ruby Grewal, Jihee Han, Beate P. Hanson, Christian Heiss, Richard Jenkinson, C. Allyson Jones, Ryan M. Khan, Guy Klein, Jennifer Klok, Hans J. Kreder Natalie Kuurstra, Susan M. Liew, Nizar Mahomed, Joy C. MacDermid, Charles T. Mehlman, Kristie More, Saam Morshed, Vanessa K. Noonan, Theodoros Pavlidis, Brad A. Petrisor, Rudolf W. Poolman, Eleanor M. Pullenayegum, Laura Quigley, Shelly-Ann Rampersad, Michel Saccone, Emil Schemitsch, Reinhard Schnettler, Lindsey C. Sheffler, Ujash Sheth, Nicole Simunovic, Gerard P. Slobogean, Holly Smith, Sheila Sprague, Sadeesh K. Srinathan, Michael Stretanski, Gabor Szalay, Steven Takemoto, Christopher Vannabouathong, Daniel Whelan, Meaghan Zehr, Rad Zdero

54 illustrations

Thieme
Stuttgart · New York

Library of Congress Cataloging-in-Publication Data
is available from the publisher.

Illustrations by Karin Baum, Paphos, Cyprus

© 2012 Georg Thieme Verlag KG,
Rüdigerstrasse 14, 70469 Stuttgart, Germany
http://www.thieme.de
Thieme Medical Publishers, Inc., 333 Seventh Avenue,
New York, NY 10001, USA
http://www.thieme.com

Cover design: Thieme Publishing Group

Typesetting by Hagedorn Kommunikation GmbH,
Viernheim, Germany

Printed in Italy by L.E.G.O., Vicenza

ISBN 978-3-13-165811-1
eISBN 978-3-13-167021-2

Foreword

Real progress in clinical care can only occur when there is solid evidence to support a change in treatment. This is especially true in surgical care, and some have estimated that up to 15 years are often required to implement a substantial positive change in orthopaedic care. Sudden changes in surgical treatment sometimes do result from aggressive commercial marketing programs or from the persuasive podium presentations of noted surgeons. Unfortunately, however, many of these changes have not been based on solid evidence and often they have proven to be no better, or even worse, than the treatment they replaced. For orthopaedic care to advance, sophisticated clinical research must be conducted to provide the foundation for effective innovations that will enhance the care of our patients.

This textbook provides an easy-to-follow road map for the orthopaedic surgeon who is interested in pursuing productive and worthwhile clinical research. In a very logical sequence, it presents a substantial number of ways to address important clinical questions, and it provides effective alternatives, in addition to conducting randomized clinical trials, that can be used to arrive at the answer to those questions in the most timely and cost-effective fashion. The text is written in a style that is very comprehensible and "reader friendly," allowing those of us who are less familiar with the concepts presented to adopt and feel comfortable with them. The research methods presented in this text are the best we currently have available, and the surgeon who employs them will discover that his or her results are more likely to be accepted as valid, be adopted in the care of patients, and endure the test of time than the results arrived at using the less effective methods of clinical investigation that we have been limited to in the past.

James D. Heckman, MD
Consulting Editor, The Journal of Bone and Joint Surgery

Preface

The purpose of this book is to provide surgical researchers with a practical and straightforward guide to understanding the advanced principles and concepts of surgical research. This book is the third book in our series on clinical research methods for surgeons. The first book in this series focused on the basic principles of health research methodology and evidence-based surgery. The second was a practical guide to preparing and publishing manuscripts in peer-reviewed journals. The present book is designed to expand upon the principles discussed in the first two, focusing on the advanced concepts relevant to surgical research.

This unique book has been written by surgical experts and is designed to provide a roadmap for the challenging concepts relevant to surgical research. The first part focuses on advanced concepts relevant to randomized controlled trials including factorial trials, expertise-based trials, randomization systems, blinding and concealment, adjudication of outcomes, subgroup analysis, and trial management. The second part details different study designs such as case–control studies, cohort studies, surveys, qualitative studies, and economic analyses. The third part of the book focuses on advanced concepts relevant to conducting systematic reviews and meta-analyses. Advanced statistical concepts are also presented, focusing on the importance of developing a statistical analysis plan, regression analysis, survival analysis, and interim analyses. The book concludes with advice on the proper reporting of surgical research, which includes discussion on conflict-of-interest reporting, modern approaches to authorship, and relevant reporting checklists. We are confident that this text will smoothly guide you to successful completion of your research initiatives.

Mohit Bhandari, MD, PhD, FRCSC
Bernd Robioneck, PhD

Acknowledgments

A special thank you to our administrative staff, Katelyn Godin, Sarah Resendes, Mike Saccone, Denise Shih, and Meaghan Zehr for all of their diligent work.

List of Contributors

Editors

Mohit Bhandari MD, PhD, FRCSC
Professor and Academic Chair
Division of Orthopaedic Surgery
McMaster University
Hamilton, Ontario, Canada

Bernd Robioneck, PhD
Research and Development Leader
Stryker Osteosynthesis
Schönkirchen/Kiel, Germany

Associate Editor

Emil Schemitsch MD, FRCSC
Department of Surgery, Division of Orthopaedics
St. Michael's Hospital
Toronto, Ontario, Canada

Managing Editor

Sheila Sprague, MSc
Program Manager
Department of Clinical Epidemiology and Biostatistics
McMaster University
Hamilton, Ontario, Canada

Contributors

Volker Alt, MD, PhD
Professor
Department of Trauma Surgery
University Hospital Giessen-Marburg GmbH
Campus Giessen
Giessen, Germany

Laurent Audigé, DVM, PhD
Senior Research Fellow
Upper Extremities
Schulthess Klinik
Zürich, Switzerland

Simrit Bains, MA, MD cand
Department of Surgery
McMaster University
Hamilton, Ontario, Canada

Lauren A. Beaupre, PT, PhD
Associate Professor
Department of Physical Therapy
Faculty of Rehabilitation
Adjunct Assistant Professor
Department of Surgery (Division of Orthopaedic Surgery)
Faculty of Medicine and Dentistry
University of Alberta
Edmonton, Alberta, Canada

S. Samuel Bederman, MD, PhD, FRCSC
Assistant Professor
Department of Orthopaedic Surgery
University of California, Irvine
Orange, California, USA

Mohit Bhandari, MD, PhD, FRCSC
Professor and Academic Chair
Division of Orthopaedic Surgery
McMaster University
Hamilton, Ontario, Canada

Dianne Bryant, PhD
Director, EmPower Health Research
School of Physical Therapy and Department of Surgery
University of Western Ontario
London, Ontario, Canada
Department of Epidemiology and Biostatistics
McMaster University
Hamilton, Ontario, Canada

Brett D. Crist, MD, FACS
Associate Professor
Co-Director of Trauma Services
Co-Director Orthopaedic Trauma Fellowship
Department of Orthopaedic Surgery
Columbia, Missouri, USA

Monica Daigl, MSc, GradStat
Clinical Data and Statistics Manager
AO Clinical Investigation and Documentation
AO Foundation,
Dübendorf, Switzerland

Ivan R. Diamond, MD, PhD
Resident, Diagnostic Radiology
Department of Medical Imaging
University of Toronto
Toronto, Ontario, Canada

Tania A. Ferguson, MD, MAS
Assistant Professor
Department of Orthopaedic Surgery
University of California
Davis, California, USA

Rajiv Gandhi, MD, MS, FRCSC
Assistant Professor
Division of Orthopaedic Surgery
Toronto Western Hospital
Toronto, Ontario, Canada

Vanja Gavranic, BHSc, MSc cand
Department of Surgery
McMaster University
Hamilton, Ontario, Canada

Anthony Gibson, MBBS
Research Specialist
Department of Orthopaedic Surgery
University of California at San Francisco
San Francisco, California, USA

Charles H. Goldsmith, PhD
Clinical Epidemiology and Biostatistics
McMaster University
Hamilton, Ontario, Canada
Faculty of Health Sciences
Simon Fraser University
Burnaby, British Columbia, Canada

Ruby Grewal, MSc, MD, FRCSC
Assistant Professor, Division of Orthopedic Surgery
University of Western Ontario
Hand and Upper Limb Center, St Joseph's Health Care
London, Ontario, Canada

Jihee Han, BSc
Department of Surgery
McMaster University
Hamilton, Ontario, Canada

Beate P. Hanson, MD, MPH
Clinical Epidemiologist
Assistant Professor
Director of AO Clinical Investigation and Documentation
AO Foundation
AO Clinical Investigation and Documentation
Dübendorf, Switzerland

Christian Heiss, MD
Professor
Department of Trauma Surgery
University Hospital Giessen-Marburg GmbH
Campus Giessen
Giessen, Germany

Richard Jenkinson, BSc, MD, FRCS(C)
Lecturer, University of Toronto
Division of Orthopaedic Surgery
Sunnybrook Health Sciences Center
Toronto, Ontario, Canada

C. Allyson Jones, PT, PhD
Associate Professor
Department of Physical Therapy
Faculty of Rehabilitation Medicine
University of Alberta
Edmonton, Alberta, Canada

Ryan M. Khan, CCRP
Orthopaedic Research Coordinator
St. Michael's Hospital
Toronto, Ontario, Canada

Guy Klein, DO
Resident, Orthopaedic Surgery
University Hospitals, Richmond Medical Center
Richmond Heights, Ohio, USA

Jennifer Klok, MD, MSc
Department of Surgery
Division of Plastic Surgery
University of Ottawa
Ottawa, Ontario, Canada

Hans J. Kreder, MD, MPH, FRCS(C)
Professor, University of Toronto
Orthopaedic Surgery and Health Policy Management
and Evaluation
Chief, Holland Musculoskeletal Program
Marvin Tile Chair and Chief, Division of Orthopaedic
Surgery
Sunnybrook Health Sciences Center
Toronto, Ontario, Canada

Natalie Kuurstra, BA
Department of Surgery
McMaster University
Hamilton, Ontario, Canada

Susan M. Liew, MBBS (hons), FRACS (Orth)
Director Orthopaedic Surgery
The Alfred
Adjunct Clinical Associate Professor
Monash University
Prahran, Australia

Nizar Mahomed, MD, ScD, FRCSC
Nicky & Bryce Douglas Chair In Orthopaedic Surgery
Smith & Nephew Chair In Orthopaedic Surgery
Professor, Department of Surgery
University of Toronto
Head, Division of Orthopaedics
Arthritis Program Managing Director
Altum Health Toronto Western Hospital
University Health Network
Toronto, Ontario, Canada

Joy C. MacDermid, PT, PhD
Professor, Assistant Dean of Rehabilition Science
School of Rehabilitation, McMaster University
Hamilton, Ontario, Canada
Co-director of Clinical Research
Hand and Upper Limb Center, St Joseph's Health Care
London, Ontario, Canada

Charles T. Mehlman, DO, MPH
Director, Musculoskeletal Outcomes Research;
Co-Director, Brachial Plexus Center
Professor, Department of Pediatric Orthopaedic Surgery
Cincinnati Children's Hospital Medical Center
Cincinnati, Ohio, USA

Kristie More, MSc
Orthopaedic Research Coordinator
University of Calgary Sport Medicine Centre
Calgary, Alberta, Canada

Saam Morshed, MD, PhD, MPH
Assistant Professor in Residence
University of California San Francisco and San Francisco
General Hospital
Orthopaedic Trauma Institute
San Francisco, California, USA

Vanessa K. Noonan, PhD, PT
Department of Orthopaedics
University of British Columbia
Blusson Spinal Cord Center
Vancouver, British Columbia, Canada

Theodoros Pavlidis, MD
Department of Trauma Surgery
University Hospital Giessen-Marburg GmbH
Campus Giessen
Giessen, Germany

Brad A. Petrisor, MSc, MD, FRCSC
Associate Professor
Division of Orthopaedic Surgery
McMaster University
Hamilton Health Sciences – General Site
Hamilton, Ontario, Canada

Rudolf W. Poolman, MD, PhD
Director of Clinical Research
Joint Research, Department of Orthopaedic Surgery
Onze Lieve Vrouwe Gasthuis
Amsterdam, The Netherlands

Eleanor M. Pullenayegum, PhD
Department of Clinical Epidemiology and Biostatistics
McMaster University
Hamilton, Ontario, Canada

Laura Quigley, MSc, MD cand
Faculty of Medicine
University of Toronto
Toronto, Ontario, Canada

Shelly-Ann Rampersad, BSc
Department of Clinical Epidemiology and Biostatistics
McMaster University
Hamilton, Ontario, Canada

Michel Saccone, BSc
Department of Clinical Epidemiology and Biostatistics
McMaster University
Hamilton, Ontario, Canada

Emil Schemitsch, MD, FRCSC
Professor of Surgery
University of Toronto
Department of Surgery, Division of Orthopaedics
St. Michael's Hospital
Toronto, Ontario, Canada

Reinhard Schnettler, MD, DVM
Professor
Director, Department of Trauma Surgery
University Hospital Giessen-Marburg GmbH
Campus Giessen
Giessen, Germany

Lindsey C. Sheffler, BS, MAS
Resident Physician
Department of Orthopaedic Surgery
University of California, San Francisco
San Francisco, California, USA

Ujash Sheth, BHSc, MD cand
Department of Surgery
McMaster University
Hamilton, Ontario, Canada

Nicole Simunovic, MSc
Department of Clinical Epidemiology and Biostatistics
McMaster University
Hamilton, Ontario, Canada

Gerard P. Slobogean, MD, MPH, FRCSC
Department of Orthopaedics
University of British Columbia
Vancouver, British Columbia, Canada

Holly Smith, BSc cand, MD cand
Research Associate
Division of Orthopaedic Surgery
Toronto Western Hospital
Toronto, Ontario, Canada

Sheila Sprague, MSc
Program Manager
Department of Clinical Epidemiology and Biostatistics
McMaster University
Hamilton, Ontario, Canada

Sadeesh K. Srinathan, MD, MSc, FRCS(C-Th), FRSC(C)
Assistant Professor of Surgery
Department of Surgery, Section of Thoracic Surgery
University of Manitoba
Winnipeg, Manitoba, Canada

Michael Stretanski, DO
Medical Director; Fellowship Director
Interventional Spine and Pain Rehabilitation Center
Mansfield, Ohio, USA

Gabor Szalay, MD
Department of Trauma Surgery Giessen
University Hospital Giessen-Marburg GmbH
Campus Giessen
Giessen, Germany

Steven Takemoto, PhD
Associate Professor
Director of Clinical Outcomes
Department of Orthopaedic Surgery
University of California, San Francisco
San Francisco, California, USA

Christopher Vannabouathong, BSc
Department of Surgery
McMaster University
Hamilton, Ontario, Canada

Daniel Whelan, MD, FRCS(C)
Assistant Professor, University of Toronto
Staff Physician, St. Michael's Hospital
Division of Orthopaedic Surgery
Toronto, Ontario, Canada

Rad Zdero, PhD
Martin Orthopaedic Biomechanics Laboratory
St. Michael's Hospital
Toronto, Ontario, Canada

Meaghan Zehr, BSc cand
Department of Clinical Epidemiology and Biostatistics
McMaster University
Hamilton, Ontario, Canada

Abbreviations

AAMC	Association of American Medical Colleges
ACE	angiotensin-converting enzyme
AMA	American Medical Association
ANOVA	analysis of variance
AAOS	American Academy of Orthopaedic Surgeons
ASA	American Society of Anesthesiologists
BMD	bone mineral density
CIHR	Canadian Institutes of Health Research
CI	confidence interval
CME	continuing medical education
CMS	Center for Medicare and Medicaid Services
CRO	contract research organization
DSMB	Data and Safety Monitoring Board
EBM	evidence-based medicine
FDA	Food and Drug Administration
HIPAA	Health Insurance Portability and Accountability Act (USA)
HLA	human leukocyte antigen
HR	hazard ratio
ICD	International Classification of Disease (in full: International Statistical Classification of Diseases and Related Health Problems)
ICMJE	International Committee of Medical Journal Editors
IRB	institutional review board (United States)
IU	international units
LCP	locking compression plate
MCID	minimum clinically important difference
MIT	Massachusetts Institute of Technology
NIH	National Institutes of Health
NPT	nonpharmacologic trial
NSAID	nonsteroidal anti-inflammatory drug
OR	odds ratio
RBC	red blood cell
RCT	randomized controlled trial
REB	research ethics board (Canada)
REC	research ethics committee
ROC	receiver-operating characteristic
ROR	ratio of odds ratios
RRR	ratio of relative risks
SAP	statistical analysis plan
SHS	sliding hip screw
SI	Système International
SMD	standardized mean difference
VAS	visual analogue scale

Table of Contents

1

Factorial Randomized Trials

Hans J. Kreder, Richard Jenkinson

Summary

Researchers have four options when faced with multiple questions or interventions that affect a particular outcome of interest: (1) run sequential randomized controlled trials (RCTs), (2) run parallel multiple RCTs, (3) test a combination of "new" treatments against the old combination of interventions, and (4) perform a factorial RCT. A factorial design involves assigning each study subject to receive a random combination of treatments, one for each study question. In this way two or more study questions can be answered with the sample size required to answer just one question. The study questions must not involve mutually exclusive treatments (e.g., operative and nonoperative interventions). Since all patients receive more than one intervention, it is possible to look specifically for interactions across treatments. However, if one hopes to power the trial sufficiently to detect an interaction, the sample size must be increased. For example, to have sufficient power to detect an interaction of the same magnitude as the main effects, the sample size would need to quadruple. Factorial RCTs represent an efficient way to answer two or more questions for the price of one when one is not expecting a clinically important treatment interaction.

Introduction

Randomized controlled clinical trials represent the best way to determine which one of two or more competing treatment options is better because this is the only design that controls for selection bias.[1]

Jargon Simplified: Selection Bias
Selection bias may occur when the study and control group subjects differ in the distribution of factors that might affect a given outcome of interest. These factors may be unknown or unmeasurable (e.g., motivation). Selection bias can only be controlled by random allocation into treatment groups such that each subject (with known and unknown characteristics) has an equal chance of being in either treatment group.

Well-powered randomized trials are generally expensive and may take years to complete. Clinical researchers and those funding research have a responsibility to ensure that important clinical questions are addressed through an efficient research design that provides timely, definitive, and implementable solutions, thus maximizing return on research investment. Most often RCTs are designed to address a question that involves a comparison of two treatments whereby subjects are simply randomized to one or the other of the two competing treatment options (e.g., to answer the question whether infection after open fracture is better prevented by high-pressure or low-pressure irrigation).

Jargon Simplified: Study Question
In the context of a clinical trial, a study question is one pertaining to the relationship between interventions and an outcome of interest. A study question usually involves two or more interventions (e.g., is intervention A better than intervention B? Is intervention A better than control?).

Jargon Simplified: Intervention
An intervention is a specific treatment (or placebo) administered to a study subject. A study question usually involves two or more competing interventions.

However, often there are additional questions that concern the same outcome (is infection after open fracture better prevented by saline or soap irrigation?), or a question may involve multiple treatment options (gravity irrigation versus low-pressure or high-pressure irrigation). There are several options when faced with multiple interventions that may affect a given outcome of interest. The factorial randomized design is a particularly efficient method in this circumstance, when applicable.

Jargon Simplified: Randomized controlled trial (RCT)
An RCT is an experiment in which individuals are randomly allocated to receive or not receive an experimental diagnostic, preventive, therapeutic, or palliative procedure and are then followed to determine the effect of the intervention.[2]

Jargon Simplified: Factorial RCT
In a factorial RCT, two or more study questions are answered at the same time within the same group of study subjects without the need for increased sample size (in the absence of interactions between the interventions to which the study questions relate).

The purpose of this chapter is to provide an overview of factorial RCT design as an option for addressing multiple interventions with respect to an outcome of interest.

Randomized Clinical Trial Design Strategies with Multiple Interventions

The rate of infection following open fractures is likely affected by multiple factors, one of which is the technique of irrigation. Let us assume that we have two specific questions regarding the irrigation procedure with respect to infection rates: a) should we use high-pressure or low-pressure irrigation, and b) is saline or soap better as an irrigating fluid? There are four possible randomized clinical study design strategies to address these two questions (involving four treatment options).

Thus question 1 (Q1) concerning the irrigation pressure has two intervention arms (P1 versus P2) and question 2 (Q2) compares two solutions (S1 versus S2). Let us assume that a power calculation suggests that Q1 requires 150 subjects in each arm and Q2 requires 100 in each arm.

Option 1: Sequential Randomized Trials

This strategy involves answering question 1 and then question 2. The second trial would standardize whatever the best treatment was from the first trial across both of the new treatment groups. The total sample size to answer both questions is the sum of patients enrolled in the two trials (N = 500 in our example). Please refer to **Fig. 1.1** for the first step in this strategy.

This trial is expected to identify the best irrigation pressure, which will subsequently be adopted as the standardized pressure to use in clinical practice (and in future clinical trials). **Figure 1.2** depicts the second step in this strategy.

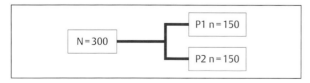

Fig. 1.1 Step 1 (Q1): clinical trial of P1 versus P2 ("Which pressure should be used?")

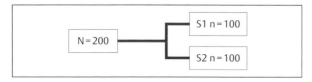

Fig. 1.2 Step 2 (Q2): clinical trial of S1 versus S2 ("Which solution should be used?")

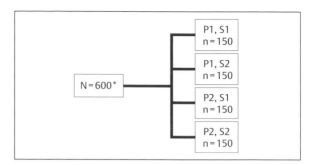

Fig. 1.3 Parallel randomized trials. *Note that adjusting for multiple comparisons would increase sample size requirements. With four groups, six comparisons are possible.

Option 2: Parallel Randomized Trials

This strategy involves comparing the possible combinations of treatments in a single trial. In the absence of more specific information, the sample size would probably need to be based on the more conservative estimate of 150 patients per treatment group. Note that the four group outcomes lead to six comparisons to identify the best group. If one adjusts for multiple comparisons, the sample size would be increased well above N = 600 (**Fig. 1.3**).

Option 3: New Treatment Combination versus Control Combination

This strategy is best applied in a situation where two or more treatments are new and can be compared to older/control treatments. It would not apply to our previous example since both high-pressure and low-pressure irrigation are commonly used and thus no "control" pressure can be identified (although saline might be considered the "control" irrigating solution type).

For a better example, let us assume that we wish to decrease length of stay as an outcome following primary total hip replacement surgery. Let us further assume that our patients have been receiving a standardized education package, a routine rehabilitation protocol, and that a standard surgical approach has been used. A new education package has been developed, a more aggressive rehabilitation protocol is being considered, and less invasive surgery has been promoted. All of these innovations may improve length of stay and they could be evaluated sequentially (best education, then best rehab, and finally best surgery) or in a parallel design with the three interventions combined into eight possible treatment groups to be assessed simultaneously. This might indeed be the best option if the new strategies were extremely costly or labor intensive, and if one would only consider using one or more of them for routine clinical practice if they were shown to be significantly superior to previous cheaper methods. However, if this is not the case, and there is no compelling reason to consider the new interventions separately, one

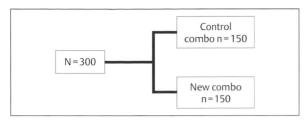

Fig. 1.4 New treatment combination versus control combination.

might simply test the new combination against the old (control) treatments. Using similar sample size considerations as in the previous example we would require N = 300 patients (**Fig. 1.4**).

Option 4: Factorial Randomized Design

Factorial randomized design represents an efficient way of answering two or more questions independently within the same overall trial without the need for increased sample size (unless one is specifically looking for an interaction —see below). The sample size is determined by the question that requires the most patients to answer. In our hypothetical example of irrigating options for open fractures, we require 150 subjects per treatment arm to evaluate the pressure (Q1) and 100 subjects per treatment arm to evaluate the solution (Q2). Using a factorial design we can answer both questions with a total of 300 subjects in a single trial, resulting in potential savings in cost and time compared to a sequential or parallel multiarm design (options 1 and 2 above) (**Fig. 1.5**).

In a factorial randomized design, the patient groups look identical to the groups formed in the parallel four-arm study design. However, the analysis is completely different in that the marginal results are the only outcomes of interest and the two questions are treated as two separate studies—but with the same subjects contributing to both study questions.

		Pressure N = 300		
		P1	**P2**	
Solution N = 300	**S1**	n = 75	n = 75	150
	S2	n = 75	n = 75	150
		150	150	

Fig. 1.5 Factorial randomized design.

Selecting a Factorial Randomized Design

Indications and Considerations

A factorial randomized clinical trial design should be considered whenever two or more questions involving the same outcome are being considered for a given patient population. Thus far we have discussed only questions with two competing treatments leading to a simple 2 × 2 factorial matrix table. For a 2 × 2 factorial design, two comparisons are made (one for each question). The factorial design can be extended in two ways: a) by increasing the number of questions and b) by increasing the number of interventions within each question beyond the minimum of two interventions.

While it is possible to consider more than two questions at the same time, the complexity of the resulting trial increases exponentially beyond a 2 × 2 factorial design. A factorial trial design with three questions (as in our total hip replacement example above: education, rehabilitation and surgical approach) results in 2 × 2 × 2 or eight cells. Four questions result in 2 × 2 × 2 × 2 = 16 cells. Nonetheless, if each question has only two interventions or levels (a term often used for ordinal variables such as drug concentration), the number of final comparisons is equal to the number of questions (old versus new education, old versus new rehabilitation, and standard versus less invasive surgery). If there are more than two interventions or levels involved in each question, the trial complexity is also increased as more cells and more comparisons are added. Our 2 × 2 example above of irrigation for open fractures is actually based on the Fluid Lavage of Open Wounds (FLOW) trial, a 2 × 3 factorial trial design where the pressure had been divided into three groups (gravity, low-pressure pulsatile lavage, and high-pressure pulsatile lavage).[3] Thus the final comparisons for this trial would be: Question 1) soap versus saline, and Question 2a) gravity versus low-pressure pulsatile, 2b) gravity versus high-pressure pulsatile, and 2c) low-pressure pulsatile versus high-pressure pulsatile lavage. If both questions had three levels there would be a total of six comparisons (three for each question). The complexity of the trial must be weighed against the expected gains in efficiency. However, one must also consider the need to adjust sample size for multiple comparisons when multiple questions and/or levels are involved.

Contraindications

To use a factorial design, the questions being considered cannot involve mutually exclusive treatments. For example, a factorial design would not be possible if any one of the intervention groups required an operative treatment for one question plus a nonoperative treatment for the other, since both cannot be effected in the same person (one cannot treat a fracture both operatively *and* nonoperatively). The questions should also concern the same outcome or outcomes. If multiple outcomes are being used, all outcomes should be relevant to all questions for the factorial design to be useful.

Design Considerations: Interactions

The basic conduct of a factorial randomized trial is similar to that of other randomized clinical trial designs with respect to the basic methodology and conduct of the trial, including the process of randomization (to one of the combined treatment groups). Block randomization and stratification can be used as required.[3,4]

Sample size calculations are generally based on the main treatment effect that requires the largest sample size. In our hypothetical example of irrigation variables for open fractures, the main treatment effects are irrigation pressure (low versus high) and the type of irrigant used (saline versus soap). An interaction occurs when the combined effect of two interventions is more than simply additive. For example, let us assume for the moment that high pressure and soap solution are better than their alternatives in our hypothetical open fracture study. If, under these assumptions, soap were much more effective at high pressure than at low pressure, this would be an example of a synergistic interaction that could increase the magnitude of the observed main treatment effect for both high pressure and soap solution (high pressure and soap still look better but they look even more so than the additive effect of either one alone). Alternatively, if soap worked very poorly in the presence of high pressure, the interaction is antagonistic and the observed magnitude of the main treatment effects for high pressure and soap are reduced (high pressure and soap still look better but much less so than the additive effect of either one alone). If a negative interaction is very strong, the main treatment effect may actually be reversed such that low pressure looks better than high pressure, or saline appears to be superior to soap, when in fact the opposite would be observed if pressure and solution were evaluated in the absence of each other. In most factorial randomized clinical trial designs, interactions are anticipated to be small and sample size may be based only on the main treatment effect.[1,5,6]

Given that study participants in a factorial randomized clinical trial receive both treatments simultaneously, it is possible to test for an interaction effect, but sample size calculations based only on the main effects will rarely elicit a statistically significant interaction effect. To look specifically for a significant interaction, one needs to increase the sample size accordingly. For a given sample size (based only on the main effects), one can only detect an interaction effect that is twice as large as the main effects. To detect an interaction that has the same effect size as the main effects, the sample size needs to quadruple.[6]

Jargon Simplified: Interaction

A statistical interaction between two variables occurs when the combined effect of two interventions is more than simply additive. If the combined effect augments the outcome, the interaction is synergistic. If the combined effect is weaker, the interaction is antagonistic.

Key Concepts: Sample Size for Detecting an Interaction

To look specifically for a significant interaction, one needs to increase the sample size accordingly.

		Pressure	Pressure	
		P1	**P2**	
Solution	**S1**	Mean primary outcome score		Mean S1 (precision)
Solution	**S2**			Mean S2 (precision)
		Mean P1 (precision)	Mean P2 (precision)	

Fig. 1.6 A 2 × 2 matrix.

Analytical Considerations and Presentation of Results

The CONSORT guidelines should be followed in the presentation of all clinical trial results to account for all participants entered into the trial.[7] A table of baseline characteristics should be presented. Given that there are generally too many relevant variables to fit into the treatment group matrix, the treatments can be presented side by side (**Table 1.1**).

Jargon Simplified: CONSORT (Consolidated Standards of Reporting Trials)

The CONSORT group has articulated various widely accepted standards for the reporting of clinical trials. The CONSORT statement can be found at http://www.consort-statement.org/.

As with all studies, the analysis for a factorial randomized clinical trial should address the principal research questions (two questions for a 2 × 2 factorial design). Given that there are usually a small number of primary and secondary research questions, it may be possible to present the crude results in a 2 × 2 matrix table, recognizing that it is only the marginal information that is useful in addressing the study questions (**Fig 1.6**). Alternatively the crude outcome information can also be presented side by side.

While a 2 × 2 factorial randomized clinical trial involves four groups of patients, it is incorrect to analyze these groups as if they were part of a parallel four-arm clinical trial (six pairwise comparisons). A factorial design is powered only to evaluate the main treatment effects (unless

sample size adjustments have been made specifically to evaluate interactions). Only two main effect comparisons should be made in a 2 × 2 factorial trial using the marginal results to address the original two questions.

The final analysis may simply involve a comparison of means, although linear and logistic regression or time-dependent analysis can also be performed, depending on the study question and whether adjustments for baseline characteristics or scores have been included in the model.[1,3,5,6] Experiments that extend beyond the 2 × 2 factorial design require multiple pairwise comparisons and should be adjusted for multiple comparisons. Presentation of the final results depends to a large degree on the specific study design, but should include some measure of the magnitude of the difference and the precision associated with the measure. Time-dependent information is often best presented graphically as a survival curve.

Finally, as noted above, unless the trial is specifically powered to detect an interaction, it is unlikely that an interaction can be detected unless it is large. Nonetheless, it is usually recommended to test for an interaction and to report the magnitude and precision (the latter expected to be poor). It is important to note that failure to detect a statistically significant interaction cannot be interpreted as showing the absence of such, given that the power to detect an interaction is low (unless the sample size was specifically developed with sufficient power in mind to detect an interaction of a specific magnitude with appropriate precision).

Table 1.1 Baseline characteristics

	Treatment	Treatment	Treatment	Treatment	Treatment	Treatment
	Pressure, N = 300	**Pressure,** N = 300		**Solution,** N = 300	**Solution,** N = 300	
	P1, n = 150	**P2**, n = 150	*P* **value**	**S1**, n = 150	**S2**, n = 150	*P* **value**
Age						
Gender						
Etc.						

Examples from the Literature: Effect of High-Dosage Cholecalciferol and Extended Physiotherapy on Complications after Hip Fracture

Below is an example of a factorial randomized controlled trial, conducted by Bischoff-Ferrari and colleagues.

Source: Bischoff-Ferrari HA, Dawson-Hughes B, Platz A, Orav EJ, Stähelin HB, Willett WC, et al. Effect of high-dosage cholecalciferol and extended physiotherapy on complications after hip fracture: a randomized controlled trial. Arch Intern Med 2010;170:813–820.

Objective: To compare both the effect of different physiotherapy (PT) regimes and different dosing regimes on rates of falls and readmission after hip fracture.

Participants: One hundred seventy-three patients older than 65 agreeing to be randomized after treatment for an acute hip fracture.

Interventions: 1. Extended physiotherapy (60 minutes/day during acute care and an unsupervised home program) versus standard physiotherapy (30 minutes per day during acute care and no home program). 2. Higher-dose vitamin D (2000 IU/day) versus standard-dose vitamin D (800 IU/day).

Design: Single-center randomized controlled trial with four groups structured according to a factorial design. Group 1: extended PT and high-dose vitamin D; group 2: extended PT and standard-dose vitamin D; group 3: standard PT and high-dose vitamin D; group 4: standard PT and standard-dose vitamin D.

Outcomes: Over 12 months of follow-up the number of falls (primary outcome), and number of hospital readmissions (secondary outcome) were recorded using monthly telephone follow-up and patient diaries. Fall and readmission rates were compared using multivariable model (Poisson) techniques to control for age, sex, body mass index, baseline vitamin D, living situation, and time enrolled in trial.

Results: Extended versus standard physiotherapy reduced fall rates by 25% (95% CI –44% to –1%). Extended versus standard physiotherapy did not affect readmission rates (95% CI –33% to 73%). High-dose versus standard-dose vitamin D did not reduce fall rates (95% CI –4% to 68%) but did reduce hospital readmissions by 39% (95% CI –62% to –1%).

Interpretation: The factorial design allowed the investigators to explore the effect of two different interventions in the same study population simultaneously within one trial. Their findings suggest that fall rates could be reduced with a more extensive physiotherapy regime but not necessarily with higher-dose vitamin D supplementation. Among these hip fracture patients, hospital readmission rates were reduced with higher-dose vitamin D supplementation but not with more extensive physiotherapy. It should be noted that, although statistically significant ($P < 0.05$), the confidence intervals are wide and include almost no difference (0%) for the outcomes of fall and readmission rates in the positive results. Further study is warranted to define more precisely the magnitude of improvement in falls and readmissions that these interventions can offer.

Conclusion

Factorial randomized clinical trials are under-utilized in orthopaedic clinical trials, and should be considered as an efficient study strategy when two or more clinical questions pertain to a given outcome of interest. The questions can involve nominal treatments or ordinal levels (such as drug concentration or irrigation pressure). While it is theoretically possible to consider multiple questions and multiple levels, extending the factorial design much beyond the minimum 2 × 2 design becomes increasingly complex. An important consideration when calculating sample size for a factorial trial design is whether or not one is specifically interested in detecting an interaction with good precision (and what effect size one is interested in). A trial powered only for the main effects will have limited ability to detect an interaction, but this is usually acceptable. Apart from the initial design considerations, conduct of the trial follows the usual protocols for all randomized clinical trials. Researchers and funders have a responsibility to maximize the return on the investment involved in each study. A factorial randomized design is a technique that, if applicable, can answer two clinical questions "for the price of one" in some cases.

Suggested Reading

Gurusamy KS, Gluud C, Nikolova D, Davidson BR. Design of surgical randomized controlled trials involving multiple interventions. J Surg Res 2011;165(1):118–127

Montgomery AA, Peters TJ, Little P. Design, analysis and presentation of factorial randomised controlled trials. BMC Med Res Methodol 2003;3:26

Torgerson DJ & Torgerson C. Designing Randomised Trials in Health, Education and the Social Sciences: An Introduction. Basingstoke [England], New York: Palgrave Macmillan; 2008

References

1. Torgerson DJ, Torgerson C. Designing Randomised Trials in Health, Education and the Social Sciences: An Introduction. Basingstoke [England], New York: Palgrave Macmillan; 2008

2. Guyatt GH, Rennie D, Meade M, Cook D, eds. Users' Guide to the Medical Literature: A Manual for Evidence-Based Clinical Practice. 2nd ed. New York: McGraw-Hill; 2008

3. Flow Investigators. Fluid lavage of open wounds (FLOW): design and rationale for a large, multicenter collaborative 2 × 3 factorial trial of irrigating pressures and solutions in patients with open fractures. BMC Musculoskelet Disord 2010;11:85

4. Bischoff-Ferrari HA, Dawson-Hughes B, Platz A, et al. Effect of high-dosage cholecalciferol and extended physiotherapy on complications after hip fracture: a randomized controlled trial. Arch Intern Med 2010;170:813–820

5. Gurusamy KS, Gluud C, Nikolova D, Davidson BR. Design of surgical randomized controlled trials involving multiple interventions. J Surg Res 2011;165(1):118–127
6. Montgomery AA, Peters TJ, Little P. Design, analysis and presentation of factorial randomised controlled trials. BMC Med Res Methodol 2003;3:26
7. Schulz KF, Altman DG, Moher D; CONSORT Group. CONSORT 2010 statement: updated guidelines for reporting parallel group randomised trials. BMC Med 2010;8:18

2

Expertise-Based Randomized Trials

Dianne Bryant, Kristie More

Summary

Conventional randomized controlled trials (RCTs) evaluating the effectiveness of surgical interventions may be biased by greater surgeon expertise or preference for one intervention over another. In an expertise-based RCT, each patient is randomized to a surgeon and that surgeon performs only the procedure for which he or she has expertise or preference. The present chapter will discuss the expertise-based RCT design as well as the challenges and benefits of this type of study.

Introduction

The conventional randomized controlled trial (RCT) randomly allocates subjects to receive one of the study interventions; each clinician participant must perform all study interventions. It is unusual, however, for a surgeon to have expertise in two or more techniques to treat the same disease; thus a preference for one procedure over the other is likely and may bias the results for that surgeon. Further, it is highly probable that, should there be a greater proportion of surgeon participants with expertise in one of the interventions over the others, the results of the study will be biased in favor of the preferred intervention. In addition, procedural crossovers (from the less preferred to the preferred intervention) are more likely, with a negative effect on the power of the study. An expertise-based RCT randomly allocates subjects to a clinician; each clinician participant performs only his or her preferred study intervention, reducing the opportunity for expertise biases and procedural crossovers. Surgeons wishing to initiate an expertise-based RCT must find a partner with a similar level of expertise for the opposite study intervention who has a similar practice, and must find a third party to screen potential participants. When interpreting the results of an expertise-based RCT, researchers must emphasize that applicability is limited to the level of expertise.

> **Key Concepts: Overcoming Bias Due to Expertise**
> - Conventional RCTs evaluating the effectiveness of surgical interventions may be biased by greater surgeon expertise in one intervention than in the other.
> - Expertise-based RCTs randomize each patient to a surgeon and that surgeon performs only the procedure for

which he or she has expertise or preference, thus overcoming biases introduced by differential expertise.
> - Expertise-based RCTs can provide information about the effectiveness of a surgical intervention if performed by an expert.
> - Surgeons who wish to participate in an expertise-based RCT must find a surgeon in close proximity with a similar practice who has expertise in the other intervention, a qualified independent clinician to screen patients for eligibility, and a well-defined and agreed-upon method of submitting referrals for trial screening.

Conventional RCT Design

Randomized clinical trials provide the most valid method of evaluating the effectiveness of interventions.[1] The strength of an RCT is its ability to limit bias. In the conventional RCT design, patients are randomized into intervention groups and the surgeon performs the allocated intervention (**Fig. 2.1a**). Thus, surgeons who wish to participate in the trial must perform both procedures.

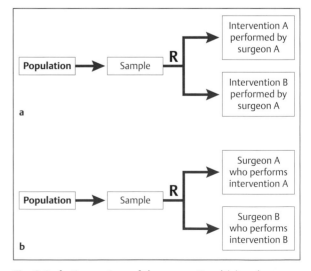

Fig. 2.1a,b Comparison of the conventional (**a**) and expertise-based (**b**) randomized clinical trial. R, randomization

Jargon Simplified: Randomized Controlled Trial (RCT)
An RCT is an experiment in which individuals are randomly allocated to receive or not receive an experimental diagnostic, preventive, therapeutic, or palliative procedure and are then followed to determine the effect of the intervention.[1]

Jargon Simplified: Bias
A bias is any trend in the collection, analysis, or interpretation of data that can lead to conclusions that are systematically different from the truth.

Jargon Simplified: Internal Validity
The internal validity of a study is the degree to which the inferences about the observed differences between two treatment groups of representative patients can be attributed only to the effect under investigation.

A lack of expertise or a stronger belief in one of the interventions than in the other will threaten the feasibility of completing the trial and may undermine the internal validity of the results. Some have suggested that equipoise, such that "there is no preference [on the part of the clinician] between treatments..."[2] is the state of mind under which a randomized trial is ethical. It is more often the case, however, that individual surgeons solely or primarily use a single surgical approach to treat a specific problem, because it takes training and experience to develop expertise in surgical interventions.[3,4] Thus, more recently, true equipoise on the part of the clinician has come to be regarded as theoretical and unlikely.

Instead, the term *equipoise* has been replaced with the term *uncertainty*, which reflects a more common state of mind: the clinician has an idea that a certain treatment is probably superior to the current standard but is uncertain whether he or she is correct. A clinical trial is initiated when there is clinical equipoise, or a "genuine uncertainty on the part of the expert clinical community about the comparative merits of two or more treatments for a defined group of patients or population."[5]

Jargon Simplified: Equipoise
Equipoise refers to the state of genuinely not knowing whether one treatment is better than another. Except where equipoise exists, ethics forces the physician to prescribe the superior treatment.[5]

Jargon Simplified: Crossover
In the case of crossover, a patient does not receive the intervention to which he or she was randomized but receives the other intervention instead.

Jargon Simplified: Differential Expertise Bias
In this form of bias a systematic effect on the results of a study is caused by an imbalance in the proportion of clinicians with expertise in one procedure over the proportion with expertise in the other.

Within the conventional RCT design, it is possible for lack of individual surgeon uncertainty to threaten the validity of the trial. For example, a different degree of expertise in one procedure over the other may influence (consciously or unconsciously) how the surgeon performs the procedure and/or the postoperative rehabilitation recommendations that he or she prescribes.[6] Surgeons may unknowingly perform their preferred procedure more meticulously or follow up patients differently (e.g., frequency, probing questions, tolerance for recommending further tests or procedures) depending on the procedure the patient underwent. There may also be an increase in the probability of crossovers (i.e., a patient randomized to the less preferred treatment receives the preferred treatment) when the surgeon is performing the procedure in which he or she has less expertise, especially in more difficult cases. Finally, a surgeon who believes that one treatment is likely to be superior to the other may experience anxiety related to the challenge this represents to professional ethics, presenting a barrier to patient recruitment both in terms of numbers[3,4] and in the representativeness of the sample.

Another source of bias, called "differential expertise bias," is introduced when there is an imbalance in the proportion of surgeons with expertise in one of the interventions. Undoubtedly, the procedure being performed by the greater number of experts has an unfair advantage over the other procedure in terms of the likelihood of its being shown to be superior.

Expertise-Based RCT Design

The expertise-based RCT is an alternative to the conventional RCT design. It was originally described by van der Linden in 1980 as the nonrandomized surgeon design,[3] but became more popular following arguments presented by Devereaux and colleagues[6] in 2005. In an expertise-based trial, a surgeon with expertise in one of the interventions is paired with a surgeon who has expertise in the other intervention. Patients are then randomized to a surgeon and that surgeon performs only the intervention that he or she has expertise in or believes is the more effective intervention (**Fig. 2.1b**).

The expertise-based design has several potential advantages over the conventional RCT. For example, it should decrease the likelihood of crossovers because the surgeon is only performing the procedure in which they have the greater expertise. There is also a low likelihood of differential expertise bias,[6] especially if there is an attempt on the part of the investigators to select surgeon partners who have a similar level of expertise but in the opposite intervention. Finally, recruitment is likely to be much more successful in terms of the numbers and variety of patients approached for participation because they are screened by a neutral party prior to randomization and can inform patients that whichever procedure they receive, it will be performed by an expert in that procedure.

Changing the Design Changes the Research Question

In a conventional RCT in which differential expertise bias is not present, the results of the trial give information about which intervention is superior. If a conventional RCT includes an imbalance in expertise or there is a lack of individual surgeon equipoise, the results of the study carry an uncertain meaning—they may (as intended) give information about the superiority of the intervention, they may reflect biases introduced by differential expertise, or both.

The results of an expertise-based RCT answer the question of which intervention is superior in the hands of a surgeon with expertise in the intervention of interest. This means that surgeons without expertise in performing the surgical procedure shown to be superior must first develop that expertise before they can achieve outcomes similar to those observed in the expertise-based trial. When evaluating the applicability of the results of an expertise-based trial, the criteria used to classify a surgeon as an expert must be explicitly stated; the more pragmatic the criteria, the more widely applicable the results of the trial.

A Potential Source of Bias: The Timing of Randomization

To be eligible for a trial, the patient must be a candidate for both interventions. If eligibility is determined with knowledge of the procedure that will be performed on that patient, a selection bias is likely. In any randomized trial, the most effective method to avoid selection bias is to ensure that eligibility is determined prior to randomization. Thus, in many orthopaedic surgical trials, randomization takes place in the operating room after the surgeon has had opportunity to view the anatomical structures, arrive at an accurate diagnosis, and confirm that the patient meets the eligibility criteria. In an expertise-based RCT, this is not always the case. Certainly intraoperative randomization to surgeon is not feasible. In most cases, eligibility will be determined by the independent assessor using the tools available to him or her outside of the operating room (e.g., history, physical examination tests, imaging). Depending on the sensitivity of these tests to diagnose the disease of interest and their specificity for ruling out concomitant diseases that would preclude participation, eligibility may not be fully assessed prior to randomization. Thus, a high rate of postrandomization exclusions is possible.

To avoid introducing a selection bias caused by postrandomization exclusions, there must be well-defined and objective criteria for excluding a randomized patient.[7] Em-

ploying an independent committee to assess eligibility is the most rigorous approach to avoiding selection bias. This committee should be blind to group allocation and have access to all information relevant to determining eligibility prior to randomization. Thus, if information becomes available during the surgery, the surgeon should photograph and document the finding to be able to present this to the committee at the time of their evaluation.

Jargon Simplified: Applicability
The applicability of trial results means the extent to which they remain valid in conditions outside the trial—that is, effectively, their usefulness in clinical practice.

Jargon Simplified: Sensitivity
The sensitivity of a test is the extent to which it correctly identifies people who have a particular disorder. It is measured as the proportion of people who truly have the designated disorder who are identified as such by the test. The test may consist of, or include, clinical observations.[1]

Jargon Simplified: Specificity
The specificity of a test is the extent to which it correctly identifies people who do not have a particular disorder. It is measured as the proportion of people who are truly free of a designated disorder who are identified as such by the test. The test may consist of, or include, clinical observations.[1]

Jargon Simplified: Selection Bias
Selection bias is present when the study and control group subjects differ in the distribution of factors that might affect a given outcome of interest. These factors may be unknown or unmeasurable (e.g., motivation). Selection bias can only be controlled by random allocation into treatment groups such that each subject (with known and unknown characteristics) has an equal chance of being in either treatment group.

Jargon Simplified: Blind
Patients, clinicians, data collectors, outcome adjudicators, or data analysts who are unaware of which patients have been assigned to the experimental or control group are referred to as "blind."

Jargon Simplified: External Validity
The external validity of a study is the degree to which the results of the study can be generalized beyond the sample studied.

Challenges of Expertise-Based RCTs

Despite the advantages of an expertise-based RCT design, there are feasibility issues that must be addressed if one is thinking of implementing an expertise-based design. First, an expertise-based design requires at least one expert in each of the interventions at each participating center or else some convenient way in which to shuffle patients from one center to another. Second, to avoid biasing the patient, it may be necessary for potential patients at a site to have their initial consultation with a neutral party (e.g., a fellow or other qualified health professional) who will determine study eligibility, explain the study and the need for its unique design (i.e., uncertainty within the surgical community regarding the superiority of either intervention), and obtain consent before randomization to a surgeon occurs. Third, an expertise-based design presents unique challenges in acute settings, where each participating facility must have two specialists on call (one with each expertise). Despite these perceived challenges, we are aware of five published expertise-based RCTs (four in orthopaedics,[8-11] one in cardiac surgery[12]) and several currently being conducted (two orthopaedic, one vascular surgery).

Examples from the Literature: Operative Treatment of Fractures of the Tibial Plafond

Wyrsch et al. conducted a quasi-randomized trial to compare complications and radiographic and functional results in patients with a displaced intra-articular fracture of the tibial plafond (pilon fracture) who underwent either open reduction and internal fixation or external fixation and limited internal fixation.[11] In this trial, the six attending orthopaedic surgeons were assigned to a treatment group according to their expertise or preference. Each patient was managed by the surgeon on call when the patient was seen in the emergency room.

Examples from the Literature: A Prospective, Randomized Study of the Management of Severe Ankle Fractures

Phillips et al. conducted a randomized trial to compare pain, function, and adequacy of reduction in patients with a closed supination–external rotation grade 4 ankle fracture or a closed pronation–external rotation grade 4 ankle fracture.[9] Patients were initially seen by the orthopaedic resident and a closed reduction was performed and a cast was applied. The adequacy of the reduction was assessed the following day. Patients who had achieved satisfactory reduction were randomized to one of two surgeons: one performed open reduction with rigid internal fixation according to ASIF (Association for the Study of Internal Fixation) techniques, the other continued closed cast treatment. Patients who had not achieved satisfactory reduction were randomized to one of two surgeons: one performed open reduction with rigid internal fixation according to ASIF techniques, the other performed open reduction with internal fixation of only the medial malleolus.

Independent Assessor

In a conventional RCT, each surgeon reviews his or her own referrals, conducts his or her own initial consultation, and explains the trial to eligible patients. Consenting patients are then randomized to undergo procedure A or procedure B performed by their own surgeon. However, in an expertise-based design, neither the research team nor the patient knows which treatment (A or B) the patient will be assigned to until the patient has consented to the study and has been enrolled and randomized. The treatment to which the patient is assigned (A or B) will then determine which surgeon that patient will see.

In our experience, having an independent assessor review referrals and conduct the first consultation is the most effective way to implement an expertise-based design. The independent assessor must have the expertise to screen patients and be willing to explain the study and both treatment options to the patient. In our study, designed to compare two methods to repair a rotator cuff tear, one expertise-based center employed a surgical fellow to fill this role, while another center recruited a sports medicine physician. Issues related to billing and how to arrange for follow-up for patients who are ineligible or who do not give consent for study participation must be addressed at the outset.

Balanced and Consecutive or Random Contributions to Screening Pool

Surgeons participating in an expertise-based trial should also agree as to how they will contribute potential participants to the screening pool for the trial. Recall that when participating in an expertise-based design, an independent assessor is screening referrals from each surgeon and determining patient eligibility. Before trial commencement, the partnering surgeons at a site must determine whether each surgeon will contribute all of their new referrals for consideration for the study or only a proportion of them. Will partnering surgeon(s) be upset if the proportion of referrals being submitted is unequal between partners (such that upon randomization, the surgeon who contributed more referrals is receiving fewer patients back into their practice)? For example, if there are four surgeons participating at a site, each surgeon should receive approximately 25% of the study patients into their surgical practice through the randomization process. If each surgeon is contributing approximately the same number of referrals into the central pool, then each surgeon will receive a similar number of patients back into their practice. However, if out of 100 referrals, one of the four surgeons is contributing 60 of those referrals, and the other three are only contributing 12–13 referrals, the randomization of those patients will see 25 patients entered into each surgeon's practice.

Further, if a surgeon elects to retain a proportion of referrals in his or her practice, the selection process must be transparent and random to avoid issues with external validity. For example, if a surgeon contributes only difficult cases into the study, the resulting study sample will contain a disproportionate number of more difficult cases and the study results will not be applicable to typical surgical practices.

Perceived Equivalence between Practices

Regardless of the procedure to which they are allocated, participants in an expertise-based RCT can be assured that their procedure will be performed by a surgeon who has expertise in performing it. Although it is rarely acknowledged, this is not the case in most conventional RCTs that evaluate a surgical intervention. Thus, participating in an expertise-based RCT should serve as a comfort to patients.

Before study commencement, however, partnering surgeons must determine whether there are other important differences between their practices that may deter a patient's decision to participate in the trial and whether anything can be done to create perceived equivalency between practices. For example, does the wait list from referral (from the independent assessor) to first appointment with the surgeon or from first appointment with the surgeon to surgery differ between practices? Is the location and accessibility (e.g., parking) similar between locations? Particularly when a study requires participants to attend several long-term follow-up visits, these issues may present an inconvenience to patients which could theoretically create challenges for long-term study follow-up.

> **Reality Check: Logistics**
> We are participating in a ten-center randomized trial to compare the quality of life, function, strength, and tendon integrity of patients who have undergone a rotator cuff repair using either an all-arthroscopic or a mini-open approach.[13] Surgeons in two of the ten centers claimed a preference for or lack of expertise in one of the procedures being compared. As a result, these two centers follow an expertise-based RCT design while the remaining eight centers follow a conventional RCT design. In both expertise-based centers, the research coordinator screens new referrals from each surgeon and seemingly eligible patients are scheduled for a first consultation appointment with an independent physician (a primary care physician at one center and a fellow at the other). The independent assessor conducts further screening and eligible patients are approached for study participation. The assessor discusses the expertise-based design, why it is necessary, and what it means for the patient (i.e., randomization to a surgeon who is expert in performing the procedure). Consenting patients are then randomized to a surgeon and are scheduled to meet the surgeon before surgery. All patients follow an identical protocol for postoperative rehabilitation and follow-up.

Conclusion

Conventional RCTs evaluating the effectiveness of surgical interventions may be biased by greater surgeon expertise in or preference for one intervention over the other. Expertise-based RCTs randomize each patient to a surgeon and that surgeon performs only the procedure for which he or she has expertise or preference. Thus, an expertise-based RCT can overcome biases introduced by differential expertise and reduce poor recruitment related to internal ethical struggles. Surgeons considering taking part in an expertise-based RCT must find a surgeon partner who is in close proximity, has a similar practice, and has expertise in the other intervention. A qualified independent clinician to screen patients for eligibility and a well-defined and agreed-upon method of submitting referrals is also recommended. An expertise-based RCT gives information about the superiority of a surgical intervention in the hands of an expert. The applicability of the results depends on how expertise was defined within the trial (pragmatic versus explanatory approach); the more pragmatic the definition, the more applicable the results.

Suggested Reading

Devereaux PJ, Bhandari M, Clarke M, et al. Need for expertise based randomised controlled trials. BMJ 2005;330:88

MacDermid JC, Holtby R, Razmjou H, Bryant D; JOINTS Canada. All-arthroscopic versus mini-open repair of small or moderate-sized rotator cuff tears: a protocol for a randomized trial. BMC Musculoskelet Disord 2006;7:25

Moher D, Hopewell S, Schulz KF, et al. CONSORT 2010 explanation and elaboration: updated guidelines for reporting parallel group randomised trials. BMJ 2010;340:c869

References

1. Guyatt GH, Rennie D, Meade M, Cook D, eds. Users' Guide to the Medical Literature: A Manual for Evidence-Based Clinical Practice. 2nd ed. New York: McGraw-Hill; 2008
2. Lilford RJ, Jackson J. Equipoise and the ethics of randomization. J R Soc Med 1995;88:552–559
3. van der Linden W. Pitfalls in randomized surgical trials. Surgery 1980;87:258–262
4. Rudicel S, Esdaile J. The randomized clinical trial in orthopaedics: obligation or option? J Bone Joint Surg Am 1985;67-A:1284–1293
5. Freedman B. Equipoise and the ethics of clinical research. N Engl J Med 1987;317:141–135
6. Devereaux PJ, Bhandari M, Clarke M, et al. Need for expertise based randomised controlled trials. BMJ 2005;330:88
7. Fergusson D, Aaron SD, Guyatt G, Hebert P. Post-randomisation exclusions: the intention to treat principle and excluding patients from analysis. BMJ 2002;325:652–654
8. Finkemeier CG, Schmidt AH, Kyle RF, Templeman DC, Varecka TF. A prospective, randomized study of intramedullary nails inserted with and without reaming for the treatment of open and closed fractures of the tibial shaft. J Orthop Trauma 2000;14:187–193
9. Phillips WA, Schwartz HS, Keller CS, et al. A prospective, randomized study of the management of severe ankle fractures. J Bone Joint Surg Am 1985;67:67–78
10. Wihlborg O. Fixation of femoral neck fractures. A four-flanged nail versus threaded pins in 200 cases. Acta Orthop Scand 1990;61:415–418
11. Wyrsch B, McFerran MA, McAndrew M, et al. Operative treatment of fractures of the tibial plafond. A randomized, prospective study. J Bone Joint Surg Am 1996;78:1646–1657
12. Machler HE, Bergmann P, Anelli-Monti M, et al. Minimally invasive versus conventional aortic valve operations: a prospective study in 120 patients. Ann Thorac Surg 1999;67:1001–1005
13. MacDermid JC, Holtby R, Razmjou H, Bryant D; JOINTS Canada. All-arthroscopic versus mini-open repair of small or moderate-sized rotator cuff tears: a protocol for a randomized trial. BMC Musculoskelet Disord 2006;7:25

3

Randomization Systems and Technology

Sadeesh K. Srinathan

Summary

When we compare treatments we want to make sure that the two groups are as alike as possible so that the comparison is a fair one. We want to be confident that any difference between the groups is due to our treatment and not to other factors that differentiate the two groups. For this reason we have to be careful about how we allocate patients into study groups, and this chapter will describe the various methods used to accomplish this.

Introduction

Is it better to ream the intramedullary canal before inserting a tibial nail or is it better not to? The best method to answer this question is to undertake a clinical trial to determine whether reaming is better than not reaming—or, more generally, if one treatment or its alternative is better. As we try to answer this question, we want to protect ourselves from making false conclusions about the effectiveness of the treatment because of biases that intrude into our study.

For example, our study may show that reamed nails lead to lower nonunion rates than nonreamed nails. However, this difference in nonunion rates may be because there are more patients with open fractures in the nonreamed group. The lower rate of nonunion in the reamed group may be due not to the treatment but to the fact that there were more patients with a high risk of nonunion (open fractures) to begin with in the nonreamed arm of the study.

To avoid this situation, and in order to make a fair comparison and be confident that the differences are due to our treatment, we must allocate subjects to the different arms of the trial in such a way that the intervention is the only differentiating factor among the groups. In other words, we must undertake a bias-free method of patient assignment.[1] By assembling comparable groups, we can ascribe with confidence any differences in outcome to the intervention alone. This is a straightforward concept in theory, but how it is implemented is a major design issue in a trial, and failure to do this with sufficient thought can jeopardize your whole study.

The response to a treatment such as an operation or drug depends on the baseline prognosis of the individual subject as it relates to the intervention and the outcome being measured. Take, for example, a study to determine differences in overall survival rates at one year after two forms of hip arthroplasty. It is obvious that the patient entering the study with renal failure, diabetes, and heart failure even before they broke their hip is likely have a shorter life expectancy than a patient without these co-morbidities; the baseline prognoses of these patients (their chances of survival after one year) are different. Now, if the study had more of these sick patients in one arm than the other, we could not be confident that the observed difference in survival was due to the intervention rather than to the differences in baseline prognosis in each of the trial arms. It is also possible that the study might fail to show a difference when one really exists; that is, one treatment really is better, but we are unable to appreciate this because of the imbalance in prognosis between the treatment groups.

These imbalances in prognosis can arise from various sources. The most important cause of imbalance, and one that we take great pains to avoid in clinical trials, is selection bias. There are a number of reasons which make it tempting to allocate subjects to either the intervention or the comparator arm: perhaps you or the resident wants more experience with one procedure over the other, or you think a particular patient will be better served by undergoing one procedure rather than another.[2,3] Allocating subjects to one arm or another in this way (even unintentionally) will lead to noncomparable groups and render the whole study unreliable.

For surgeons, it is already very difficult to undertake the "ideal" trial such as those seen in fields like cardiology, for example. It can be difficult or impossible to blind surgeons or patients, and it is also difficult to deal with the differences in surgical expertise which may account for differences in outcomes rather than the intervention itself. It can be difficult to achieve a sufficiently large sample size, and it may be difficult to assure that the co-interventions such as physiotherapy or nursing care are the same in different arms of the study.[4–6] For these reasons, it is especially important to pay attention to patient allocation, since this is one aspect of a clinical trial that can and should be done well in surgical trials and one reason it is considered an important marker of quality in surgical trials.

Methods of Patient Allocation

There are a myriad of methods to allocate patients to study arms. These methods can be broadly classified as deterministic—that is, one can *always* determine with certainty the study arm a subject will be assigned to ahead of time; or random—that is, one cannot predict which study arm a patient will be assigned to.

Deterministic Allocation

Examples of deterministic methods are study group assignment by date of birth, day of admission to hospital, or hospital numbers. Although these systems may appear to be random since people don't usually their choose birth dates, the investigator can determine with certainty which treatment assignment a participant is going to receive. Theoretically these systems may also result in unbiased comparison groups; however, the ability to predict allocation will lead to selection bias that will jeopardize the trial.[7] For example, if patients admitted on odd days receive treatment A and those admitted on even days receive treatment B, it is clear that the opportunity to choose who will be eligible to enter the trial on those days is made that much easier.

> **Key Concepts: Avoiding Selection Bias**
> To have a fair test of an intervention we must not bias the results by *selecting* subjects to treatment or control arms.

Random Allocation

The defining feature of simple random allocation is that each eligible participant in the trial has the same fixed probability of entering either study arm. Even if there is an allocation ratio greater than one (i.e., nonequal sample sizes for each arm), each individual has the same probability of entering either study arm (e.g., 1/2 for a 1:1 allocation ratio or 2/3 if there is a 2:1 allocation ratio). Most of the statistical tests of significance used in the analysis of trial data assume that the study sample is randomly selected from the population of interest.

Another feature of simple random allocation, which is of great practical importance, is that randomization balances prognostic factors among the treatment arms. Prognostic factors can be either known or unknown. Although deterministic allocation systems can deal with the known prognostic factors, only random methods can balance the unknown prognostic factors with certainty, and no other system is as unpredictable or free of bias.[8,9]

Among the random methods, allocation schemes can be divided into fixed or adaptive schemes. Fixed schemes such as simple randomization ensure that each participant in the trial has the same probability of allocation to each arm as the next participant throughout the entire study. In adaptive schemes, the probability of being allocated to a particular arm changes during the study.

There are three types of adaptive systems to consider.

1. **Adaptive response:** Treatment-adaptive response is where the number of subjects already assigned to each study arm determines the probability of being assigned to that study arm. For example, if the starting probability of allocation is 1/2, and in the course of the study there are 15 patients in study arm A and 5 in study arm B, the probability of assignment can be altered to increase the probability of being assigned to treatment B from 1/2 to 3/4 for example. This system still maintains randomness—one cannot actually predict with certainty where the next patient is to be placed, but the probability of being assigned to a particular arm varies.

2. **Response adaptive:** The second system is response adaptive, in which allocation of one participant relies on the previous participant's response to the intervention. Thus, for example, if a person allocated to a particular treatment does well (e.g. survives), the next person is allocated to the same treatment, whereas if the person dies, the next person is allocated to the alternative treatment. A version of this is also called the "modified play the winner" rule for allocation. Although this system has been used in cases where the intervention is extreme with high mortality,[10] it has a number of disadvantages. You need to wait for a response each time before enrolling the next subject, and serious imbalances in numbers in each arm are expected, which requires very complex analysis in order to adequately interpret the results.[11] These two adaptive methods have restrictions and complexities that do not readily lend themselves to use in surgical trials and will not be discussed further, but the reader is referred to Pocock or Chow and Liu[11,12] for further details.

3. **Covariate adaptive randomization:** Covariate adaptive randomization adjusts the probability of allocation depending on the balance of *known* important prognostic factors—this is also termed the "minimization method" and is of particular interest and value in surgical trials. It has been referred to as the "platinum standard"[13] and will be discussed further.

Drawbacks of Random Allocation

It is intuitively obvious that simple randomization is the method that is least susceptible to selection bias and the most "fair," so why is this method rarely used in surgical trials?

As already stated, the major goal of random allocation is to balance prognostic factors and end up with comparable groups. However, despite the potential for simple random allocation to *eventually* balance prognostic factors, this does not usually happen in the early stages of a large trial or at any time in a small trial. It is perfectly possible for an imbalance of prognostic factors to occur purely due to random chance. Consider the following: if two males and two females are randomized to two treatment arms A and B, the probability of both females being randomized to treatment arm B is 25%. If this occurs, clearly these will not be comparable groups. Even in relatively large studies, such imbalances can occur purely due to chance, although the likelihood of this decreases as the sample size increases and the imbalances become less of a factor (see Reality Check: Worked Examples for an illustration). These imbalances can lead to uncertain or uninterpretable results from a trial if they are of prognostically important factors. Simple random allocation can also result in unequal sample sizes, which can present problems in statistical analysis and be a major problem if the study does not reach the intended recruitment target.

Reality Check: Worked Examples

Below are some worked examples to demonstrate how the allocation systems work for a two-armed trial. The treatment and control arms are labeled Treatment A and Treatment B. A random number generator (http://www.random.org/integers/) was used to generate the random number sequences.

Simple Randomization

We establish a rule that an even number corresponds to Treatment A and an odd number corresponds to Treatment B. Two runs of random sequences are generated.
First run generates 6 As and 5 Bs:

2	A
8	A
2	A
8	A
3	B
0	A
3	B
1	B
7	B
8	A

Second run generates 7 As and 3 Bs:

2	A
0	A
6	A
2	A
8	A
1	B
8	A
9	B
4	A
1	B

Note that in these sequences, there were imbalances in the number of subjects in each of the trial arms. If the trial terminated after the first five patients in the first run there would only be one patient in Treatment B, while there would have been no patients allocated to Treatment B in the second run.

Block Randomization

The permutations of Treatment A and Treatment B are listed below for block sizes of two or four.
For a block size of two there are two permutations:

1	AB
2	BA

For a block size of four there are six permutations:

1	AABB
2	ABAB
3	BBAA
4	BABA
5	ABBA
6	BAAB

To generate a random allocation scheme, generate a random number sequence from 1 to 6, which will be used to select the corresponding blocks as listed. The following sequence was generated: 5, 3, 1, 6, 5, 6, 4, 6, 4.
These correspond to the blocks below:

5	ABBA
3	BBAA
1	AABB
6	BAAB
5	ABBA
6	BAAB
4	BABA
6	BAAB
4	BABA

Note that, if the study were not blinded with fixed block sizes, it would be easy to predict the remainder of the allocations within the block at the end of the block; for example, after BAB, you will know for certain that the next patient will be allocated to A.
To use random block sizes of two or four, list the eight permutations:

1	AB
2	BA
3	AABB
4	ABAB
5	BBAA
6	BABA
7	ABBA
8	BAAB

A random sequence with numbers from 1 to 8 directly corresponds to above list.
Here the random sequence generated is: 6, 8, 6, 1, 4, 3, 1, 2, 2, 7.

6	BABA
8	BAAB
6	BABA
1	AB
4	ABAB
3	AABB
1	AB
2	BA
2	BA
7	ABBA

The allocation visible to the investigator is:
BABABAABBABAABABABAABBABBABAABBA.
Even if the study terminates after the 20th patient, the imbalance is half the block size at most. In this case, there are two more As than Bs at the end of the trial. With random block sizes, it is difficult to predict the next allocation as you will be unaware of which block size is being used.

Minimization: Pocock and Simon Method
The prognostic factors which are considered important are listed and categorized. In this example (**Table 3.1**) the factors are split into two categories.
So far in the study after recruiting 40 patients, the distribution of each factor is described in the table (**Table 3.2**). Note that the categories are not mutually exclusive except within each characteristic.
If the next patient to be allocated (patient #41) is a 64-year-old with an open fracture and diabetes from Hospital X, the current totals for each treatment after 40 patients are:
Total for A = 12 + 5 + 12 + 10 = 39
Total for B = 11 + 6 + 13 + 10 = 40
If this patient is allocated to Treatment A, then the total for A will become: 13 + 6 + 13 + 11 = 41 and the difference between A and B will be 1.
If the patient is allocated to Treatment B, then the total for B will become: 12 + 7 + 14 + 11 = 44 and the difference between A and B will be 5.
Therefore to minimize the differences in overall distribution of prognostic factors, the patient is allocated to Treatment A. This allocation could be with a probability of 1 (always allocated to minimize the difference) or have a rule that increases the probability to more than 0.5 but less than 1 and maintains a random component.

Stratified Randomization
If a study is stratified according to study center (X, Y, or Z) and fracture type (open or closed), the cells or subgroups formed by this combination are:

X, open	X, closed
Y, open	Y, closed
Z, open	Z, closed

Within each cell, the subjects undergo simple randomization.
Note that for only two factors there are already 6 cells. If another factor such as diabetes (classified as yes or no, i. e., two levels) was added, the number of subgroups would increase to 3 × 2 × 2 = 12.

Table 3.1 Pocock and Simon method of minimization: factors of interest

Factors of interest	Levels	
Age, years	>65	≤65
Fracture type	Open	Closed
Diabetes	No	Yes
Hospital	X	Y

Table 3.2 Pocock and Simon method of minimization: distribution of factors

Characteristic	Levels	Treat-ment A	Treat-ment B	Marginal total
Age, years	>65	8	9	17
	≤65	12	11	23
Fracture type	Open	5	6	11
	Closed	15	14	29
Diabetes	No	8	7	15
	Yes	12	13	25
Hospital	X	10	10	20
	Y	10	10	20

Problems with Random Allocation—An Example
To illustrate these problems, consider a hypothetical multicenter trial that compares two types of knee prosthesis where pain at one year is the primary outcome of interest. The trial compares the ACE Knee to the SuperDuper Knee. In the study, patients are to be recruited at different sites over a period of three years. It eventually turns out that during the study, there were changes in co-interventions (for example, a new anesthetic technique) from the beginning to the end of the study. Further, the study was terminated early at two years because of difficulties with funding and recruitment. It also became apparent during the study that one site had a very different referral pattern for the patients, with an unusually large number of patients with pre-existing chronic pain. These and other factors that affect the prognosis of the patients in relation to the outcome being measured (pain at one year) have implications for how the trial eventually plays out in terms of the balance of prognosis of patients at the end of the trial. With only simple randomization, we could have ended up with a large number of patients with chronic pain allocated to Site 1, where there were more patients allocated to the ACE Knee at the time the study was terminated early. These imbalances in prognostic factors such as the presence of chronic pain prior to surgery and the disproportionate number of patients receiving the ACE Knee at Site 1 could have rendered the whole trial uninterpretable, resulting in a huge waste of effort and resources.

Key Concepts: Random Imbalances

Because imbalances in prognostic factors can occur at random, steps may need to be taken to counter this; however, this is done at the cost of increasing complexity and increased chances of deciphering allocation and selection bias.

As the above example illustrates, when considering allocation of subjects to the arms of a clinical trial a number of factors must be taken into consideration. The factors that should be considered when deciding upon the method of patient allocation during the design of a clinical trial are discussed below. This is not an algorithm as it is up to the individual investigators and their particular circumstances how best to balance the competing demands of these factors.

Reality Check: Nothing is Perfect

There is no perfect system of randomization, and in the real world finding equilibrium between the conflicting demands of balancing prognostic factors and ensuring freedom from bias requires careful thought and compromises including taking into consideration the "optics" of the final study (i.e., will it be believable to the average reader).

Other Considerations

Unit of Randomization

The first consideration is the unit of randomization. Will individual subjects be randomized or will it be surgeons or hospitals? It is also possible to consider randomizing one of a paired structure such as a knee, where the other serves as the control. It would make sense to randomize individual patients to an experimental or control arm of a surgical procedure, but it may make more sense to randomize physiotherapy clinics in studies examining the effectiveness of a physiotherapy treatment plan after knee replacement.

Sample Size

The number of subjects in the study is important when considering allocation strategy. As stated earlier, the most important consideration is the balance of prognosis with minimal bias. In a study with a large number of patients (more than 100 in each arm), it is likely that there will be good balance with a simple random allocation method.[9] However, when the numbers are smaller, as is often the case in orthopaedic trials where the average number is 113 ± 102,[14] there is a risk of prognostic imbalance with simple randomization.

Key Concepts: Small Trial

The issue of imbalances in prognosis is most acute in small trials.

Number and Frequency of Important Prognostic Factors

It is important to be aware of important prognostic factors and their frequency. These factors could either be related to the treatment, such as bone density in arthroplasty, or unrelated to treatment, such as the study site. It would be generally unwise to undertake a trial where the response to intervention is likely to vary widely or qualitatively, that is, some subjects improve with an intervention while others become worse. If this is the case, it is better to adjust the inclusion and exclusion criteria to make the population more homogenous.[15] If an important prognostic factor remains, then stratification based on this factor must be considered, especially if the factor is common. A special case is center effects with multicenter trials, since the study center is certain to be an important source of variation that we would want to correct for to increase the power of the study. Stratifying for center also allows dumping of a stratum (i.e., a center)[16] if a center withdraws without a major effect on the remainder of the study. Analysis will have to take into consideration the stratification undertaken at the design stage—"analyze the way you randomize."[17] However, the benefits of stratification on power disappear once a trial is above 100 or so.[9,16–18] Another important point to consider in using prognostic factors in the design of the study is the precision with which they can be classified. It is easy to determine sex or location of a fracture accurately and with minimal judgment. On the other hand, the stability of a knee joint or degree of disability is much harder to classify for use in stratification.[15,18]

Number of Arms in a Trial

In most trials, there are two arms—an intervention and a control arm. Other designs, such as multiple arm parallel trials or factorial trials, may also be considered and this will affect the methods of allocation chosen, particularly with regard to the ease of implementing the allocation scheme.

Allocation Ratio

Allocation ratios are, in general, left at a 1:1 ratio of experimental to control in two-armed parallel trials. However, this does not always have to be the case, and there are often good reasons to alter this ratio. Although statistical tests of significance are usually most powerful (able to detect a difference when one exists), with equal sample sizes among treatment arms (an allocation ratio of 0.5), the drop in efficiency is quite small until the allocation ratio moves beyond 0.7.[9,12] There are instances where it would be advantageous or even more ethical for the study as a whole to have unequal allocation.[19]

We may want to allocate patients to experiment versus control in a 2:1 ratio to improve recruitment since participants then have a greater likelihood of receiving the treatment which is expected to be "better." Alternatively, there could be more recruitment to the control arm for a secondary objective of the study, such as to determine the natural history of those who are untreated in a placebo or non-treatment arm. Going outside of the 1:1 ratios may lead to changes in statistical analysis and sample size calculations that need to be considered, but these adjustments are unlikely to be particularly difficult and may be worth the effort.

Length of Recruitment Period

The time frame of recruitment is important because it is possible that the subjects and their prognosis may change during the course of the trial. For example, it can be expected that perioperative care changes over time so that a patient's likelihood of certain complications decreases. This will have important implications if the recruitment period were so long that those patients recruited at the beginning of the study faced a different risk of perioperative complications than those recruited at the end of the study. It is also important to consider that there can be seasonal variations in those being recruited into a study. In studying an intervention for injuries to the anterior cruciate ligament, one would have to bear in mind that there may be differences in the type of patients presenting with these ligament injuries during the winter ski season than during the summer soccer season. A difference in the nature of the injury that follows a seasonal pattern may have an impact on the effectiveness of the intervention.

Time from Randomization to Intervention

One must consider the timing of the randomization process in relation to the intervention. It is important to analyze the results on an intention-to-treat basis in order to preserve the benefits of random allocation in the first place.[20] If there is too long a gap between allocation and intervention, it is possible for there to be significant crossover of subjects to the other arm, which will lead to difficulty in interpretation and amelioration of detectable treatment effects. This cannot be dealt with by analysis according to treatment received because of the possibility that the reason for the crossover itself may be of prognostic significance.[20] In surgical trials, it is ideal to randomize just prior to the operation as the chance of crossover is very low if the intervention immediately follows randomization, although even this may not be enough.[21] Contrariwise, if a subject is allocated to one arm a few weeks prior to the intervention because of necessary preoperative work-up or because of expertise-based trial design,[6,22] the opportunity for crossover increases.

Resources Available

All studies have to be carried out within the constraints of limited resources of both time and money. A complex allocation scheme with a large number of strata, although theoretically ideal for minimizing bias and increasing the power of the study, may be so costly in terms of resources and complexity that the entire study becomes impossible. Compromises must always be made, and these factors must be taken into consideration.[18] Therefore, unless subjects are allocated appropriately, the validity of the whole study can come into question.

Time from Recruitment to Randomization

The method of randomization must take into account the time from recruitment of subjects to randomization. For example, if the study is addressing acute treatment of open fractures, where the time from recruitment of eligible patients to the intervention is short, the ease of accessing the randomization system is very important as randomization will have to be done during the nights and weekends. If, by contrast, the study is comparing different hip prostheses for degenerative disease, the requirement for ease and speed of implementation of randomization may be less important. In the first example, a complex system such as minimization might be too cumbersome, but in the second example this is not an issue.

Allocation Concealment

Allocation concealment, although separate from randomization, is an integral part of appropriate allocation of subjects to the treatment and control arms and must be considered carefully when deciding on randomization procedures. As mentioned earlier, even if a balance of prognosis can be achieved (at least for known prognostic factors), a deterministic allocation scheme or one that is easy to predict—for example, small and fixed block sizes with block randomization—will allow selection bias because one can predict the allocation of the next patient and thus choose not to allocate a patient to that arm. Failure in concealment of the random allocation will negate any benefits accrued by random allocation in the first place.

Allocation concealment is important to maintain blinding in blinded studies, but is arguably even more important in unblinded studies. The number of tools for reducing bias is reduced if the study is unblinded. Random allocation with adequate concealment of allocation to protect against selection bias takes on a more important role in overall bias reduction.

On this basis, some methods of randomization, such as a centralized system with random block sizes, may be preferable to others because of advantages in concealment compared to a system with a predetermined allocation schedule administered by someone at the study site.

Mechanics of How to Randomize

Despite the large number of methods available, ultimately, four methods of allocation will suit most studies likely to be carried out in orthopaedic surgery (**Table 3.3**). A summary of these methods is listed below with examples illustrated in the boxes.

Table 3.3 Comparison of allocation schemes

System	Pro	Con	Comments
Simple randomization	Least chance of bias and completely unpredictable	Can lead to imbalances in numbers in each arm and prognostic factors	Most of these drawbacks disappear with large sample sizes (>200 subjects)
Block randomization	Ensures even numbers in each arm Some protection against early stops or loss of centers	Can be predictable at the end of a block Does not balance prognostic factors	Can randomly vary sample sizes to deal with predicting allocation Central randomization will help in adequate concealment of allocation
Stratified randomization	Accounts for important prognostic factors Allows for easier subgroup analysis at a later stage	Assumes one knows that the prognostic factors are indeed important Often cumbersome if more than one or two factors are used Can lead to more strata than subjects	Center is an important stratifying factor which should be used in multicentered trials Block randomization must be carried out within each stratum, otherwise imbalance in numbers within strata defeats the purpose of stratification Must analyze with stratification factor as a covariate
Minimization	Balances prognostic factors throughout the study Can use many more prognostic factors than in stratification Very useful in small sample sizes	Not strictly random, but can add random components Possible to predict if able to keep track of prognostic factors, but this is very difficult and cumbersome	Works best with centralized computer system to both determine and conceal allocation Not well understood or well used

1. **Simple randomization:** the simplest method of allocating, analogous to a coin toss. Because one cannot create an audit trail with a coin toss, however, the use of a random number table is preferred. This is the ideal method if the study is large enough to assure balance in prognosis at the end of the trial or sometime earlier.

> **Jargon Simplified: Randomization**
> Randomization is the allocation of participants to groups by chance, usually done with the aid of a table of random numbers. Not to be confused with systematic allocation, quasi-randomization (e.g., on even and odd days of the month), or other allocation methods at the discretion of the investigator.[20]

2. **Block randomization:** assures similar numbers of patients in each arm of the study—but does not balance prognosis. With this method, "blocks" of allocations are randomized, where each block is one permutation of treatment arms depending on the block size. So if block size is two in a two-armed trial, there are two permutations or two blocks, while if the block size is four, there are six permutations. Smaller block sizes are easier to decipher, while too large a block size is sensitive to changes over time and in extremes and defeats the purpose of assuring equal numbers in each arm of the study.

> **Jargon Simplified: Block Randomization**
> Block randomization is a technique to ensure equal distribution of study subjects across treatment

groups over time. Blocks of either varying (most common) or equal sizes are created such that each block contains an equal number of treatment and control (or treatment A and treatment B) allocations. The order of treatment allocation within each block is random, and the order of blocks, once they have been created, is also random.

3. **Stratified randomization:** balances known prognostic factors which may impact the outcome. We want to assure that these are distributed evenly across the trial arms, and this will theoretically decrease variability within the strata, enabling better detection of an effect. However, the gain in efficiency may not be worth the cost once the sample size becomes large. This is very useful in multicenter trials where the center will obviously be an important factor. One would want to limit the number of strata to very important factors that are frequent enough not to leave strata with too few subjects or events.

> **Jargon Simplified: Stratification**
> The stratification process groups individuals into strata based on an important known and measurable characteristic (such as study site or patient sex or age) to ensure that these characteristics are equally represented across the intervention groups.

4. **Minimization**[12,13,23]**:** allows for balancing of known risk factors. It can balance unknown factors to an extent, but not as much as simple randomization. The benefits of minimization do decrease after a suffi-

ciently large sample size is achieved, but this system is very good for small trials, which are the norm in surgery. Unlike stratification, minimization works at reducing the total imbalance of factors in the study rather than considering mutually exclusive subgroups, for example comparing young patients to old or young patients with open fractures to old patients with closed fractures.[23] Although theoretically it may not balance the unknown factors well, in practice it performs well enough to be considered equivalent to the other randomized allocation procedures.

Jargon Simplified: Minimization
Minimization adjusts the probability of allocation depending on the balance of known important prognostic factors.

Reality Check: Resources
1. http://www.random.org/
This online randomizer is useful for generating a variety of random numbers. Not ideal for carrying out a study, but very useful for planning.
2. http://www-users.york.ac.uk/~mb55/guide/rand-sery.htm
This is a fantastic resource to identify web-based services which can be used to allocate patients to a study.

Conclusion

Appropriate allocation to intervention and control is a fundamental aspect of clinical trials and requires a great deal of thought at the design stage. It is important to consider how the allocation sequence is generated and how it will remain concealed. Failure to address these issues will jeopardize the integrity of the study.

Regardless of the actual method of random allocation selected, the mechanics of patient allocation must ensure that the process is free of bias and must be able to provide an audit trail of patient allocation. As the techniques become more complex, these requirements also become more complex. The complexities, which must be appreciated at the outset of the trial design, illustrate the importance of obtaining sound statistical advice during the design phase of these studies as well as during the conduct and analysis stage.

The ultimate aim of a trial is to have a fair test of an intervention and appropriate allocation; that is why minimizing bias is the first step toward the goal.

Suggested Reading

Altman DG, Bland JM. Treatment allocation by minimisation. BMJ 2005;330:843

Altman DG, Bland JM. How to randomise. BMJ 1999;319:703–704

Altman DG, Bland JM. Statistics notes. Treatment allocation in controlled trials: why randomise? BMJ 1999;318:1209

Chow S, Liu J. Design and Analysis of Clinical Trials: Concepts and Methodologies. 2nd ed. Hoboken, New Jersey: John Wiley & Sons, Inc; 2004

Moher D, Hopewell S, Schulz KF, et al. CONSORT 2010 explanation and elaboration: updated guidelines for reporting parallel group randomised trials. BMJ 2010;340:c869

Pocock SJ. Clinical Trials: A Practical Approach. 1st ed. Toronto: John Wiley & Sons Ltd; 1983

References

1. Meinert CL. Essential design features of a controlled clinical trial. In: Clinical Trials: Design, Conduct and Analysis. Chapter 8. New York: Oxford University Press; 1986: 65–70
2. Schulz KF. Subverting randomization in controlled trials. JAMA 1995;274:1456–1458
3. Schulz KF, Grimes DA. Allocation concealment in randomised trials: defending against deciphering. Lancet 2002;359:614–618
4. Boutron I, Moher D, Tugwell P, et al. A checklist to evaluate a report of a nonpharmacological trial (CLEAR NPT) was developed using consensus. J Clin Epidemiol 2005;58:1233–1240
5. Devereaux PJ, Bhandari M, Clarke M, et al. Need for expertise based randomised controlled trials. BMJ 2005;330:88
6. Devereaux PJ, McKee MD, Yusuf S. Methodologic issues in randomized controlled trials of surgical interventions. Clin Orthop Relat Res 2003;413:25–32
7. Chalmers I. Assembling comparison groups to assess the effects of health care. J R Soc Med 1997;90:379–386
8. Lachin JM. Properties of simple randomization in clinical trials. Control Clin Trials 1988;9:312–226
9. Lachin JM, Matts JP, Wei LJ. Randomization in clinical trials: conclusions and recommendations. Control Clin Trials 1988;9:365–374
10. Bartlett RH, Roloff DW, Cornell RG, Andrews AF, Dillon PW, Zwischenberger JB. Extracorporeal circulation in neonatal respiratory failure: a prospective randomized study. Pediatrics 1985;76:479–487
11. Chow S, Liu J. Randomization and blinding. In: Design and Analysis of Clinical Trials: Concepts and Methodologies. 2nd ed. Hoboken, NJ: John Wiley & Sons, Inc; 2004:120–166
12. Pocock SJ. Methods of randomization. In: Clinical Trials: A Practical Approach. 1st ed. Toronto: John Wiley & Sons Ltd; 1983:66–89
13. Treasure T, MacRae KD. Minimisation: the platinum standard for trials? Randomisation doesn't guarantee similarity of groups; minimisation does. BMJ 1998;317:362–363
14. Chan S, Bhandari M. The quality of reporting of orthopaedic randomized trials with use of a checklist for nonpharmacological therapies. J Bone Joint Surg Am 2007;89:1970–1978

15. Meinert CL. Randomization and the mechanics of treatment masking. In: Clinical Trials: Design, Conduct and Analysis. Chapter 10. New York: Oxford University Press; 1986:90–112

16. Kernan WN, Viscoli CM, Makuch RW, Brass LM, Horwitz RI. Stratified randomization for clinical trials. J Clin Epidemiol 1999;52:19–26

17. Lachin JM. Statistical properties of randomization in clinical trials. Control Clin Trials 1988;9:289–311

18. Meier P. Stratification in the design of a clinical trial. Control Clin Trials 1981;1:355–361

19. Avins AL. Can unequal be more fair? Ethics, subject allocation, and randomised clinical trials. J Med Ethics 1998;24:401–408

20. Guyatt G, Rennie D, Meade MO, Cook DJ, eds. Users' Guide to the Medical Literature: A Manual for Evidence-Based Clinical Practice. 2nd ed. Toronto: The McGraw-Hill Companies; 2008

21. SPRINT Investigators, Bhandari M, Guyatt G, et al. Study to prospectively evaluate reamed intramedullary nails in patients with tibial fractures (S. P. R. I.N.T.): study rationale and design. BMC Musculoskelet Disord 2008;9:91

22. Cook JA. The challenges faced in the design, conduct and analysis of surgical randomised controlled trials. Trials 2009;10:9

23. Scott NW, McPherson GC, Ramsay CR, Campbell MK. The method of minimization for allocation to clinical trials. A review. Control Clin Trials 2002;23:662–674

4

Blinding and Concealment

Daniel Whelan, Ryan M. Khan

Summary

The use of blinding and concealment in a clinical trial helps to eliminate bias in a variety of ways. The use of allocation concealment prevents researchers from influencing which study group participants are assigned to. Blinding, on the other hand, prevents bias following treatment allocation. This chapter will discuss types of allocation concealment, methods of blinding, and the strengths and limitations of these techniques.

Introduction

In any randomized trial, investigators are constantly trying to limit the effects of bias. Two important tools in that process are allocation concealment and blinding. The goal of randomization is to provide groups of similar prognosis, thereby limiting the effect of confounding. "Confounding" refers to the bias that occurs when groups are unevenly balanced with respect to factors that affect the relationship between the intervention and the outcome of interest. Allocation concealment and blinding are employed both before and after randomization to reduce biases that occur during the conduct of a trial.

> **Key Concepts: Difficulty of Blinding in Surgical Trials**
> While it is possible to have proper allocation concealment in all clinical trials, it is not always possible to blind the investigator or patients to treatments received. This is of significant importance for a surgical trial, where it is all but impossible to blind surgeons to the procedures they perform.

Concealment

Simply put, allocation concealment refers to the practice of preventing the randomization sequence from being known (to either investigators or patients) prior to assignment. Allocation concealment is an essential part of a quality study as it prevents selection bias on the part of investigators. If those responsible for enrolling participants know, or can detect, the upcoming treatment allocations, then theoretically they can direct participants with a better prognosis to the experimental group and those with a poorer prognosis to the control group, or vice versa. In a systematic review of randomized controlled trials, Schulz et al. demonstrated that failure to employ proper allocation concealment can lead to an overestimation of treatment effects in comparison to trials with adequate concealment.[1] The differences were not small: odds ratios were exaggerated by as much as 40% in inadequately concealed trials. This is likely because investigators direct lower-risk patients with a more favorable prognosis (and suspected higher responsiveness) to experimental groups. The finding that improperly concealed allocation exaggerates treatment effects has been observed subsequently in several other investigations across various fields of medicine.[2,3]

Allocation concealment is possible in all types of trials, including unblinded trials, and is therefore universally recommended and a crucial part of a quality study protocol. There are several different methods that can be implemented to achieve allocation concealment, ranging from very basic and affordable to large-scale web-based applications that can carry a substantial cost.

Types of Allocation Concealment

The most widely used and discussed practical methods for ensuring allocation concealment are sealed opaque envelopes, telephone randomization, and web-based randomization systems. The envelope method is the easiest and most cost-effective way of creating allocation concealment and—if carried out correctly—can be very effective. It is ideal for single-center sites where "centralization" of the randomization process is neither practical nor necessary.

There are some pitfalls that can detract from the effectiveness of the envelope method and may introduce possibilities of a loss of concealment or fraudulent randomization. As an example, consider a study comparing a nonsurgical treatment to an emergent surgical procedure. For both surgeons and patients in these studies the temptation can be strong to direct patients to the nonoperative group, especially during evening hours and on weekends. Imagine you are the surgeon on call and a patient comes in late at night that fits the eligibility criteria for the study. The limited personnel and resources available during "off hours"—as well as the extra work involved in performing the operative procedure—make it understandable that some surgeons would be tempted to either not randomize patients or "choose" nonsurgical treatments at night. Knowing which treatment group the patient will be directed to ahead of time may have a direct influence on whether or not randomization is attempted. There have been numerous publications describing scenarios where investigators or study personnel have held envelopes up to light sources to subvert concealment.[4,5] A straightforward way around this is to cover the contents of the envelope with a dark-colored paper or foil so that the content is not visible even when held up to a strong light.

Another important safeguard to consider in the concealment process when using envelopes is to ensure that the person who is creating the envelopes is not a part of the study team. In general, all those individuals who may have access to the allocation sequence should be impartial as they could be tempted to alert the investigators to the next treatment allocation if in doubt about enrolling a particular patient. Serially numbering envelopes is essential to avoid treatments being given out of sequence. Even if all of the proper precautions and steps are taken in order to have good-quality, sealed envelope allocation concealment, it is still not the ideal method for concealment.

> **Reality Check: Temptations of Sealed Envelope Allocation**
> Sealed envelopes can be opened or transilluminated to reveal the treatment assignment. The temptation to do this is strong if investigators or patients are biased or if one of the treatments is more difficult or time-consuming. In this situation the biased investigator may exclude the patient or choose a new (and more desirable) envelope out of sequence.

The second most common form of allocation concealment is a telephone-based system. Over time these systems have become easier to set up and administer, but they do introduce an increased cost compared to the envelope method. Phone systems are slightly different from one another in that some have different levels of security and access for different study personnel. However, they all typically involve a member of the study team telephoning a central number and receiving the treatment group allocation only after it is determined that the subject meets the inclusion/exclusion criteria and has been deemed suitable for enrollment into the study. The fact that all randomization is handled centrally at an impartial site ensures that study personnel are not able to identify which treatment group a potential patient would be randomized to, thereby eliminating any selection bias.[6] Furthermore, because potential patients have to be registered as part of the randomization telephone call, it is not possible for investigators to subsequently exclude those patients if a "favorable" (to either the patient or the investigator) randomization allocation is not assigned. Telephone systems are a good option for large multicenter trials whereas a single-site study may find it unnecessary or too costly and opt for using the envelope method.

Today, most trials employ a central randomization service that is internet based. Online systems have the advantage of allowing investigators to enter demographic and prognostic baseline data more quickly and efficiently compared to telephone systems. Reliable and consistent access to a computer and internet connection is mandatory, however, and may be an issue in remote sites. For surgical trials requiring intraoperative randomization this requirement might also provide a unique challenge. Whether by telephone or computer, centralized randomization is essential for larger multicenter trials due to the ability to oversee multiple randomization strata and ensure balance within these strata across multiple sites. Cost is obviously the major drawback of these types of systems.

A note of caution must be made regarding the use of block randomization schemes and preservation of concealment. Dividing the randomization sequence into smaller blocks can be advantageous as it helps to preserve the allocation ratio of treatments, particularly in larger trials with a number of study sites and randomization strata.[7] The use of blocking can subvert randomization concealment, however, if the block sizes are small and fixed throughout the trial. For this reason it is recommended that block sizes for each site be sufficiently large and of variable lengths so that investigators cannot easily predict the sequence order.

Blinding

Investigators utilize allocation concealment to eliminate any bias that might occur at the initiation of patients into a trial during the process of randomization. Thereafter, blinding is employed to reduce the bias that may occur in the conduct of the trial itself. Investigators, patients, and outcomes assessors may change their behavior in a systematic way (whether consciously or subconsciously) over the course of a trial if they are aware of treatment allocation and have preconceived attitudes about efficacy.

> **Examples from the Literature: Does Blinding of Outcome Assessors Matter?**
> Poolman et al. conducted a systematic review of 32 randomized, controlled trials published in *The Journal of Bone and Joint Surgery* (American volume) and found that unblinded outcomes assessment was associated with significantly larger treatment effects than blinded outcomes assessment. The ratio of odds ratios (unblinded to blinded outcomes assessment) was 0.31, suggesting that the unblinded outcomes assessment was associated with a potential for a significant exaggeration of the benefit of the effectiveness of a treatment.[8]

Blinding is a very simple yet effective method of preventing both conscious and unconscious bias in research. Beyond allocation concealment—which is a form of early blinding and is directed only at those individuals assigning the treatment allocation—blinding during the trial is usually directed at three different groups: treatment providers, participants, and outcomes assessors. An important part of any trial design is deciding on the level of blinding. Generally it is preferable to use the highest level of blinding possible within the trial constraints (i.e., to blind as many groups as possible).

> ### Key Concepts: Blinding of Outcomes Assessors in Surgical Trials
> Complete or "double" blinding is impossible in surgical trials, as surgeons can never be truly blind to the procedures they perform. Blinding of outcomes assessors becomes even more essential in surgical trials as a way to reduce bias.

Levels of Blinding

A trial without blinding of caregivers, patients, or assessors is called an unblinded study. The potential for bias is obviously highest in the unblinded situation. In these "open label" study designs, everyone involved in the trial knows which treatment group each subject has been randomized to. Trials comparing surgical and nonsurgical treatments are often unblinded due to the presence or absence of incisions. Outcomes assessors may be blinded in these situations, but extra levels of effort are necessary to cover incisions or hide x-rays during assessments, etc.

The next level of blinding is termed "single-blind," where at least one of the patient, caregiver, or outcomes assessor is blinded to treatment group allocation. The usual scenario is that the patient is blinded. Trials of medications, medical products or devices, or policy and procedures are usually of this nature. Again, it is often more difficult to conduct single-blind surgical trials, the usual requirement being that the two surgical procedures be nearly identical in terms of incisions, pain profiles, postoperative protocols, and even the x-ray appearance. Any variation between the procedures could lead to "unmasking." An example of a single-blind trial would be one which compares two different bearing surfaces in total hip replacement. Provided the incisions for the two implants are the same and the x-ray appearance is similar, patients can usually be blinded to treatment allocation (e.g., what type of "bearing" they have in their hip) in these situations. An obvious shortcoming of the single-blind study design is that several groups remain unblinded. The treating physician or surgeon is aware of allocation and therefore could—knowingly or unknowingly—introduce "performance bias" at the time of the surgical procedure. Performance bias occurs when one treatment is systematically performed differently (perhaps technically more proficiently or carefully) than the other. Furthermore, caregivers such as physiotherapists in this "single-blind" study may introduce co-intervention bias by providing different modalities of therapy to one group more frequently than the other. Finally, the outcomes assessor may introduce "detection biases" in more rigorously or efficiently adjudicating outcomes in one of the experimental groups.

The third and highest level of blinding is the "double-blind" study, where neither the patient nor the clinician knows which treatment the patient is randomized to. Placebo-controlled drug trials are usually double-blinded as it is easy to blind both the patient and physician as to whether the pill taken was the medication or the placebo. As mentioned previously, it is impossible to conduct a double-blinded surgical trial, as the surgeon can never be truly unaware of the procedure that was performed.

> ### Examples from the Literature: A Controlled Trial of Arthroscopic Surgery for Osteoarthritis of the Knee
> An example of a surgical trial which approached the "double-blind" ideal was conducted on patients undergoing knee arthroscopy for osteoarthritis. In the investigation by Moseley et al., three groups of patients were compared: those who underwent arthroscopy and débridement of the knee as per the usual standard of care, another group in whom the surgical incisions were made for arthroscopy and a saline irrigation was performed only (without débridement of cartilage lesions or meniscal tears), and a third, "sham" group who had only the incisions and neither irrigation nor débridement.[9] In all groups a general anesthetic was given and patients and outcomes assessors remained blinded throughout the course of the trial. As the surgical incisions were identical in all groups and there were no major changes in the x-ray appearance of the knees pre- and postoperatively, patient and outcome assessor blinding was well preserved in this study. For most surgical trials, however, sham surgery (the surgical "placebo") is not an option as it poses significant challenges to achieving institutional ethics approval and is unpalatable to many patients. Furthermore, there are usually differences in pain, incisions, rehabilitation protocols, or x-ray appearances amongst surgical procedures being compared in trials that make patient blinding difficult or impossible. In surgical trials then, it is essential to have blinded outcomes assessors whenever possible.

Blinding can take on a heightened importance depending on the type of outcome measures that are used in a trial. Objective or "hard" outcomes (such as blood tests, x-ray parameters, or mortality) are often less prone to bias in their assessment and therefore more easily blinded than more subjective or "soft" outcomes.[10] For example, an orthopaedic study assessing mortality after two types of hip fracture surgery may be less apt to detection bias, despite being poorly blinded, than the same study with "time to painless ambulation" as a primary outcome. In the latter situation, the unblinded (and biased) outcomes assessor has more latitude to allow for variations in the interpretation of the outcome. The situation becomes even

Table 4.1 Potential benefits accruing dependent on those individuals successfully blinded

Individuals blinded	Potential benefits
Participants	Less likely to have biased psychological or physical responses to intervention More likely to comply with trial regimens Less likely to seek additional adjunct interventions Less likely to leave trial without providing outcome data, leading to "lost to follow-up"
Trial investigators	Less likely to transfer their inclinations or attitudes to participants Less likely to differentially administer co-interventions Less likely to differentially adjust dose Less likely to differentially withdraw participants Less likely to differentially encourage or discourage participants to continue trial
Assessors	Less likely to have biases affect their outcome assessments, especially with subjective outcomes of interest

Reproduced with permission from Schulz KF, Grimes D.[15]

more difficult in surgical trials utilizing patient-assessed outcomes. As is the case in most of these "open label" designs, patient blinding is either difficult or impossible because of the nature of the procedures being compared, and therefore utilizing patient-assessed outcomes measures, such as functional outcome scores, will always be subject to some degree of detection bias.

It is an unfortunate fact that—despite utilizing study resources in attempts to blind caregivers, patients, and/or assessors—many investigators do not report these efforts in published manuscripts.[11–13] This leaves the reader unsure of the risk of bias and less secure in adopting the study results. It has been further suggested that the terms "single" and "double" blinding may be confusing to both readers and investigators.[14] The simplest, most transparent approach, then, is to list those individuals who were blinded and the methods undertaken to do so. **Table 4.1** outlines some of the benefits of blinding the different people involved with the study.

Conclusion

Both allocation concealment and blinding have as their goal the reduction of bias. Allocation concealment is employed by investigators to eliminate selection bias and preserve the equality of experimental groups provided by randomization. Allocation concealment can be reliably achieved by a number of methods including sealed envelopes and central randomization services. Blinding is applied after allocation and is used to limit bias that may arise during the conduct of the trial. This can include performance bias on behalf of investigators, co-intervention bias as introduced by caregivers, and/or detection bias on the part of outcomes assessors. Achieving blinding in surgical trials is particularly challenging as surgeons can never be truly "blind" to the procedures they perform.

Suggested Reading

Bhandari M, Guyatt GH, Swiontkowski MF. Users guide to orthopaedic literature: how to use an article about surgical therapy. J Bone Joint Surg Am 2001;83:916–926

Haynes RB, Sackett DL, Guyatt GH, Tugwell P. Clinical Epidemiology: How to Do Clinical Practice Research. 3rd ed. Philadelphia: Lippincott, Williams and Wilkins; 2006

Schulz KF. Assessing allocation concealment and blinding in randomized controlled trials: why bother? Evid Based Med 2000;5:36–38

Schulz KF, Grimes DA. Blinding in randomized trials: hiding who got what. Lancet 2002;359:696–700

References

1. Schulz KF, Chalmers I, Hayes RJ, et al. Empirical evidence of bias. Dimensions of methodological quality associated with estimates of treatment effects in controlled trials. JAMA 1995;273:408–412
2. Pildal J, Hróbjartsson A, Jórgensen KJ, Hilden J, Altman DG, Gøtzsche PC. Impact of allocation concealment on conclusions drawn from meta-analyses of randomized trials. Int J Epidemiol 2007;36:847–857
3. Schulz KF, Grimes DA, Altman DG, Hayes RJ. Blinding and exclusions after allocation in randomized controlled trials: survey of published parallel group trials in obstetrics and gynaecology. BMJ 1996;312:742–744
4. Hansen JB, Smithers BM, Schache D, Wall DR, Miller BJ, Menzies BL. Laparoscopic versus open appendectomy: prospective randomized trial. World J Surg 1996;20:17–20
5. Schulz KF. Subverting randomization in controlled trials. JAMA 1995;274:1456–1458
6. Haag U. Technologies for automating randomized treatment assignment in clinical trials. Drug Inf J 1998;32:11
7. Higgins JPT, Green S (eds). Cochrane handbook for systematic reviews of interventions version 5.0.0. Available at: http://www.cochrane-handbook.org. Accessed July 22, 2010
8. Poolman R, Struijs P, Krips, R, et al. Reporting of outcomes in orthopaedic randomized trials: does blinding of outcome assessors matter? J Bone Joint Surg Am 2007;89:550–558
9. Moseley JB, O'Malley K, Petersen NJ, et al. A controlled trial of arthroscopic surgery for osteoarthritis of the knee. N Engl J Med 2002;347:81–88
10. Wood L, Egger M, Gluud LL, et al. Empirical evidence of bias in treatment effect estimates in controlled trials with different interventions and outcomes: meta-epidemiological study. BMJ 2008;336:601–605
11. Montori VM, Bhandari M, Devereaux PJ, Manns BJ, Ghali WA, Guyatt GH. In the dark: the reporting of blinding status in randomized controlled trials. J Clin Epidemiol 2002; 55:787–790

12. Chan AW, Altman DG. Epidemiology and reporting of randomised trials published in PubMed journals. Lancet 2005;365:1159–1162

13. Gøtzsche PC. Methodology and overt and hidden bias in reports of 196 double-blind trials of nonsteroidal antiinflammatory drugs in rheumatoid arthritis. Control Clin Trials 1989;10:31–56

14. Devereaux PJ, Manns BJ, Ghali WA, Quan H, Lacchetti C, Guyatt GH. In the dark: physician interpretations and expert definitions of blinding in randomized controlled trials. JAMA 2001;285:2000–2003

15. Schulz KF, Grimes D. Blinding in randomized trials: hiding who got what. Lancet 2002;359:696–700

5

Composite Outcomes in Orthopaedics: Understanding the Concepts

Lauren A. Beaupre, C. Allyson Jones

Summary

In this chapter, we discuss methods to deal with multiple study outcomes through the use of a composite outcome. Four different types of composite end points are described, as well as the rationale for their use and potential limitations. Guidelines for constructing and interpreting composite outcomes are provided to give clinicians the tools to both create clinically sensible composite endpoints and also assess their appropriateness and utility when reported in the literature.

Introduction

When investigators design a clinical research trial, they must define their primary outcome or end point prior to implementing the study. Typically, the selected outcome will be meaningful to both clinicians and patients and be biologically plausible. The outcome must not only have the potential to be affected by the intervention of interest but also be measurable.[1] Perhaps more importantly, the outcome must be aligned with the research question. In some cases, researchers are faced with a myriad of potential outcomes associated with a medical condition. When these outcomes are of similar importance or the most important end point occurs infrequently, they may choose to combine multiple clinically important end points to make a single "*composite*" *end point* or *outcome*.[2]

Although the definition of a composite outcome is still evolving, there is general consensus that a composite end point is the occurrence of any one or more predefined events in a given set of events after a certain period of follow-up.[3] Components consist of a variety of measures that are aligned with the research question. Different types of composite end points can be reported. The first type of end point is a *total score*, which typically sums the occurrence of the components. A second type of composite end point is an *event rate*, which is the occurrence of any one of a predefined set of events over a specified time period. Another type of composite end point is *time to first event*, which is commonly reported in large clinical trials.[4] A fourth type of end point is when no single component that defines an outcome exists. In this case, investigators may choose to create a set of criteria in which a specified number of component outcomes must occur to attain the composite end point.

Jargon Simplified: Composite Outcome (or End Point)
A composite outcome (or end point) consists of a combination of multiple selected outcomes that are counted and reported as a single "composite" outcome. For example, rather than reporting each fracture type separately, investigators report the total number of fractures occurring as the study outcome, regardless of anatomical site.

Key Concepts: Types of Composite Outcome
Total score composite outcome: The cumulative number of events occurring from a predefined set of outcomes (e.g., number of fractures occurring, regardless of anatomical site).
Event rate composite outcome: The rate of occurrence of any out of a predefined set of events over a specified time (e.g., 1-month failure rate, in which the total number of occurrences of any of periprosthetic fracture, dislocation, or infection is counted).
Time to event composite outcome: The time to any one of the selected component outcomes (e.g., time to either nonunion or deep infection).
Criteria-based composite outcome: When no single criterion provides evidence of an event occurring, criteria are set as to what number or combinations of criteria must occur for an event to be deemed to have occurred (see example below).

Examples from the Literature: How a Composite Outcome Can Be Used When No Gold Standard Exists
A randomized, controlled trial conducted by Jones and colleagues that examined the impact of two different bone grafting strategies in tibial fractures used fracture healing as the primary outcome.[5] As there is no single clinical or radiographic measure that defines when a fracture has healed, the authors created a composite outcome consisting of both clinical and radiographic parameters. For a fracture to be considered healed, there had to be radiographic evidence of cortical bridging callus on three of four cortices as well as at least one of the following two clinical parameters: pain-free full weightbearing and lack of tenderness on palpation of the fracture site. This definition is clinically sensible as clinicians make decisions regarding fracture healing based on multiple features—both radiographic and clinical.

Rationale for Use of a Composite Outcome

There are a number of reasons why investigators may choose to combine multiple outcomes into a single composite measure. One of the most commonly cited reasons for support of composite outcomes is to increase the statistical power and improve the efficiency of a study.[2,3,6] An adequate number of events that are attributable to the intervention under study need to occur. Combining multiple outcomes has a number of potential ramifications: more "events" are likely to occur, and the number of subjects required in the study is reduced. Consequently, the time and costs required to complete a clinical trial can be reduced by the use of a primary composite outcome. This decision is frequently made when one of the important outcomes is a relatively rare event.

Examples from the Literature: Use of a Composite Outcome to Increase Statistical Efficiency
The effect of an intravenously administered bisphosphonate, zoledronic acid, was examined in a randomized, controlled trial of 2127 patients with hip fracture conducted by Lyles and colleagues.[7] The investigators chose the rate of new clinical fractures as their primary composite outcome. New clinical fractures were defined as any one of nonvertebral, vertebral, or hip fractures. Although the treatment did not affect the rate of new hip fractures, which occurred relatively infrequently over the first two postoperative years, treatment with zoledronic acid did significantly reduce the rate of nonvertebral fracture, vertebral fracture, and any new fracture. The difference for any fracture type was significant at $P = 0.001$; while nonvertebral and vertebral fractures were both significantly different at $P < 0.05$.[7] For hip fractures no significant difference arose between treatment arms. Had the investigators chosen only hip fracture occurrence as their outcome, they would have needed substantially more subjects to be able to show a significant difference. Using any new fracture as the end point allowed them to demonstrate the impact of the medication more efficiently.

Using a composite outcome also allows us to determine the net effect of an intervention across a set of clinical outcomes. This can assist clinicians and decision makers in assessing the "net clinical benefit" of a treatment across a spectrum of clinically relevant outcomes. When the overall magnitude of effect for a specific treatment can be examined, rather than looking at each clinical issue separately, a fuller picture is presented to determine the impact of an intervention as a whole.

Examples from the Literature: Use of a Composite Outcome to Demonstrate the Net Clinical Benefit of an Intervention
In a randomized study that examined a case manager intervention to improve osteoporosis care following a hip fracture, Morrish et al. used a composite outcome that they defined as "appropriate care".[8] If, following a hip fracture, a subject underwent bone mineral density (BMD) testing and was found to have low BMD, and subsequently started bisphosphonate treatment, he/she was deemed to have received appropriate care. If, however, after having had BMD testing performed, a subject was found to have normal BMD and was *not* started on bisphosphonate therapy, he/she was also deemed to have received appropriate care. By combining two outcomes of interest (BMD testing and medication use) into a single composite outcome (BMD testing and medication where indicated), the investigators were able to show the net benefit of their osteoporosis intervention (see **Fig. 5.1**).

Another common reason given for creating and using a composite outcome is when multiple important outcomes can potentially be affected by the treatment under study; this approach avoids speculation among a number of meaningful outcomes. By creating a composite primary outcome at the study onset, investigators do not have to select the "most" important outcome or the one that is likely to be "most" affected by the intervention. In this case, a composite outcome is a practical way to deal with a situation where there is no obvious single important outcome. A composite outcome is also useful when there is no single

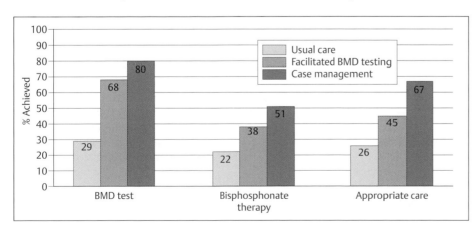

Fig. 5.1 Osteoporosis management 12 months after hip fracture. Reproduced with permission from Morrish et al.[8]

measurement that reflects the outcome of interest, as seen in our initial example of different bone grafting interventions for tibial fractures.[5]

Further, when there are multiple important outcomes, using a composite outcome also deals with the statistical problem of *multiple testing*. If investigators allot multiple outcomes to be tested separately without defining which is the primary outcome, statistical adjustments need to be performed.[9] Multiple outcome reporting is a common issue in orthopaedic clinical research, which to date has not frequently used composite outcomes as a methodological approach.

Jargon Simplified: Multiple Testing

Multiple testing occurs when investigators report the statistical significance of multiple outcomes being tested on the same set of participants. If we test enough outcomes, the chance of seeing a difference increases just due to chance alone. Caution is needed when a single difference among many nonsignificant findings is reported.

Reality Check: Risk of False-Positive Results with Multiple Testing

In a systematic review of orthopaedic surgical trials, Bhandari et al. found that only 33.3% of orthopaedic surgery trials specified the primary study outcome.[10] In the studies that did not specify the primary outcome, the mean number of outcomes reported in each study was 12.5 (range 2–30). Of 182 outcomes that were initially reported as significant, only 108 (59%) remained significant after correcting for multiple testing. The risk of reporting false-positive results could be substantially reduced by considering a composite outcome approach when designing a study.

Key Concepts: Advantages of Using Composite Outcomes

Increases statistical efficiency and power of a study: The cumulative number of events occurring will be higher when multiple outcomes are added together, so fewer subjects will be required to determine if there is a significant difference between interventions.

Determines the net clinical benefit of an intervention: A composite outcome allows us to look at how a single intervention may affect multiple clinical outcomes as a whole.

Combines multiple important clinical events into a single outcome: If there are multiple clinical events that are of similar importance, or multiple criteria need to be met to determine when an outcome has occurred, a composite outcome is an efficient way to manage this issue.

Avoids multiple testing issues: A single *P* value is produced for each composite outcome rather than multiple *P* values from each separate component.

Limitations of Using Composite Outcomes

The use of a composite end point presents both clinical and statistical deliberations. Although the use of composite outcomes may appear to be clinically sensible, there is also the potential to misinterpret the results of a study when a composite outcome has been reported. This is the most common disadvantage attributed to composite outcomes and can arise if the selected combined components occur at highly differing rates or vary substantially in their relative clinical importance.[3]

Jargon Simplified: Qualitative Heterogeneity

If individual components of a composite outcome are substantially different in clinical importance, the composite outcome is qualitatively heterogeneous.

Jargon Simplified: Quantitative Heterogeneity

If individual components of a composite outcome occur at substantially different rates, the composite outcome is quantitatively heterogeneous.

Quantitative heterogeneity occurs when one or more of the components that make up the composite outcome changes at a differential rate or in terms of number of events relative to the other components being measured. *Qualitative heterogeneity* occurs when outcomes occur differentially among components that are deemed more or less important. The other concern in terms of component heterogeneity is if the components do not move in the same direction (i.e., the intervention does not have the same effect on all components). In this case, the effect of one component could be masked by the stronger effect of another component moving in the opposite direction. In pharmaceutical randomized, controlled trials where both mortality and major morbidity are of interest, the primary composite outcome will frequently include mortality with other important nonfatal outcomes.[4,11] In these cases, investigators and readers must ensure that the impact of mortality is not being masked by other components in the composite outcome.

Reality Check: Quantitative Heterogeneity in the Zoledronic Acid Trial

Returning to the zoledronic acid trial discussed above, there was quantitative heterogeneity among the selected components.[7] Nonvertebral and vertebral fractures occurred more commonly than hip fractures, the worst of the osteoporotic fractures. Some might argue that in achieving statistical efficiency, the authors limited their ability to talk about the effect of the trial medication on the incidence of subsequent hip fracture.

**Examples from the Literature: An Example
of Qualitative Heterogeneity**
In the recently published SPRINT trial that compared reoperation rates between patients with reamed and unreamed tibial intramedullary nails, the investigators
used a composite outcome that included bone grafting,
implant exchange, or dynamization within 12 months
of fracture.[12] In patients with closed fractures, the
authors reported a benefit for reamed nails over unreamed nails (relative risk 0.67; 95% confidence interval
0.47–0.96; P = 0.03). However, the difference between
the two groups was primarily due to different rates of
dynamization, particularly autodynamization, which
was the least important of all the measured outcomes.

In orthopaedics, we often report "clinician-driven" outcomes. If outcomes where clinicians make a judgment
about the occurrence of an outcome are included as a component of the composite outcome, we may allow a single
component that is subject to *clinical bias* to unduly influence the reported outcome.[13,14] One common clinician-driven outcome is reoperation following surgical intervention. Often the decision to perform additional surgery is
left to the discretion of the participating surgeons rather
than based upon a prespecified set of criteria for reoperation. The aforementioned SPRINT trial had much lower
overall reoperation rates than previous studies of the
same intervention; the authors speculated that their prespecified reoperation criteria forced clinicians to delay reoperation to meet the study requirements rather than relying solely on their clinical preferences.[12]

Jargon Simplified: Clinical Bias
Clinical bias can occur when the decision about when an
outcome has occurred is left to the clinician's discretion
(e.g., deciding when to readmit patients to hospital or
perform additional surgical procedures). Reported
study outcomes may then be biased, as clinical decisions
by clinicians may not directly relate to the intervention,
but to clinical preferences instead.

**Key Concepts: Disadvantages of Using
Composite Outcomes**
Heterogeneity in occurrence of components: Components vary in importance, frequency, or direction, making the clinical interpretation of the composite outcome
difficult or less clinically meaningful.
Risk of bias from clinically driven events: Inclusion of
components that are rated by clinician judgment may influence the number of events reported in the composite
outcome.

Guidelines for Creating a "Good" Composite Outcome

First and foremost, the composite outcome should be
guided by a specific research question. The events that
comprise the composite outcome can include one or a
combination of different perspectives that are congruent
with the theoretical construct. Further, components that
make up a composite outcome should be measurable
events that can sensibly be added together as representing
aspects of the same process or outcome of interest.[3]
Although composite outcomes typically increase the precision of the statistical estimate of treatment effect, precision often comes at the cost of greater uncertainty in interpreting the result.[2]

Several authors have suggested three main issues to consider when constructing a composite outcome.[2,3,6,15]

1. **Is each of the selected components that make up the
   composite outcome of similar importance to the
   clinicians and patients?**
   There are instances where two or more outcomes may
   be deemed to be similarly important. Both nonunion
   and deep infections following fracture have serious negative ramifications for patients' quality of life, clinicians' ongoing patient management, and health service
   utilization. More often, however, when selecting components for composite outcomes, there are gradients
   of importance among components, with the most important component often occurring with the least frequency (e.g., death) and less serious outcomes occurring more frequently (e.g., reoperation or hospital readmission).[15] In these instances, investigators must be
   careful that the study interpretation is not that each individual component has the reported impact on outcome, but rather, the reported impact on outcome is a
   synthesis of all the components' effects.[16]

2. **Does each of the components occur with similar frequency?**
   Ideally all of the selected components should have a similar likelihood of occurring. In reality, most composite
   outcomes include serious adverse outcomes that occur
   infrequently along with less serious adverse outcomes
   that occur more frequently. In most trials that report
   composite outcomes, the majority of participants experienced the less serious events.[6] Therefore, the estimated effect of the intervention will often be weighted
   toward the less important outcomes. Whenever possible, investigators should try to combine events that are
   likely to occur at similar rates.

3. **Is each of the components likely to show similar
   effects?**
   When selecting components for a composite outcome,
   investigators need to ensure that each component is
   likely to be influenced by the intervention under
   study. The more apparent it is that a composite end
   point is linked to a disease process, the less challenging

the interpretation of the end point, as the components will likely respond similarly to the intervention. In fact, much of our confidence in a composite outcome rests in our belief that all components are similarly affected by the intervention.[3,15] Further, when selecting outcomes, it must be anticipated that all components are likely to move in the same direction as a result of the intervention. If components move in opposite directions, the composite outcome will be difficult to interpret clinically.

There are other important issues to consider when constructing a composite outcome. The first of these relate to determining when an outcome has occurred. If the selected outcome involves clinical judgment (e.g., need for reoperation or readmission), the outcome likely will depend upon the clinician's expertise or usual care and is inherently subject to bias. To ensure a standardized evaluation, investigators should consider how the outcome can be objectively measured or implement strategies to minimize variation such as utilizing Data Safety and Monitoring Boards (DSMB), assessors blinded to group allocation, blinded adjudication committees, prespecified definitions of outcomes, or a combination of these techniques.[14] Even mortality may be subject to bias as there are differing views on the type of mortality to be included in a composite end point. General consensus is that all-cause mortality should be used rather than cause-specific mortality, to prevent a censoring bias.[2,4,11]

Finally, a composite outcome should not consist of too many components. There are two important reasons; the first is *outcome ascertainment*—the more components that researchers use to create a composite outcome, the more work they must do to validate that all outcomes have occurred. Perhaps, more importantly, as the number of components in a composite outcome increase, the ability to clinically interpret the outcomes becomes more uncertain. It has been proposed that composite outcomes be composed of no more than three or four individual components.[17]

Jargon Simplified: Outcome Ascertainment

Outcome ascertainment is determining when or if the outcome has occurred. To standardize ascertainment among investigators and study centers, the definition of what constitutes an "outcome" needs to be defined at study outset.

Reporting and Interpreting Composite Outcomes

Transparent reporting is required so that interpretation of the outcome is comprehensible. To achieve this, a number of steps should be followed. Firstly, the composite outcome needs to be prespecified at the study onset.[9] If the composite outcome is the primary study end point, then it should be reported as such at completion of the study. Each of the component outcomes should also be reported, so that readers can determine if any one component has dominated and/or examine for consistency of effect among components.[3] Accordingly, all patients should be followed to the completion of the study for all components, with the frequency of each component for each composite outcome reported. Accounting for the components will also minimize the bias of censored data and improve the precision of the analysis. Finally, authors and journal editors need to ensure that the interpretation of the composite outcome is of the "net effect" of the components rather than as the impact of each individual component. If emphasis is placed on reporting the components of the composite outcomes, investigators should adjust for multiple testing prior to making conclusive statements about the components.

Reality Check: Beware of Bait and Switch

Readers should be aware of the "bait and switch" strategy, when the focus of reporting results changes from the composite outcome to one or more of its components.[6] The use of composite outcomes is not to allow researchers to find a significant finding through endless combinations of outcomes, but rather to make the net effect of an intervention clearer to the clinician.

Key Concepts: Interpreting Composite Outcomes

1. What is the research question? Is the composite outcome clinically sensible and biologically plausible?
2. How many components are included in the composite outcome? Are the components of similar importance to patients and clinicians?
3. Are the components likely to occur with similar frequency? Is each component likely to be similarly affected by the intervention?
4. What is the follow-up of the composite outcome? Are all components followed for the same amount of time?
5. Do the authors report the outcomes of each individual component in addition to the composite outcome?

Conclusion

Composite outcomes have frequently been used in pharmaceutical trials, but their use in orthopaedics has been more limited. However, such outcomes may be useful when used appropriately. A recent examination of outcomes used in fracture healing trials suggested that composite outcomes that combine patient-reported and clinician-assessed outcomes may provide the "best available" outcome in studies where no clearly defined primary outcome currently exists.[14]

The development and implementation of a composite end point is challenging due to issues surrounding selection of components, which can lead to contradictory results if not carefully done. Until standardized methods are developed to define the optimal number and type of items to include in a composite end point, investigators should provide a judicious rationale for using a composite outcome and the selection of each component. Likewise, users of clinical evidence should consider carefully their clinical relevance and appropriateness prior to applying study findings in practice.

Suggested Reading

Bhandari M, Whang W, Kuo JC, Devereaux PJ, Sprague S, Tornetta P III. The risk of false-positive results in orthopaedic surgical trials. Clin Orthop 2003;413:63–69

Ferreira-Gonzalez I, Permanyer-Miralda G, Busse JW, et al. Methodologic discussions for using and interpreting composite endpoints are limited, but still identify major concerns. J Clin Epidemiol 2007;60:651–657

Kooistra BWB, Sprague SM, Bhandari M, Schemitsch EHM. Outcomes assessment in fracture healing trials: a primer. J Orthop Trauma 2010;24:S71–S75

References

1. Neaton JD, Gray G, Zuckerman BD, Konstam MA. Key issues in end point selection for heart failure trials: composite end points. J Card Fail 2005;11:567–575

2. Freemantle N, Calvert M, Wood J, Eastaugh J, Griffin C. Composite outcomes in randomized trials: greater precision but with greater uncertainty? JAMA 2003;289:2554–2559

3. Ferreira-Gonzalez I, Permanyer-Miralda G, Busse JW, et al. Methodologic discussions for using and interpreting composite endpoints are limited, but still identify major concerns. J Clin Epidemiol 2007;60:651–657

4. Chi GY. Some issues with composite endpoints in clinical trials. Fundam Clin Pharmacol 2005;19:609–619

5. Jones AL, Bucholz RW, Bosse MJ, et al. Recombinant human BMP-2 and allograft compared with autogenous bone graft for reconstruction of diaphyseal tibial fractures with cortical defects. A randomized, controlled trial. J Bone Joint Surg Am 2006;88:1431–1441

6. Tomlinson G, Detsky AS. Composite end points in randomized trials: there is no free lunch. JAMA 2010;303:267–268

7. Lyles KW, Colon-Emeric CS, Magaziner JS, et al. Zoledronic acid and clinical fractures and mortality after hip fracture. N Engl J Med 2007;357:1799–1809

8. Morrish DW, Beaupre LA, Bell NR, et al. Facilitated bone mineral density testing versus hospital-based case management to improve osteoporosis treatment for hip fracture patients. Arthrit Care Res 2009;61:209–215

9. Pocock SJ. Clinical trials with multiple outcomes: a statistical perspective on their design, analysis, and interpretation. Control Clin Trials 1997;18:530–545

10. Bhandari M, Whang W, Kuo JC, Devereaux PJ, Sprague S, Tornetta P III. The risk of false-positive results in orthopaedic surgical trials. Clin Orthop 2003;413:63–69

11. Lubsen J, Kirwan BA. Combined endpoints: can we use them? Stat Med 2002;21:2959–2970

12. Bhandari M, Guyatt G, et al. Study to prospectively evaluate reamed intramedullary nails in patients with tibial fractures. J Bone Joint Surg Am 2008;90:2567–2578

13. Corrales LA, Morshed S, Bhandari M, Miclau T, III. Variability in the assessment of fracture-healing in orthopaedic trauma studies. J Bone Joint Surg Am 2008;90:1862–1868

14. Kooistra BWB, Sprague SM, Bhandari M, Schemitsch EHM. Outcomes assessment in fracture healing trials: a primer. J Orthop Trauma 2010;24:S71–S75

15. Montori VM, Permanyer-Miralda G, Ferreira-Gonzalez I, et al. Validity of composite end points in clinical trials. Br Med J 2005;330:594–596

16. Freemantle N, Calvert M. Weighing the pros and cons for composite outcomes in clinical trials. J Clin Epidemiol 2007;60(7):658–659

17. Lauer MS, Topol EJ. Clinical trials multiple treatments, multiple end points, and multiple lessons. JAMA 2003;289:2575–2577

6

Adjudication of Outcomes—Systems and Approaches

Jihee Han, Simrit Bains, Natalie Kuurstra, Christopher Vannabouathong, Sheila Sprague, Mohit Bhandari

Summary

Outcomes assessment in clinical trials is a critical yet subjective process, leading to the increasing use of adjudication committees to evaluate outcomes. Adjudication committees have the potential to provide a systematic and unbiased method of evaluating endpoints. In order to introduce greater efficiency to this adjudication process, web-based systems have been developed to serve as both an electronic data capturing system and a data management system. This chapter demonstrates the benefits of using an adjudication committee to assess study outcomes, and how using a web-based adjudication system facilitates this process.

Introduction

Outcomes assessment is a critical component of all clinical research. When properly and diligently planned, it yields an abundance of insightful information for health care in terms of policy making and treatment options.[1,2]

Jargon Simplified: Outcome
The outcome is the end result or consequence of interest in a clinical trial.

Jargon Simplified: Outcome Variable
The outcome variable is the target variable of interest— the variable that is hypothesized to depend on or be caused by another variable (the independent variable).[3]

The primary objective when conducting randomized controlled trials is to use empirical evidence to gain a valid understanding of how the intervention of interest affects patient outcomes. Such interventions often involve surgical procedures or pharmaceutical drugs. However, establishing appropriate end points is often difficult; this is due to the complexity that is introduced as a consequence of the fact that there is usually a degree of subjectivity involved in the evaluation process.[1,4–6]

Jargon Simplified: End Point
The end point of a study is an event or outcome that can be measured objectively to determine whether the intervention being studied is beneficial.

This process is further complicated by the fact that most clinicians are not trained to make decisions based on the principles of evidence-based medicine. The focus of evidence-based medicine is to base clinical practice on the results of scientific studies as opposed to personal preference. The lack of this philosophy in health care is a problematic issue as end points must be impartially evaluated. Careful planning of outcomes assessments is of the utmost importance in a clinical trial as this process has a direct impact on the validity of the study results.

Jargon Simplified: Evidence-Based Medicine
The term "evidence-based medicine" refers to health care policies and practices that are derived from the systematic, scientific study of the effectiveness of various treatments.

Jargon Simplified: Outcome Ascertainment
Outcome ascertainment is determining when or whether the outcome has occurred. To standardize ascertainment among investigators and study centers, the definition of what constitutes an "outcome" needs to be defined at study outset.

Importance of Adjudication

Many researchers are recognizing the significance of outcomes assessment; as a result, there is a growing trend toward assessing outcomes by means of an independent adjudication committee.

An adjudication committee consists of a group of independent experts who are not otherwise involved in the study.[6] The adjudication committee members should be blinded to treatment allocation, as well as any other factors that may introduce bias. For example, if an adjudication committee member is aware that the attending physician is a respected colleague of theirs, then the adjudicator may be biased to assess the subject's outcome more positively.

The use of an independent adjudication committee helps to standardize the evaluation process and achieve consistency in outcomes assessment. This is important as many assessments in the medical field are subjective. For example, multiple physicians can view the same x-ray of a fractured tibia and have diverging opinions on whether the fracture is healed. Having study participants assessed by the same group of individuals reduces the amount of subjectivity involved by limiting the assessment to a smaller pool of qualified persons.

> **Jargon Simplified: Adjudication Committee**
> An adjudication committee is a group of clinical experts who determine end point assessment in a standardized and unbiased manner.[7]

> **Jargon Simplified: Adjudication**
> In clinical research studies, adjudication is the determination of an outcome by an independent person or group of individuals who are not otherwise involved in the study.

Multiple studies have demonstrated the benefits of using an adjudication committee in clinical trials.[5,8] This suggests that the adjudication committee members are at less risk than those immediately involved in the study of being reliant on raw data in conducting clinical assessments, and that they therefore evaluate the evidence more objectively. In recognition of the importance of assessing patient outcomes accurately, at appropriate intervals, and in manners which minimize the risk of bias, the use of adjudication committees has become the current clinical standard.[4,6,9]

> **Examples from the Literature: The Impact of an End-Point Committee in a Large Multicenter, Randomized, Placebo-Controlled Clinical Trial**
> A double-blinded, multicenter clinical trial (the TRIM study) used an independent end-point committee and found that disparities existed between the decisions by the local site investigators and adjudication committee members leading to statistically significantly different study results.[5,8] The same study identified as its most important finding that "in a clinical trial, the number of events may change significantly during data processing" due to reasons such as inadequate documentation of patients' progress by the site investigator.[8]

> **Key Concepts: Using an Adjudication Committee**
> Using an adjudication committee is the most reliable method of assessing study outcomes.

Process of Adjudication

An adjudication committee will consist of a handful of experts in the relevant field, which will depend on the research being performed. Ideally, the adjudication committee should be comprised of at least three physicians. An uneven number of adjudicators prevents a tie from occurring in the case that a vote is required. The primary responsibility of an adjudication committee member is to provide an unbiased assessment of specific end points outlined in the study protocol.[2,6] Adjudication committee members should be experienced clinicians who lack direct involvement in the study and do not have any motivation to influence the results in a particular manner.[2] This is so as to minimize the effects of bias.

Before initiating the adjudication process, the adjudication committee members should attend training meetings in which they will be instructed on the study protocol and will discuss the end point definitions with each other. Major decisions reached by the adjudication committee may be relayed to the steering committee by the methods center, and these decisions may even be influenced by the steering committee.[2] It is of particular value to have a system in place to deal with undefined areas. This is important because adjudicators and local site investigators are clinicians who are accustomed to making clinical decisions autonomously and who may find it challenging to come to consensus within the definitions outlined in the study protocol.[2] It is also likely that disagreements among adjudicators will arise, especially during the initial stages of the adjudication process. Such situations should be regarded as excellent opportunities to clarify and expand on study protocols and the adjudication guidelines.[2] Site investigators and the data monitoring committee may also be consulted by the methods center on behalf of the adjudication committee.[2,8] **Figure 6.1** presents the relationship between the adjudication committee, the steering committee and the data monitoring committee.

> **Jargon Simplified: Methods Center**
> The methods center is the main facility that captures, stores, and manages data pertaining to the trial.

> **Jargon Simplified: Steering Committee**
> A study's steering committee is comprised of investigators, physicians, and other experts not actively involved in the conduct of the study. This committee serves to oversee the data collection processes, direct the implementation of changes in procedures, and evaluate study progress.[2]

> **Jargon Simplified: Data Monitoring Committee/Data and Safety Monitoring Board (DSMB)**
> The primary role of the DSMB is to ensure the safety of the study participants by reviewing interim reports for evidence of adverse or beneficial treatment effects. The DSMB also makes decisions regarding the frequency, timing, and manner in which interim data are analyzed.[2,5]

Before the adjudication committee can participate in adjudication, the materials needed for adjudication must be prepared. The preparation of these materials and, by virtue of that, the adjudication process depend greatly on an efficient system of data collection, verification, and validation.[2,4] To prepare for adjudication and consensus meetings, supporting staff are required to check the received materials for completeness and consistency, blind received documents to maintain anonymity, enter and track re-

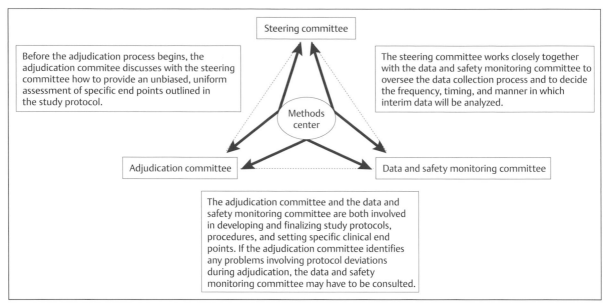

Steering committee

Before the adjudication process begins, the adjudication commitee discusses with the steering committee how to provide an unbiased, uniform assessment of specific end points outlined in the study protocol.

The steering committee works closely together with the data and safety monitoring committee to oversee the data collection process and to decide the frequency, timing, and manner in which interim data will be analyzed.

Methods center

Adjudication committee

Data and safety monitoring committee

The adjudication committee and the data and safety monitoring committee are both involved in developing and finalizing study protocols, procedures, and setting specific clinical end points. If the adjudication committee identifies any problems involving protocol deviations during adjudication, the data and safety monitoring committee may have to be consulted.

Fig. 6.1 Relationship between the adjudication committee, steering committee, and data and safety monitoring committee.

ceived documents into a tracking database, and ask site investigators for missing materials and clarifications. Preparation of adjudication materials can absorb a substantial amount of time and is labor-intensive.[2,4,5] Researchers and research coordinators need to take into consideration that the process of gathering clinical data requires careful planning. A possible trade-off between the depth of evaluation and feasibility should also be acknowledged.[1] Multisite clinical studies often require a significant amount of time to send and receive necessary materials. Consequently, it takes longer to process the adjudication materials, perform the subsequent analysis, and gather the study results.[5]

Once these materials have been prepared, the actual process of adjudication can begin. If there is more than one adjudication committee member, then the individual members must adjudicate the outcomes independently so as not to influence each other's answers.[4] At each study visit, the adjudication committee members will have specific questions to answer. The adjudication committee members' individual answers are based on the clinical evidence provided, which is usually in the form of x-rays or clinical notes. The individual answers are then tabulated and any disagreements are discussed during a consensus meeting.[5] It is quite possible to have the final consensus be completely different from most adjudicators' initial assessments. Regular consensus meetings provide adjudicators with the opportunity to discuss the reasoning behind their decisions. An added benefit of discussion is that the committee members may realize that they initially missed something in the evidence that is significant enough to alter their previous decision. It is also at the consensus meeting that the adjudication committee members

may decide to ask the site investigator for additional materials and clarifications as appropriate. **Figure 6.2** presents the basic steps of the adjudication process.

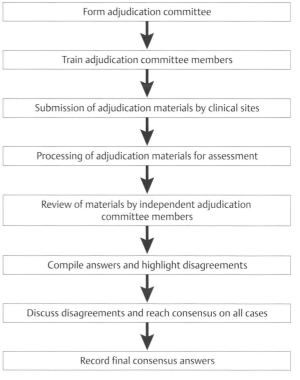

Form adjudication committee

Train adjudication committee members

Submission of adjudication materials by clinical sites

Processing of adjudication materials for assessment

Review of materials by independent adjudication committee members

Compile answers and highlight disagreements

Discuss disagreements and reach consensus on all cases

Record final consensus answers

Fig. 6.2 Basic steps of the adjudication process.

Existing Methods of Adjudication

In the past, it was much more difficult to conduct multisite randomized clinical trials, owing to the lack of technological and logistical options that are available to researchers today. Communication via email, sending and receiving of adjudication materials via fax or in electronic forms, and the development of sophisticated software systems to aid in the entering and tracking of materials have made conducting clinical studies much more efficient.

Since the use of adjudication committees has become a common practice, there have been some developments to facilitate the adjudication process. As previously mentioned, collecting adjudication materials can be time consuming. It may also take time to obtain the results from the adjudication committee members. Systems and approaches to simplify the process, thereby increasing efficiency and reducing time and errors, are certainly warranted and desirable.

Web-Based Adjudication

The Global Adjudicator is an online system that aids clinical researchers and supporting staff with the efficient organization, analysis, and storage of adjudication related materials and data. As the system can be used to adjudicate study outcomes, subject eligibility, and protocol deviations, many different parties (clinical researchers, pharmaceutical companies, medical device companies, etc.) will find the Global Adjudicator system to be of immense benefit. Advantages include increased accessibility, reduced time and cost, and easier data extraction.[5] The Global Adjudicator website (www.globaladjudicator.ca) can tailor the study visits and adjudication questions to each specific trial requirement.

Examples from the Literature: A Web-Based End-Point Adjudication System for Interim Analyses in Clinical Trials

Nolen et al. developed a web-based end-point adjudication system (WebEAS) to study the efficiency and capability of web-based adjudication; the system automatically notified adjudication committee members upon validation of a subject's data, electronically captured and compared the results, and stored the adjudicated results for future use. The authors concluded that WebEAS expedited the adjudication process greatly and proposed a web-based end-point adjudication system as a plausible solution for future clinical trials.[5]

Examples from the Literature: Is the Future for Clinical Trials Internet Based? A Cluster Randomized Clinical Trial

A study by Litchfield et al. randomly allocated study centers to use either the internet or paper case report forms for data collection. They found that the time from the last patient completing the study to the release of the database was shorter in the internet group even though a much larger number of patients were enrolled in the internet group.[10] They also found that the data gathered at a patient visit were entered into the electronic (internet) database much quicker than into paper-based case report forms. The transfer of data over the internet to the sponsor was faster as well.[10]

Conclusion

The process of outcomes assessment is critical as it is the basis on which the therapeutic techniques under investigation are evaluated. Using an adjudication committee to determine study outcomes has been shown to have tremendous benefits, such as standardizing assessments and minimizing bias. The adjudication process has become the clinical standard; however, it can also be time consuming and costly. Due to the importance of adjudication, web-based systems such as the Global Adjudicator have been developed to make this process as simple and straightforward as possible.

Suggested Reading

Dijkman BG, Sprague S, Schemitsch EH, Bhandari M. When is a fracture healed? Radiographic and clinical criteria revisited. J Orthop Trauma 2010;24:S76–80

Hanson B. The art of choosing sound study endpoints. Injury 2008;39:656–658

Kooistra BW, Sprague S, Bhandari M, Schemitsch EH. Outcomes assessment in fracture healing trials: a primer. J Orthop Trauma 2010;24:S71–S75

Lopez-Carrero C, Arriaza E, Bolanos E, et al. Internet in clinical research based on pilot experience. Contemp Clin Trials 2005;26:234–243

Mahaffey KW, Harrington RA, Akkerhuis M, et al. Disagreements between central clinical events committee and site investigator assessments of myocardial infarction endpoint in an international clinical trial: review of the PURSUIT study. Curr Contr Trials Cardiovasc Med 2001;2:187–194

Morshed S, Corrales L, Genant H, Miclau T. Outcome assessment in clinical trials of fracture healing. J Bone Joint Surg Am 2008;90:62–67

References

1. Dawson J, Carr A. Outcomes evaluation in orthopaedics. J Bone Joint Surg Br 2001;83–B:313–315
2. Isaacsohn JL, Khodadad TA, Soldano-Noble C, Vest JD. The challenges of conducting clinical endpoint studies. Curr Atheroscler Rep 2003;5:11–14
3. Guyatt GH, Rennie D, Meade M, Cook D, eds. Users' Guide to the Medical Literature: A Manual for Evidence-Based Clinical Practice. 2nd ed. New York: McGraw-Hill; 2008
4. Walter SD, Cook DJ, Guyatt GH, King D, Troyan S. Outcome assessment for clinical trials: how many adjudicators do we need? Control Clin Trials 1997;18:27–42
5. Nolen TL, Dimmick BF, Ostrosky-Zeichner L, et al. A web-based endpoint adjudication system for interim analyses in clinical trials. Clin Trials 2009;6:60–66
6. Bhandari M, Petrisor B, Schemitsch E. Outcome measurements in orthopedic. Indian J Orthop 2007;41:32–36
7. European Medicine Agency. Pre-authorisation Evaluation of Medicines for Human Use. Guideline on Data Monitoring Committees. London, England: European Medicine Agency; 2005
8. Naslund U, Gript L, Fisher-Hansent J, Gundersen T, Lehtol S, Wallentin L. The impact of an end-point committee in a large multicenter, randomized, placebo-controlled clinical trial. Eur Heart J 1999;20:771–777
9. Dechartres A, Boutron I, Roy C, Ravaud P. Inadequate planning and reporting of adjudication committees in clinical trials: recommendation proposal. J Clin Epidemiol 2009;62:695–702
10. Litchfield J, Freeman J, Schou H, Elsley M, Fuller R, Chubb B. Is the future for clinical trials internet based? A cluster randomized clinical trial. Clin Trials 2005;2:72–79

7

Subgroup Analyses

Shelly-Ann Rampersad, Sheila Sprague

Summary

Subgroup analyses are useful for detecting differences that may otherwise be overlooked when data are pooled. The practical utility of a subgroup analysis lies in its ability to decipher which patients will benefit the most from a particular treatment. Poorly designed subgroup analyses will have severe limitations in drawing conclusions. In this chapter, the design, reporting, and interpretation of a sound subgroup analysis is presented. The advantages and disadvantages of subgroup analyses are highlighted.

Introduction

Clinicians are often faced with the task of deciding which patients will benefit the most from a particular treatment. To discern differences in treatment effects across different types of patients, subgroup analyses can be conducted. Results of subgroup analyses may have implications in providing some patients with benefits while protecting others from harm. To this end, researchers need sensible recommendations on how to critically examine subgroup analyses to determine their validity and utility. This chapter will discuss the design, reporting and interpretation of a reliable subgroup analysis.

Subgroup Analysis Defined

A subgroup analysis is any evaluation of treatment effects in subgroups for a specific end point defined by baseline characteristics.[1] Subgroup analyses aim to identify inconsistencies or large differences in the magnitude of treatment effects on the basis of specific patient characteristics.[1,2] This can aid in identifying which particular patients will benefit most from a treatment under study.[3] Such an analysis must always be conscientious in design, reporting, and interpretation, but in practice they seldom actually fulfill the criteria that apply.[2] As a result, critics complain of "spurious inferences" while advocates maintain that important differences can be missed when results are pooled.[4] In reality, a subgroup analysis can fall in either of these categories depending on its execution.

Design of a Subgroup Analysis

A sound subgroup analysis begins with proper design. Four considerations in design will be discussed in this section: (1) the rationale, (2) the hypothesis, (3) stratified randomization, and (4) statistical power. Subgroup analyses considered unreliable are normally deficient in one or more of these areas. One of the most notorious examples of a false subgroup analysis that affected practice incorrectly was the observation that aspirin was ineffective in preventing stroke and death in women.[5,6] As a consequence of this, women were not treated with aspirin for at least a decade, until subsequent trials correctly suggested benefit.[7] Other examples of false subgroup analysis observations that were later corrected include (**Table 7.1**):[4]

- Antihypertensive treatment is ineffective or harmful in the elderly (refuted by 38 references).
- Thrombolysis is ineffective when administered later than 6 hours after an acute myocardial infarction (refuted by 45 references).
- Ticlopidine is superior to aspirin for the prevention of recurrent stroke, myocardial infarction, or vascular death in black people but not in white people (refuted by 56 references).

The Rationale

The first step in starting a subgroup analysis is to develop a sensible rationale in line with the main study. A strong justification and well-thought-out rationale will maximize the practical utility and will help to inform the design. According to Rothwell, there are four clinical indications for conducting a subgroup analysis:[7]

1. Potential heterogeneity of treatment effect related to risk;
2. Potential heterogeneity of treatment effect related to pathophysiology;
3. Clinically important questions related to the practical application of a treatment;
4. Underuse of a treatment in clinical practice due to uncertainty about benefit.

It is important to consider choosing variables, such as demographics and co-morbidities, that can be easily applied to common patient populations. A subgroup analysis that fails here will have little true utility.

Table 7.1 Examples of subgroup analyses subsequently shown to be false

Observation	No. of refuting references
Aspirin is ineffective in secondary prevention of stroke in women	33
Antihypertensive treatment for primary prevention is ineffective in women	36
Antihypertensive treatment is ineffective or harmful in elderly people	38
ACE inhibitors do not reduce mortality and hospital admission in patients with heart failure who are also taking aspirin	40
β-Blockers are ineffective after acute myocardial infarction in elderly people and in patients with inferior myocardial infarction	43
Thrombolysis is ineffective > 6 h after acute myocardial infarction	45
Thrombolysis for acute myocardial infarction is ineffective or harmful in patients with a previous myocardial infarction	46
Tamoxifen citrate is ineffective in women who have breast cancer and are aged <50 years	48
Benefit from carotid endarterectomy for symptomatic stenosis is reduced in patients taking only low-dose aspirin because of an increased operative risk	50
Amlodipine reduces mortality in patients with chronic heart failure caused by nonischemic cardiomyopathy but not in patients with ischemic cardiomyopathy	52
Platelet-activating-factor-receptor antagonist reduces mortality in patients with Gram-negative sepsis but not in other patients with sepsis	54
Ticlopidine is superior to aspirin for preventing recurrent stroke, myocardial infarction, or vascular death in black but not in white people	56
Angiotensin-receptor blockers increase mortality in patients with New York Heart Association functional class II–IV heart failure who also take both ACE inhibitors and β-blockers but lower mortality in patients not already taking drugs in both of these classes	58
Lamifiban lowers 6-month mortality and nonfatal myocardial infarction at 6 months in patients whose plasma concentrations are between 18 and 42 ng/mL but not in patients whose plasma concentrations are outside of this range	61

ACE, angiotensin-converting enzyme.

The Hypothesis

Following the development of a sound rationale, the hypothesis should be formulated a priori. A priori means that the hypothesis is generated and focuses on differences at the start of the study. Exact definitions and categories of variables should also be specified at this time, as well as the end point, baseline characteristics, statistical methods, and expected direction and magnitude of subgroup effects.

A hypothesis developed after the study has begun is termed "post hoc" and is generally considered unreliable (although not automatically untrue). Such analyses are common as unexpected results often yield new research questions. There is a significant difference in the hypothesis depending on when it is formulated. Post hoc hypotheses are problematic since they are based on outcome-dependent data, and thus an effect may be the result of one subgroup having a better prognosis rather than the result of the treatment.[2] A detailed and methodical a priori hypothesis will avoid criticisms that definitions were subsequently used to make data statistically significant.

In addition, the number of hypotheses should be limited to decrease the probability of false-positive findings. This problem, known as "multiplicity," states that false-positive results (type I errors) will be erroneously reported in about 5% of the tests performed.[2,8] The risk of false-positive results will be particularly high when many factors, such as sex, age, race, and co-morbidities, influence the outcome.[8] Multiplicity increases the probability that positive findings are based on chance. It should be noted that this problem is not limited solely to post hoc hypotheses. Even a priori hypotheses, if numerous, will be subjected to the inflated risk of false-positive findings associated with multiplicity. In addition, from a reader's standpoint, multiplicity will also make results confusing and difficult to follow.

> **Key Concepts: Multiplicity**
> Multiplicity is the challenge associated with testing multiple hypotheses. When many hypotheses are specified, the risk of false-positive results is inflated.

Stratified Randomization

During the design stage of subgroup analyses, stratified randomization should also be considered. For instance, it may be advantageous to investigate low-risk patients separately, since potentially harmful interventions may actually provide no benefit to them.[2] Moreover, surgical skill may be of importance in determining treatment results when comparing operative interventions.[2]

Stratified randomization must always be planned in advance. It leads to a greater similarity between treatment groups with regard to prognostic factors that influence treatment effect, so that treatment assignments within groups are balanced.[2] Further, stratified randomization makes each subgroup similar to a small trial, allowing valid inferences about treatment efficacy to be drawn.[2]

Statistical Power

If important subgroup–treatment effect interactions are anticipated, trials should ideally be powered to detect them reliably. Having an underpowered subgroup analysis can lead to false-negative results (type II errors): the risk of concluding that there is no effect when in fact one is present. Usually, the sample size of a trial is just large enough to detect treatment effect with a power of 80%. With fewer patients, as in a subgroup analysis, treatment effect is significantly harder to detect; therefore, for effects of interactions of the same size and power as the overall treatment effects, sample sizes should be inflated four-fold.[2]

> **Key Concepts: Design Phase**
> A sound subgroup analysis begins with four important considerations during the design phase:
> • The rationale
> • The hypothesis
> • Stratified randomization
> • Statistical power

Reporting

Reporting should begin with the four considerations of design. The rationale, hypothesis, stratified randomization, and power should all be reported in the methods section of the report. Specifically, details of how and why subgroups were selected should be provided, along with the number and type (a priori or post hoc) of hypotheses. Multiplicity should be addressed if several hypotheses were tested. If formal adjustments were made, these should also be indicated. Finally, imbalances regarding prognostic factors should be reported if they are still present after stratified randomization.

Next, interaction effects should be reported (i.e., whether treatment efficacy differs between the subgroups). The efficacy of treatment given to subgroups separately should not be reported since heterogeneity cannot be claimed this way. For example, testing a hypothesis in women and then separately in men will not address the question of whether treatment differences vary according to sex.[1]

In general, there are two ways to report the magnitude of an observed treatment effect: absolute and relative risk reductions. Dijkman et al. suggest the favored measure should be relative risk reduction, as it gives an estimate of the proportion of risk that is removed by the treatment.[2] Meanwhile, Rothwell suggests that both absolute and relative risk reductions should be reported, with statistical significance of difference in absolute risk reductions tested

where relevant.[7] The absolute risk reduction is the difference in the absolute risk for a certain outcome between the patient group with and the patient group without the treatment.[2] Naturally, the magnitude of reduction will habitually be greater in groups with higher baseline risk. This is problematic for interpretation since one may conclude the existence of a difference between subgroups on the basis of a reduction of absolute risk, even when no difference in relative risk reduction actually exists.[2]

Finally, subgroup analyses should not be reported in a way that would affect the conclusions of a trial, since they are exploratory in nature.[2] The emphasis of the discussion and conclusion should remain on the overall treatment effect and not on the subgroup analysis results.[2]

> **Example from the Literature: Reporting a Subgroup Analysis**
> The SPRINT Investigators performed a multicenter randomized trial comparing reamed and unreamed intramedullary nailing of tibial shaft fractures with regard to rates of reoperations and complications.[9] The following excerpt from the methods section illustrates the manner in which the design of subgroup analyses can be reported:
> "Subgroup analyses were conducted with use of tests for interactions; all were specified a priori. Our subgroup analysis of primary interest was the comparison between open fractures and closed fractures. Additional subgroup hypotheses included the impact of treatment in patients with multiple trauma as compared with those with isolated fractures; OTA classification type C as compared with types B and A; operations performed by surgeons as compared with fellows and residents; and fracture gaps of >1 cm as compared with <1 cm as compared with no gap."

Interpretation

After the analysis is performed and results obtained, it is up to the researcher to decide the applicability of the observed subgroup effect or interaction.

Replication

Replication of the subgroup treatment effect is sometimes considered to contribute even more to the validity of the analysis than the significance of the effect. Along with a sound design, replication of results will combat criticisms that findings may be based on chance. However, comparisons of subgroup analyses across studies should be performed with caution since (1) most subgroup analyses are generally small in size and thus underpowered, and (2) studies may be incomparable since they almost always vary in design, population, intervention, and outcome.[2]

Key Concepts: Replication
Due to lingering skepticism with regard to subgroup analyses, replication is considered a strong indicator of validity.

Alternatively, a meta-analysis combining the results of many trials may have improved power to document subgroup effects, but published data seldom provide adequate information to allow a consistent subgroup analysis.[4] Strict inclusion and exclusion criteria will be of benefit here.

Example from the Literature:
Using a Meta-analysis to Find Subgroup Effects
Source: Eppsteiner RW, Shin JJ, Johnson J, van Dam RM. Mechanical compression versus subcutaneous heparin therapy in postoperative and post-trauma patients: a systematic review and meta-analysis.[10]
Background: The risk of postoperative venous thromboembolic disease is as high as 30%, with an associated fatality risk of 1%. Therefore, prophylaxis is essential, but the optimal regimen remains controversial. This study was designed to systematically review and quantitatively summarize the impact of mechanical compression versus subcutaneous heparin on venous thromboembolic disease and post-treatment bleeding in postsurgical and posttrauma patients.
Methods: Computerized searches of the MEDLINE and EMBASE databases through November 2008 were performed and supplemented with manual searches. We included studies that had: (1) a patient population undergoing surgery or admitted immediately post-trauma, (2) a randomized comparison of prophylaxis with mechanical compression versus subcutaneous heparin, (3) outcome measured in terms of deep vein thrombosis, pulmonary embolism, or bleeding.
Results: Two reviewers independently extracted data from the original articles, which represented 16 studies, including a total of 3887 subjects. Meta-analysis was performed using a random effects model. The pooled relative risk for mechanical compression compared with subcutaneous heparin was 1.07 (95% confidence limits [CI] 0.72–1.61) for deep vein thrombosis, and 1.03 (95% CI 0.48–2.22) for pulmonary embolism. Mechanical compression was associated with a significantly reduced risk of postoperative bleeding compared with subcutaneous heparin (risk ratio 0.47; 95% CI 0.31–0.70). Subgroup analyses by heparin type suggested that low molecular weight heparin may reduce risk of deep vein thrombosis, compared with compression (relative risk 1.80; 95% CI 1.16–2.79) but remains similarly associated with an increased risk of bleeding.
Conclusions: These results suggest that the overall bleeding risk profile favors the use of compression over heparin, with the benefits in term of venous thromboembolic disease prophylaxis being similar between groups. Subgroup analyses suggest that low molecular weight heparin may have a differential effect; this observation should be further evaluated in future studies.

Applicability

The question of applicability of results deals with whether subgroup patients are comparable to your own patients. Since randomized controlled trials often have stringent inclusion and exclusion criteria, the patients in the study will rarely be similar to your patients.[2] Subgroup patient characteristics should be critically assessed before their results are applied to any population of patients. A researcher thinking about applicability of results should also consider whether interactions found are biologically plausible.

Guidelines for Interpretation

When interpreting a subgroup analysis, a number of questions should be considered by the researcher. The researcher should ask whether:

• The hypothesis preceded rather than followed the analysis.
• The subgroup difference was only one of a small number of hypothesized effects tested.
• The subgroup difference is suggested by comparisons within studies rather than between studies.
• The magnitude of the subgroup difference is large.
• The subgroup difference is consistent across studies and statistically significant.
• There is external evidence to support the hypothesized subgroup difference.

Conclusion

To discern differences in treatment effect across different types of patients, subgroup analyses can be conducted. Researchers must be aware of the challenges associated with subgroup analyses, which may increase the risk of both type I and type II errors. In this chapter we have suggested guidelines for design, reporting, and interpretation of reliable subgroup analyses.

Suggested Reading

Dijkman B, Kooistra B, Bhandari M. How to work with a subgroup analysis. Can J Surg 2009;52:515–522

Guyatt G, Wyer P, Ioannidis J. When to Believe a Subgroup Analysis. In: Guyatt G, Rennie D, Meade MO, Cook DJ. Users' Guides to the Medical Literature. 2nd ed. New York: McGraw-Hill; 2008:571–593

Rothwell PM. Subgroup analysis in randomized controlled trials: importance, indications, and interpretation. Lancet 2005; 365:176–186

References

1. Wang R, Lagakos SW, Ware JH, Hunter DJ, Drazen JM. Statistics in medicine—reporting of subgroup analyses in clinical trials. N Engl J Med 2007;357:2189–2194
2. Dijkman B, Kooistra B, Bhandari M. How to work with a subgroup analysis. Can J Surg 2009;52:515–522
3. Groenwold RHH, Donders ART, van der Heijden GJMG, Hoes AW, Rovers MM. Confounding of subgroup analyses in randomized data. Arch Intern Med 2009;169:1532–1534
4. Guyatt G, Wyer P, Ioannidis J. When to Believe a Subgroup Analysis. In: Guyatt G, Rennie D, Meade MO, Cook DJ. Users' Guides to the Medical Literature. 2nd ed. New York: McGraw-Hill; 2008:571–593
5. The Canadian Cooperative Study Group. A randomized trial of aspirin and sulfinpyrazone in threatened stroke. N Engl J Med 1978;299:53–59
6. Fields WS, Lemak NA, Frankowski RF, Hardy RJ. Controlled trial of aspirin in cerebral ischaemia. Stroke 1977;8:301–314
7. Rothwell PM. Subgroup analysis in randomized controlled trials: importance, indications, and interpretation. Lancet 2005;365:176–186
8. Cook DI, Gebski VJ, Keech AC. Subgroup analysis in clinical trials. Med J Aust 2004;180:289–291
9. SPRINT Investigators. Bhandari M, Guyatt G, Tornetta P III, et al. Randomized trial of reamed and unreamed intramedullary nailing of tibial shaft fractures. J Bone Joint Surg Am 2008;90:2567–2578
10. Eppsteiner RW, Shin JJ, Johnson J, van Dam RM. Mechanical compression versus subcutaneous heparin therapy in postoperative and posttrauma patients: a systematic review and meta-analysis. World J Surg 2010;34:10–19

8

Trial Management—Advanced Concepts and Systems

Meaghan Zehr, Christopher Vannabouathong, Sheila Sprague, Mohit Bhandari

Summary

Clinical trials are designed to determine the effects of an intervention on patient health and safety outcomes. This chapter will outline the four phases of a clinical trial and describe ideal sample sizes, participant characteristics, and methods of eliminating bias. Some common barriers to completing a successful clinical trial are difficulties in obtaining funding, ethics approval, and lack of qualified staff. This chapter will explore these concerns in detail and provide some guidelines on how to overcome these challenges.

Introduction

A clinical trial is "any research study that prospectively assigns human participants or groups of humans to one or more health-related interventions to evaluate the effects on health outcomes."[1] In other words, clinical research involves testing the effects of a new drug or medical procedure on human subjects. A clinical trial can be either industry-initiated or investigator-initiated. The aim of a clinical trial is to prove that an intervention has a desired outcome on patients and is safe to use. Some barriers to completing a successful clinical trial are lack of funding, lack of ethics approval, and lack of qualified staff. Without proper guidance, conducting a clinical trial can be time-consuming and yield few useful results. In this chapter, we will define each of the stages of a clinical trial and discuss strategies for success.

> **Jargon Simplified: Industry-Initiated vs. Investigator-Initiated Trials**
> An industry-initiated trial is a study that is developed, sponsored, and coordinated by a pharmaceutical or medical device company.[2] An investigator-initiated trial is a study developed and directed by a researcher.[2]

Phases of Clinical Trials

Phase 1

The goal of a phase 1 clinical trial is to determine if an intervention is safe for human use.[3] In drug trials, it is during this phase that an Investigator determines the highest dose of the drug that can be safely administered.[3] The sample size, or number of participants, is small, typically 15 to 50 participants. Participants are selected who have minimal co-morbidities and they may not be representative of the target population.[3] Single blinding and placebos may be appropriate here, although they may be unnecessary.[3]

> **Jargon Simplified: Blind**
> Patients, clinicians, data collectors, outcome adjudicators, or data analysts who are unaware of which patients have been assigned to the experimental group and which to the control group are referred to as "blind" or "blinded." In blinding in the case of diagnostic tests, those interpreting the test results are unaware of the result of the reference standard and vice versa.[4]

> **Examples from the Literature: Phase 1 Trial**
> In a study conducted by Suntharalingam et al., six healthy, young male participants were recruited to test a novel antibody that directly stimulates T cells. Within 12–16 hours after infusion, pulmonary infiltrates and lung injury, renal failure, and disseminated intravascular coagulation were observed. Severe and unexpected depletion of lymphocytes and monocytes occurred within 24 hours after infusion.[5]

Recruiting Participants for Phase 1 Trials

Investigators may not be able to recruit healthy participants for phase 1 trials if the intervention is invasive. For example, current therapeutics for the possible treatment of spinal cord injuries involve direct infusion into or around the injured spinal cord; participants without a spinal cord injury will not be recruited for this type of study.[6]

Phase 2

The goal of a phase 2 clinical trial is to determine if there is any benefit associated with the intervention. If the intervention is a drug, the participants are given the maximum dose with the least risk (established during phase 1). The duration and sample size can vary widely depending on the intervention, but phase 2 trials generally include a larger number of participants (25–100). Blinding, randomization, and placebos may be used during this phase.[3]

Jargon Simplified: Randomization
Randomization is the "allocation of individuals to groups by chance, usually done with the aid of table of random numbers. [...] Not to be confused with systematic allocation (e.g., on even and odd days of the month) or allocation at the convenience or discretion of the Investigator."[7]

Reality Check: Comparing Apples to Oranges
During phase 1 and 2 clinical trials, participants should be selected who have similar prognostic factors.[5] Certain conditions are associated with different rates of recovery and levels of severity regardless of the allocated treatment. These outcomes may increase the recorded variability of recovery time if they are compared together. For example, suppose a clinical trial investigates the rate of fracture healing after the administration of a drug. The protocol does not exclude patients with osteoporosis. Each participant is randomized to receive either the drug treatment or a placebo. Irrespective of any drug administration, however, patients diagnosed with osteoporosis typically take a longer time to heal than do patients without osteoporosis.[8] This is why the inclusion and exclusion criteria specified in the study protocol should be such that only patients with similar prognostic factors are eligible for study. This produces a more accurate representation of the true results of the intervention.

Phase 3

If an intervention proves to have beneficial effects after completing phase 2, the Investigator must now compare this treatment method to current standard therapies.[3] In phase 3 clinical trials, the sample size is generally large and it should be representative of the target population. The number of participants and the duration of the trial must be sufficient to show a clinically relevant and statistically significant difference between the intervention and the current standard of care. Blinding, randomization, and placebos are typically used.[3]

Key Concepts: Clinical Relevance vs. Statistical Significance
Statistical significance refers to the likelihood that an event occurred by chance.[2] An intervention may demonstrate statistical significance, but the potential benefits may not actually be meaningful. For example, suppose an Investigator shows that the use of a new surgical device can lead to increased range of motion after surgery. If the range of motion only increases by less than one degree, it may not be worth abandoning the current therapy in favor of a lesser known and possibly more expensive one.

Phase 4

In a phase 4 clinical trial, the intervention has already been approved for public use and the Investigator begins to explore clinical observations, rare side effects, or long-term health outcomes.[3] Due to the nature of the research questions, the duration and sample size required are generally very large. Instead of the narrow inclusion criteria typical of a phase 3 trial, the patient eligibility criteria tend to be very broad.[9] This is because during this phase the goal is to determine whether the results from the phase 3 trial are externally valid.[9] Blinding and randomization can be employed, depending on the nature of the study question, whereas some Investigators choose to analyze already-published studies for results. For example, Bongartz et al. conducted a systematic review and meta-analysis to establish the occurrence of rare harmful events in randomized trials of anti-tumor necrosis factor (TNF) therapy. This review included 3493 patients who received anti-TNF antibody treatment and 1512 patients who received a placebo.[10] Conducting a meta-analysis should be considered when the time and resources required to initiate a large-scale clinical trial are not available.

Key Concepts: Clinical Trials
- Clinical trials can be either industry-initiated or investigator-initiated.
- Clinical trials can be categorized into four phases.
- Clinical trials should use blinding, randomization, and placebos whenever possible.
- Conducting a meta-analysis is an option to be considered if resources are limited.

Common Considerations in Conducting a Clinical Trial

This section of the chapter highlights common considerations in conducting investigator-initiated trials and industry-initiated trials such as the role of research ethics review boards, the importance and considerations of budgeting, available funding sources and how to strengthen a funding application, as well as the resources necessary for a successful trial.

Research Ethics

All Investigators must comply with the regulations specific to their local research ethics review boards, which will relate to things such as submitting study documents for review and maintaining communication with the review board. In Canada, these review boards are referred to as Research Ethics Boards, or REBs, and are unaffiliated with the research group. In the United States, these review boards are called Institutional Review Boards, or IRBs, and are authorized through the Food and Drug Administration and the Department of Health and Human Services.[11] In some other countries, such as in Europe and Africa, they are called Research Ethics Committees, or RECs, and, likewise, provide third-party review.[11] An REB typically includes professionals with a working knowledge of law, ethics, and sciences, and members of the lay community.[12]

Procedures for ethics approval vary internationally and institutionally. Generally, the application for initial ethics approval is the most comprehensive and includes questions related to:

- Whether the study has industry sponsorship
- Whether the study is multicentered
- What medical records the study will require access to
- The phase of the trial and if the trial is randomized or blinded
- Placebo use
- How equipoise is maintained
- Trial characteristics such as the rationale, objectives, design, population, procedures, sample size, and data analysis
- Whether a Data Monitoring Committee will review safety data
- What patient risks exist and what efforts have been made to minimize them
- How patient consent is obtained and how patients are recruited

After initial approval is obtained, the Investigator must complete an annual ethics renewal form, which is less extensive. It may be necessary to notify the REB of any protocol deviations, study amendments, and adverse events. A protocol deviation is a failure to adhere to the procedures specified in the protocol.[12] An example of a protocol deviation is the enrollment of an ineligible patient. In addition, all amendments to the protocol, case report forms, or consent forms require ethics approval before they can be administered to study participants. Adverse events must also be reported to the REB. For example, in Canada, serious adverse events must be reported within 24 hours of occurrence and nonserious adverse events must be reported within 48 hours.[13] After patient recruitment, patient follow-up, and statistical analysis are completed, the Investigator must complete a study termination report and submit it to the ethics review board.[14]

Jargon Simplified: Equipoise

Equipoise refers to genuine uncertainty in the literature and medical community as to whether a treatment is better than another—otherwise the physician must prescribe the superior treatment.[15]

Key Concepts: Equipoise Applications

Equipoise relates to both subjective (quality of life) and objective (morbidity and mortality rates) elements. Some experts argue that placebos should only be administered if no pre-established treatment exists.[15] Some physicians hesitate before enrolling patients into clinical trials because they do not believe the treatments considered are equal.[15]

Jargon Simplified: Adverse Event

An adverse event is "any untoward medical occurrence in a research participant, which does not necessarily have a causal relationship with the treatment."[13] Serious adverse events result in death, are life-threatening, require in-patient hospitalization, or result in persistent or significant disability or incapacity, or birth defect. Adverse events which are nonserious do not meet any of these criteria.[13]

Budgeting

The budgeting needs of a trial will vary depending on whether it is industry-initiated or investigator-initiated.

Industry-Initiated Trials

Initially, the Investigator may be asked to create a preliminary budget, or be allocated an amount within which to operate.[16] It is important to be accurate and to negotiate a feasible budget in order to cover all costs associated with conducting the trial. Investigators should also consider price increases at the beginning of each fiscal year. The final budget is usually negotiated between the Sponsor and the Investigator.[16] Investigators can determine the adequacy of a budget by reviewing the protocol, developing a cost estimate, and then comparing the estimate with the Sponsor's initial offer.[16] When developing a cost estimate, consider the following:[16]

- If the Sponsor agrees to pay for screened subjects, is the definition of a potential subject clear?
- What is required by the Investigator during the follow-up visits?
- If the study is terminated before any patients are enrolled, will the Sponsor pay for prestudy activities such as time spent on the ethics application and meetings?
- Will the Sponsor pay for a study coordinator or for time spent on unanticipated activities such as:
  - Protocol amendments?
  - Re-consenting subjects?
  - Unanticipated monitoring visits?
  - Audits?

– An unexpectedly large number of adverse events (as this requires additional time to document and communicate to the local ethics board)?

- Are payments made according to the amount of work required by the study protocol?
- Will the Sponsor pay for off-site storing fees?
- Will the Sponsor pay for excluded patients?
- What other hospital resources are required?

Personnel for Industry-Initiated Trials

The Investigator is responsible for obtaining ethics approval from the local ethics committee, obtaining patient consent, randomizing patients, completing case report forms, scheduling patient follow-up appointments, and responding to data queries. Generally, the Investigator hires a Study Coordinator to assist with the coordination of the trial.[3] Additionally, a Study Monitor, who works for the Sponsor, will monitor the study to ensure all patient data and study-related information are recorded on time and accurately.[17] The Investigator should budget for the time required to complete all these tasks, including communication with the Study Monitor.

Investigator-Initiated Trials

Developing the budget for an investigator-initiated clinical trial demands more time and effort from the Investigator because it must include the costs of all participating sites plus the costs of operating a Central Methods Center. A Central Methods Center is responsible for the day-to-day activities required to manage a clinical trial, which include protocol development, maintaining a centralized randomization system, data management, coordination of trial committees, and overall management of the clinical centers participating in the study.[2] The Central Methods Center can be a private contract research organization or may be coordinated through an academic institution under the direction of the Nominated Principal Investigator.[2] Generally, the budget should be prepared after the study protocol is finalized and before research funding is applied for. The format should reflect the specifications of the funding agency to which the Investigator will apply.[18]

> ### Jargon Simplified: Central Methods Center
> A Central Methods Center can be a private contract research organization or it can be an academic institution under the direction of the Nominated Principal Investigator. It is responsible for the day-to-day activities of managing a clinical trial, which include protocol development, maintaining a centralized randomization system, data management, organization of trial committees, and communication with the clinical centers participating in the study.[2]

Methods Center Costs

Administrative costs can include computer hardware, the clinical database system, communication (conference calls, communication with clinical sites), randomization system (programming, maintenance, telephone costs), printing and center supplies (manual of operations, protocol, pocket protocol, study posters, study patient binders, adjudication binders, patient identification sheets, incentives, photocopying, office supplies), and postage and couriers (study-related material, mailings to the clinical centers, center payments, mailing to the Outcomes Adjudication Committee members, mailings to the Steering Committee members, mailings to the Data Monitoring Committee members).[18]

Site Investigator Costs

Site Investigator costs include personnel costs and meeting and travel costs. The budget should consider the number of hours each team member will dedicate to the trial as well as their wages. Meeting costs include the costs of attending Investigators' meetings, Data Monitoring Committee meetings and conference calls, Steering Committee meetings and conference calls, and Central Outcomes Adjudication Committee meetings and conference calls.[18]

Personnel for Investigator-Initiated Trials

A clinical trial requires the collaboration of key personnel from the Central Methods Center and participating clinical sites to ensure proper conduct of the trial.

Personnel for the Central Methods Center

The Nominated Principal Investigator's duties may include the design and conduct of the trial, finding funding, applying to funding agencies, locating sufficient clinical sites to enroll patients, and organizing trial committees.[2]

The Co-Principal Investigator can be an expert in health research methodology, in epidemiology, or in clinical trials. He or she may be responsible for the conduct of the clinical trial in a geographical region. Specifically, his or her duties may include maintaining frequent communication with participating sites, ensuring sites are using current protocol and consent forms, ensuring sites are ethics approved, and checking participant enrollment rates.[18]

Co-Investigators can also be health research methodology experts, economists, senior biostatisticians, or medical experts. They can act as consultants and members of the Steering Committee or Central Outcomes Adjudication Committee. They should all be involved in the design, organization, and conduct of the trial. Economists are involved in overall economic analysis and the planning, execution, and analysis of data. Biostatisticians are responsible for planning statistical analyses, performing the sample size calculation, and overseeing all analyses. Economists and biostatisticians should be blinded to treatment allocation.[18]

Collaborators are identical to Co-Investigators but have a much smaller time commitment. Some examples of their responsibilities include acting as consultants, Steering Committee members, or Adjudication Committee members. These experts may be involved in the design, organization, or conduct of the trial.[2]

The Study Coordinator or Coordinators play a major role in the clinical trial. They communicate frequently with the Nominated Principal Investigator and provide updates on recruitment, data submission, upcoming meetings, and problems. They help design case report forms, the database, and the randomization system. They also develop the manual of operations and standard operating procedures. This is the first line of communication for all clinical sites. They hire and supervise Research Assistants, participate in study meetings and conference calls, and prepare training and audit visits with the funding agency.[2]

Data Analysts prepare statistical reports of the data during and at the end of the trial, in addition to working with the Study Coordinator and Senior Biostatistician. However, the bulk of their responsibilities occur after the trial. Common duties include conducting data analyses, completing reports for the Data Monitoring Committee, preparing consensus tables for the Central Outcomes Adjudication Committee, and summarizing data for monthly newsletters. Data Analysts should be familiar with common statistical software such as the Statistical Package for the Social Sciences or Statistical Analysis Software.[2]

The Data Manager is responsible for setting up and maintaining the randomization system in a randomized controlled trial, designing case report forms, and programming and maintaining the database system. Most of the Data Manager's time is spent at the beginning of the trial; it then decreases gradually.[2]

The Financial Manager can be one of the Study Coordinator's duties if the trial is small. The Financial Manager drafts the study budget, prepares financial reports, conducts financial projections, ensures funding is spent within the Sponsor's guidelines, sets up contracts with clinical sites, and ensures that the funding for clinical sites is transferred. This person can be responsible for setting up a payroll of other members. The time commitment is small and is continuous throughout the trial.[2]

Research Assistants are involved in data validation, contacting clinical sites to discuss data queries and overdue follow-up visits, preparing adjudication packages, preparing binders of case report forms, and taking minutes at meetings. They have a large time commitment which is continuous throughout the trial.[2]

The Administrative Assistant works closely with the Study Coordinator to schedule meetings and conference calls. Typical duties include filing, mailing, issuing payments to clinical centers, photocopying, and typing study material.[2]

Clinical Research Monitors are responsible for reviewing all patient data and study-related information from source documents and records.[19] Additionally, the Clinical Research Monitor assists in maintaining regulatory files and ensures that all records are completed and documented in an accurate and timely manner.[19]

Key Concepts: Key Personnel for Central Methods Center
- Nominated Principal Investigator
- Co-Principal Investigator(s)
- Co-Investigator(s)
- Collaborator(s)
- Study Coordinator(s)
- Data Analyst(s)
- Data Manager(s)
- Financial Manager(s)
- Research Assistant(s)
- Administrative Assistant(s)
- Clinical Research Monitor(s)

Personnel for Clinical Sites

One Investigator from each site is designated the Site Principal Investigator, who serves as the primary contact for the Central Methods Center. The Site Principal Investigator protects the rights and safety of study participants, ensures informed consent is obtained from each participant, ensures that the trial adheres to the protocol and all other regulations, is accountable for all products in the study, ensures staff are appropriately trained and provide documentation of training, ensures case report forms and hospital records are documented correctly, is available for monitoring visits, and reports adverse events according to regulations.[2]

Site Investigators are responsible for enrolling patients, following the study protocol, completing patient follow-up, and communicating with the Methods Center to discuss any problems that may arise.[2]

The Clinical Research Coordinator communicates with the local ethics committee and the Central Methods Center, obtains patient consent, assists with patient randomization, completes case report forms, schedules patient follow-up appointments, submits data to the Central Methods Center, and responds to data queries.[2]

Key Concepts: Key Personnel for Clinical Sites
- Site Investigators
- One Investigator is designated the Site Principal Investigator
- Clinical Research Coordinator

Trial Committees

Steering Committee

Industry-initiated trials are guided and directed by the industry Sponsor's Steering Committee, which generally does not include the Site Investigator.[16] Investigator-initiated studies are directed by a Steering Committee that may include the Nominated Principal Investigator, Co-Principal Investigators, Senior Biostatistician, and Trial Methodologist. The Steering Committee determines the overall design and conduct of the trial and discusses and approves amendments to the protocol and case report forms. Steering Committee members communicate regularly with the Central Methods Center, Data Monitoring Committee, Central Outcomes Adjudication Committee, and Site Principal Investigators. They are also responsible for the final data analysis and manuscript preparation on behalf of all the study Investigators and sites.[2]

Data Monitoring Committee

The Data Monitoring Committee is an independent body common to both investigator-initiated trials and industry-initiated trials. It is required primarily for large, randomized multicenter studies that evaluate interventions intended to prolong life or reduce risk of a major adverse health outcome. If a study does not have a Data Monitoring Committee, it will still require safety monitoring. The Data Monitoring Committee acts in an advisory capacity to a national funding body to monitor patient safety and progress. The chairperson is responsible for overseeing meetings and is the primary contact person. The Data Monitoring Committee reviews the research protocol, informed consent documents, and the Investigator's plan for data safety and monitoring. It also evaluates the progress of a trial (data quality and timeliness, participant recruitment, participant risk and benefit), considers current relevant literature that may impact the safety of the participants, reviews study performance and makes recommendations, assists in resolving problems reported by the Principal Investigator, and protects the safety of the study participants.[2]

> **Examples from the Literature: Importance of Data Monitoring Committees**
> In an editorial, DeAngelis et al. identified the importance of an independent Data Monitoring Committee. They discussed a particular industry-sponsored clinical trial that appeared to be more concerned with preserving market share than with the potential to cause harm to patients.[20] DeAngelis et al. stated that industry-sponsored studies involving misleading reporting and misrepresentation of results have become increasingly common.[20] The involvement of a Data Monitoring Committee would help prevent such an occurrence.

Central Outcomes Adjudication Committee

The Central Outcomes Adjudication Committee reviews clinical end points to determine whether they meet protocol-specified criteria. This committee may request radiographs, chart notes, operative reports, and other material to guide their decision making. Although this committee is not necessary in a clinical trial, it is desirable when the assessment of clinical end points requires an element of judgment or subjectivity or when the Investigator cannot be blinded to the intervention. In investigator-initiated trials, the Steering Committee must weigh the expected benefit of adjudication for accurate determination of outcomes against the cost. In industry-initiated trials, it is the responsibility of the Sponsor to organize the adjudication process.[2] Please refer to Chapter 6 for additional information concerning adjudication.

> **Key Concepts: Trial Committees**
> • The Steering Committee determines the overall design and conduct of the trial and discusses and approves amendments to the protocol and case report forms.
> • The Data Monitoring Committee acts in an advisory capacity to a national funding body to monitor patient safety and progress.
> • The Central Outcomes Adjudication Committee reviews clinical end points to determine whether they meet protocol-specified criteria.

The Search for Funding

Investigators participating in industry-initiated clinical trials will receive funding from the industry Sponsor to support the conduct of the trial at their site.[16] However, depending on the size and scope of the trial, funding needs for investigator-initiated clinical trials can vary substantially. It may be necessary to obtain funding from several sources.

Internet

Investigators can search the internet for government funding agencies, foundations, professional organizations, and online databases. Websites such as The Community of Science (www.cos.com) allow Investigators to customize their searches to their specialties. The government may also make special incentives available periodically to Investigators, which can be explored online.[2]

Institutions

Investigators can also approach institutions for support by contacting the administrative staff in the grants and contracts department. Institutions may also post a summary list of research funding opportunities. Local sources of funding, such as hospitals, tend to offer small amounts of funding that may be sufficient to support a pilot study. Pilot studies can demonstrate feasibility in applications for larger government grants.[2]

Government

The government can provide a large amount of funding, sufficient for a multisite clinical trial; however, the application process is very formal and time consuming. In Canada, the primary conduit for government funding is the Canadian Institutes of Health Research (CIHR). In the United States, the primary conduit for government funding is the National Institutes of Health (NIH).[21] Investigator-initiated applications for NIH funding are evaluated by peer review groups composed of scientists from outside the NIH, who evaluate the scientific and technical merit of the proposed research.[21] Both organizations favor study designs that could improve the health of the global community. Generally, it is useful to start preparing an application well ahead of time, noting submission deadlines and application requirements, budgeting the time that will be needed to complete the application, and checking for common errors, as incomplete applications may not be considered. It may also be useful to contact an experienced colleague who could act as a mentor throughout the process. Investigators can contact the government agency personnel for advice on completing applications. Conducting a pilot study in advance of the application can strengthen an application by demonstrating the ability to successfully enroll patients, to follow a study protocol, and to adhere to a budget.[2]

> **Key Concepts: Tips for Government Funding Applications**
> - Plan for admission deadlines and budget time.
> - Check for common errors, which can be found on the agency website.
> - Check whether the application meets all requirements.
> - Contact a mentor.
> - Contact agency personnel.
> - Conduct a pilot study.

Conclusion

Conducting a clinical trial involves a significant amount of time and commitment from all involved parties. The goals of a clinical trial will vary depending on the phase of the trial. Since clinical trials involve human participants, applying for ethics approval can be a demanding process. Initially, Investigators may only be able to obtain a limited amount of funding, but this can be resolved by obtaining funding from multiple sources. Designing an accurate budget and conducting a pilot study can strengthen applications for larger grants. Finally, the Investigator alone is not responsible for the overall success of a clinical trial; it requires the collaboration of many individuals with different areas of expertise.

> **Key Concepts: Trial Management**
> - Know the requirements instituted by your local research ethics review board.
> - Identify key personnel and consider all the costs associated with conducting a clinical trial, whether it be industry-initiated or investigator-initiated.
> - Identify the importance of developing a budget
> - Identify the importance of obtaining funding and funding agencies
> - Establish Trial Committees prior to the onset of the study

Suggested Reading

Bhandari M, Joensson A, eds. Clinical Research for Surgeons. New York, NY: Georg Thieme Verlag; 2009

Bhandari M, Schemitsch EH. Beyond the basics: the organization and coordination of mulitcenter trials. Tech Orthop. 2004;19:83–87

References

1. World Health Organization. International clinical trials registry platform. Available at: http://www.who.int/ictrp/en/. Accessed February 2, 2010
2. Altman R, Brandt K, Hochberg K, et al. Design and conduct of clinical trials in patients with osteoarthritis: recommendations from a task force of the Osteoarthritis Research Society. Osteoarthritis Cartilage 1996;4:217–243
3. Bhandari M, Joensson A, eds. Clinical Research for Surgeons. New York, NY: Georg Thieme Verlag; 2009
4. Guyatt GH, Rennie D, Meade M, Cook D, eds. Users' Guides to the Medical Literature: A Manual for Evidence-Based Clinical Practice. 2nd ed. New York: McGraw-Hill; 2008
5. Suntharalingam G, Perry MR, Ward S, et al. Cytokine storm in a phase 1 trial of the Anti-CD28 Monoclonal Antibody TGN1412. N Engl J Med 2006;355:1018–1028
6. Steeves JD, Lammertse D, Curt A, et al. Guidelines for the conduct of clinical trials for spinal cord injury (SCI) as developed by the ICCP panel: clinical trial outcome measures. Spinal Cord 2007;45:206–221
7. Guyatt GH, Rennie D, eds. Users' Guides to the Medical Literature: A Manual for Evidence-Based Clinical Practice. Chicago, IL: AMA Press; 2002
8. Singh AP. Factors Affecting Fracture Healing. Available at http://boneandspine.com/fractures-dislocations/factors-affecting-fracture-healing/. Accessed March 22, 2010.
9. Farahani P, Levine M, Gaebel K, Thabane L. Clinical data gap between phase III clinical trials (pre-marketing) and phase IV (post-marketing) studies: evaluation of etanercept in rheumatoid arthritis. Can J Clin Pharmacol 2005;12:254–263
10. Bongartz T, Sutton AJ, Sweeting MJ, Buchan I, Matteson EL, Montori V. Anti-TNF antibody therapy in rheumatoid arthritis and the risk of serious infections and malignancies: systematic review and meta-analysis of rare harmful effects in randomized controlled trials. JAMA 2006;295:2275–2285
11. Kass NE, Hyder AA, Ajuwon A, et al. The structure and function of research ethics committees in Africa: a case study. PLoS Med 2007;4:e3

12. Health Canada. Drugs and health products: definitions. Available at: http://www.hc-sc.gc.ca/dhp-mps/prodpharma/activit/consultation/clini-rev-exam/definition-eng.php. Accessed February 9, 2010

13. Flather M, Aston H, Stables R. Handbook of Clinical Trials. London: ReMedica Publishing; 2001

14. Hamilton Health Sciences Research Ethics Board. Available at http://www-fhs.mcmaster.ca/healthresearch/reb/forms.html. Accessed February 26, 2010

15. Freedman B. Equipoise and the ethics of clinical research. N Engl J Med 1987;317:141–145

16. University of Washington School of Medicine. Clinical trials administrative start-up handbook. Available at http://depts.washington.edu/clinres/clinicaltrialshandbook/1getting.html#FinancialPlanning. Accessed April 10, 2010

17. Clinical Trials Knowledge Center. Available at http://www.washington.edu/research/guide/clinical.html. Accessed January 28, 2012

18. Bhandari M, Schemitsch EH. Beyond the basics: the organization and coordination of multicenter trials. Tech Orthop 2004;19:83–87

19. Clinical Research Jobs. Available at http://www.clinical-research-jobs.net/For-Clinicians/Clinical_Research_Monitors.html. Accessed April 10, 2010

20. DeAngelis CD, Fontanarosa PB. Ensuring integrity in industry-sponsored research. JAMA 2010; 303:1196–1198

21. US Department of Health and Human Services. Available at http://www.nih.gov/about/researchplanning.htm. Accessed April 11, 2010

9

Case–Control Studies

Gerard P. Slobogean, Vanessa K. Noonan

Summary

Case–control studies are used to examine the association between one or more exposures and a particular outcome.[1] The defining feature of this type of study design is that the investigator first identifies persons with the outcome of interest and then finds a suitable control group —i.e., it works backward.[2] This type of study design offers the advantages of being cost effective and efficient, since the investigator does not have to wait for the outcome of interest to develop and it can be conducted with fewer subjects than cohort studies. However, the investigator must use caution, especially when selecting the controls, because of the opportunities for sampling and measurement bias.[2] This chapter will first describe a case–control study design, discuss the strengths and limitations of case–control studies, describe how to deal with sampling and measurement bias, and then highlight some variations of case–control study designs including a nested case–control study and a case–cohort study.

Introduction

Imagine that you are interested in determining whether the use of statins reduces the risk of having a revision following total hip arthroplasty. Thilleman and colleagues conducted a nested case–control study to determine the answer to this very question.[3] These authors could have used a cohort study design where the investigators would first identify and sample individuals from the population (those undergoing a primary total hip arthroplasty), measure relevant risk factors (statin use), and then follow the cohort over time to determine whether they develop the outcome of interest (revision of a primary total hip arthroplasty). Answering this research question using a cohort study design would require enrolling a large number of individuals to ensure that there are enough individuals who develop the outcome of interest (revision of a primary total hip arthroplasty). Furthermore, using a cohort study design could take a considerable amount of time to complete since the investigators would have to wait for the outcomes of interest to develop. Because of these challenges, Thilleman et al. opted to conduct a nested case–control study where they first identified individuals who had a revision following a primary total hip arthroplasty and then assembled appropriate control groups to effectively deter-

mine that the use of statins was associated with a lower risk of revision after primary total hip arthroplasty.[3]

Definition of a Case–Control Study

A case–control study is a type of observational study.[4] The defining feature of a case–control study is that the investigator works backward by first identifying persons with the outcome of interest (the cases) and then identifies a sample of persons who do not have the outcome (the controls) to serve as a reference or comparative group (**Fig. 9.1**).[2] Factors are then examined among these two groups to identify possible associations. Case–control studies have several advantages as a study design. According to Busse and Obremskey, a case–control study:[1]

1. Facilitates the study of rare outcomes and conditions with substantial time between exposure and outcome;
2. Allows for control groups to be matched according to known (or suspected) confounding variables;
3. Permits the study of multiple potential causes of an outcome of interest;
4. Is relatively inexpensive and can be completed over short time periods.

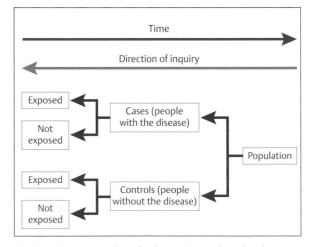

Fig. 9.1 Case–control study design. Reproduced with permission from Bhandari and Joensson.[4]

Despite its many strengths and advantages, the case–control study design also has several limitations:[1]

- It is inefficient when the exposure is rare.
- Information derived from interviews is subject to recall bias.
- Selection of an appropriate control group may be challenging.
- Lack of randomization means that groups may suffer from an imbalance of confounding factors.
- Only one outcome of interest can be studied and causality cannot be established.
- Validation of exposure information is often difficult.
- It cannot provide information on prevalence of the outcome of interest.
- Methodology and correct interpretation of results may be challenging.

> **Key Concepts: Case–Control Studies**
> Case–control studies are retrospective in design. Cases and controls are identified first, then exposures or risk factors are compared between the groups.

Case–Control Methodology

Selecting Cases

Cases are selected based on the presence of the disease or health state of interest. Since the case–control study design works "backwards" from identifying the cases, this is often the easiest step; however, researchers must recognize that the nature of the disease influences the type of cases identified and the accuracy of obtaining exposure data. Recently identified cases are described as incident cases, whereas subjects who have experienced the disease for a long time are known as prevalent cases. Depending on the nature of the disease, using prevalent cases can threaten the internal validity of the study because other potential cases may have been missed if they are already cured or have died from the disease.[5] Furthermore, in a prevalent case the subject may have difficulty remembering exposures from many years ago and is more likely to demonstrate recall bias.

> **Jargon Simplified: Incident Cases**
> Incident cases "are new occurrences of a condition (or disease) in a population over a period of time. Incidence refers to the number of new cases of disease occurring during a specified period of time, expressed as a percentage of the number of people at risk."[4,6]

> **Jargon Simplified: Prevalent Case**
> The term "prevalent case" "refers to the total number of people with a disease or condition in a certain population at a certain time. This includes both people who are newly diagnosed and those who have had the disease or condition for a long time. Prevalent cases must have been incident cases at some earlier point."[4]

> **Jargon Simplified: Recall Bias**
> Recall bias "occurs when patients who experience an adverse outcome have a different likelihood of recalling an exposure than the patients who do not have an adverse outcome, independent of the true extent of exposure."[4,7]

Selecting Controls

Selecting appropriate controls is crucial to ensuring the internal validity of a study. The control group is used to estimate the distribution of the exposure in the source population; therefore, defining the source population is important.[8] The source population can be defined by geographic region, referrals to a subspecialty practice, or a hospital's catchment area. Once the source population has been identified, one must ensure that potential controls are representative of the source population and selected independently of their exposure status.

Several strategies can be used for selecting controls. If the population can be accurately defined and a roster of all members of the population exists, then random sampling of the roster can be employed. For hospital or clinic-based controls, it is important to consider the referral pattern for subjects that will comprise the control group to ensure a representative sample of the desired source population. Other potential sources of control groups include neighborhood controls, random-digit dialing, or deceased controls.[9]

> **Key Concepts: Controls**
> Controls do not have the disease of interest and are used to estimate the distribution of exposure in an underlying source population. Controls must be selected independent of their exposure status.

Data Analysis

Case–control studies provide an estimate of the strength of association between an exposure and the disease. The odds ratio is the commonly reported measure of association for case–control data. It represents the odds of exposure in the disease group (cases) compared to the odds of exposure in the nondisease group (controls) (**Table 9.1**). The odds ratio is a less precise estimate of the risk ratio, which can only be obtained by directly measuring the entire source population (cohort study design). The loss in precision from performing a case–control study is offset by the benefits of time and resource savings compared to performing a larger prospective cohort study.

Table 9.1 Calculation of the odds ratio

Exposure	Disease Yes (cases)	No (controls)
Yes	a	b
No	c	d
Odds of exposure	a/c	b/d

Reproduced with permission from Bhandari and Joensson.[4]

Examples from the Literature:

Outcomes That Occur over a Long Period of Time

The case–control study design is an excellent method for investigating outcomes that take several years to develop. Kohatsu and Schurman investigated risk factors for the development of osteoarthrosis (OA) of the knee using this study design.[10] Forty-six cases were identified and defined as subjects with severe OA treated with total knee arthroplasty. An equal number of control subjects were randomly selected from a larger community sample and matched on the basis of age and gender. Detailed information of lifetime work and leisure-time physical activity, history of significant knee injury, and demographic variables were collected by questionnaire from all participants. These questionnaire data provided the authors with exposure data to quantify risk factors for the eventual development of knee OA. The results were reported using odds ratios, and identified that subjects with OA were two to three times more likely than controls to have performed moderate to heavy work during their lifetime. Also, OA case subjects were 5.3 times more likely than controls to be obese at age 40 years. Additionally, OA case subjects were 4.6 times more likely than controls to have suffered a significant knee injury.

Key Concepts: Case–Control Design to Study Outcomes that Occur Long after Exposure

Case–control design is a time-efficient method for studying outcomes that occur many years after an exposure. Since exposure data are collected retrospectively, they are subject to issues of reliability and recall bias.

Reality Check: Time-Efficient Study of Risk Factors Associated with Osteoarthritis

The aforementioned study conducted by Kohatsu and Schurman demonstrates that a case–control design is more time efficient than a prospective cohort. The authors were able to identify and quantify certain risk factors associated with developing OA many years after their exposure. These results provide clinicians with early evidence to support exposure hypotheses and can also be used to plan prospective study designs. For certain clinical questions, it may not be worthwhile to spend the time and resources to answer the question

prospectively, and therefore, the case–control design is an excellent alternative.

The primary limitation in many case–control studies, and in the study by Kohatsu and Schurman, is that it relies on retrospective collection of exposure data. Determining participants' body mass index at age 20 years through hospital records may be reliable; however, determining the intensity of their work or the extent of a knee injury 50 years after the exposure is at risk of significant recall bias.

Examples from the Literature: Rare Outcomes

Case–control studies also provide an efficient method for studying rare outcomes. Garcia Mata and colleagues used the case–control design to determine whether children exposed to passive smoking are at higher risk for developing Legg-Calvé-Perthes disease (LCPD).[11] Since the incidence of LCPD is quite low, using a cohort study design would require substantial resources to identify cases of LCPD and it would therefore be difficult to address the authors' research question.

The authors identified 90 subjects ages 2 to 14 years old treated for LCPD during a 3-year period at their center.[11] They then selected two controls per case from similar-age patients seen at their center for non-hip-related diagnoses. All participants and their families were then interviewed about family smoking habits around the child. Seventy-eight percent of children in the LCPD group were passive smokers, compared to only 43% in the control group. Using logistic regression to adjust for age and gender, passive smoking was shown to be strongly associated with LCPD (odds ratio 5.32; 95% confidence interval 2.92–9.69; $P < 0.0001$).[11]

Key Concepts: Case–Control Design to Study Rare Outcomes

Case–control design is a resource-efficient method for studying rare outcomes.

Reality Check: Statistical Modeling Controls for Other Associated Variables

Beyond demonstrating the obvious efficiency of the case–control design for investigating rare outcomes, the example above also illustrates how most investigators are now using logistic regression models to adjust for differences in age, gender, or other potentially influential variables that may affect their outcome. The benefit of regression modeling is that it provides an adjusted odds ratio for the exposure of interest as well as all other independent variables included in the model. Finally, since the control group was made up of similar-age patients referred to the center for non-hip-related diagnoses, it is important to know whether the referral patterns for the control group and cases are similar. For example, the investigators' center may be the only hospital that treats LCPD and therefore has a wide referral base for hip conditions, while their catchment area for non-hip-related diagnoses may be limited.

Jargon Simplified: Logistic Regression

Logistic regression is a popular regression technique used to model the relationship of several predictor variables to a dichotomous dependent variable. In case–control studies, the dependent variable is the disease state (present or absent); the independent variables include the exposure of interest.

Case–Control Studies within a Cohort Study

Case–control studies in theory occur within a cohort and the challenge to the investigator is to characterize the study cohort.[12] Two common variations of the case–control study, the nested case–control design and the nested case–cohort design, have been introduced to address this challenge. In the nested case–control design, cases are identified within an established cohort study and controls consist of those persons who are at risk at the time the case is identified but have not developed the outcome. Multiple controls can be selected for each case or matching can be used to account for known or suspected confounding variables.[1,2] Factors which are hypothesized to contribute to the development of the outcome (e.g., patient-reported variables or clinical measures) are then examined in both the cases and controls.

Jargon Simplified: Nested Case–Control Study Design

A case–control study is incorporated or "nested" into a cohort study. The cases include the persons with the outcome of interest that occurred during a cohort study. In a similar way to a case–control study, the controls are the individuals who are at risk in the cohort at the time the case develops but who do not develop the outcome.

A nested case–cohort study is similar to a nested case–control study in that the cases are obtained from a cohort study. The controls, however, include a random sample of all the members of the cohort (both those who do and those who do not develop the outcome of interest), and unlike the nested case–control study they can be selected immediately (sample from the cohort at baseline).[1,2] Randomly selecting controls from all persons in the cohort ensures that the controls are representative of the persons included in the cohort, and estimates of incidence and prevalence can be determined.[2] In addition, this allows the investigator to use the individuals in the cohort as a comparison group for more than one type of case, as long as the cases of interest are not too common.[2]

Jargon Simplified: Nested Case–Cohort Study Design

When a case–control study is incorporated or "nested" into a cohort study, the controls are a random sample selected from the entire cohort (cases and controls) and can be selected immediately (no requirement to wait until a case occurs).

Examples from the Literature:
A Nested Case–Control Study

Puisto et al. conducted a nested case–control study to examine the association between the severity of vertebral fractures and the risk of subsequent hip fractures.[13] The cohort used in this study consisted of 3280 men and 3815 women in the Mini-Finland Health Survey in 1978–1980 who had chest radiographs completed at baseline. The cases were 182 individuals who had been hospitalized and treated for a hip fracture by the end of 1994. Eligible controls included individuals who were alive at the end of 1994 and did not have a hip fracture. For each case two to three controls of the same sex were selected by matching on age (within 9 years) and municipality. There were 13 cases for whom no control could be identified and these were therefore subsequently removed. A total of 169 cases and 485 controls were finally included in the analysis. The investigators reviewed the chest radiographs and identified vertebral fractures at the levels of T3 to T12. The severity of the vertebral compression was graded as normal, mildly deformed, moderately deformed, or severely deformed. A conditional logistic regression model was used to estimate the strength of the association between vertebral fractures and the risk of hip fracture. The following variables were considered to be potentially confounding or effect modifying and entered into the model: level of education, physical activity, smoking, alcohol consumption, and self-rated general health. Hip fracture was strongly associated with the presence of severe vertebral compression. The adjusted relative odds was 12.06 (95% confidence interval 3.80–38.26) after controlling for the variables described above.

Typically in case–control studies, sampling bias can arise from cases and controls being selected from different populations, and it is often difficult to obtain accurate estimates of exposure because of the measurement bias introduced when individuals have to recall information (recall bias).[2] Puisto et al. avoided issues with selection bias by obtaining controls from the same cohort.[13] They also took advantage of the detailed and standardized health data collected at baseline during the Mini-Finland Health Survey. Accurate estimates of exposure (severity of vertebral fractures) were available for 89% of the original sample who had chest radiographs taken at baseline. This study highlights how a nested case–control design can be used very effectively to answer research questions within established registries or cohort studies.

Reality Check: Benefits of Matching

The study by Puisto et al. illustrates some points to consider when implementing a case–control study.[13] First, each hip fracture case was matched to two or three controls. Matching more than one control to each case is a frequently used technique to increase precision; however, one must be careful not to overmatch controls by matching on variables that are not risk factors, and matching should not be conducted on variables that are of scientific interest.[2] By matching on gender, age, and municipality the investigators ensured that the cases and controls were similar on these potential confounding variables. Other advantages of matching include controlling for unmeasured confounders and increasing the power to identify a real association by balancing the number of cases and controls at each level of the confounder.[2]

Secondly, the investigators also adjusted for potential confounding or effect-modifying variables in the statistical analysis. The results included univariate relative odds and multivariate odds, along with the 95% confidence interval. A conditional logistic regression model was used since the cases were matched to controls and ordinary statistical techniques assume that the groups are sampled independently.[2,14] The univariate analyses are "unadjusted" and the multivariate analyses are "adjusted" for level of education, physical activity, smoking, alcohol consumption, and self-rated general health. Puisto et al. reported both the univariate and multivariate odds ratio (**Table 9.2**).[13] The univariate odds ratio for risk of hip fracture in individuals with severe vertebral compression was 10.53 (95% confidence interval 3.46–32.02) and the multivariate odds ratio increased to 12.06 (95% confidence interval 3.80–38.26). By including these variables in their analysis, the researchers were able to identify a stronger association between vertebral fracture severity and hip fracture than had been previously reported.[13]

Jargon Simplified: Matching

Matching involves selecting a control or controls that have the same or a similar value for identified confounding variables (e.g., age, gender) as the case.

Jargon Simplified: Overmatching

Overmatching is matching on variables that are not risk factors. This leads to decreased variance in the exposure variables, but does not control for any additional confounding.

Jargon Simplified: Conditional Logistic Regression

Conditional logistic regression is used when there is one or more matched control for each case.

Conclusion

A case–control study design offers the advantages of being able to study a rare outcome in a short amount of time. Due to these advantages, this type of study design is often preferable to using a cohort study design and has been frequently used in the orthopaedic literature. A case–control study design was selected to determine whether children exposed to passive smoking are at greater risk of developing LCPD, a very rare outcome.[11] Similarly, this type of study design was used to examine risk factors for developing OA of the knee since the time between the exposure and the outcome was close to 50 years.[10] Often investigators will examine the strength of the association between the exposure and the outcome using an odds ratio, which is the odds of exposure in the group with the disease or outcome of interest (cases) compared to the odds of exposure in the group who do not have the outcome (controls).

When using a case–control study design it is important to select the cases and the controls carefully to avoid sampling biases. To maintain the internal validity of the study it is often preferable to use incident cases as opposed to prevalent cases because of the risk that missing cases might have already died from the disease. In addition, controls are selected to estimate the distribution of the exposure in the underlying source population, and the internal validity of the study can also be threatened by not carefully defining the source population. There are numerous sources for control groups, including hospital clinics, neighborhoods, and deceased persons, and it is important to consider the potential sources of bias introduced by each. Case–control studies are also susceptible to measurement bias because of the retrospective nature of the data collection. In particular, recall bias is often a concern due to the prolonged time interval between the outcome and the time of exposure.

More recently a nested case–control study and a nested case–cohort study have been utilized in the orthopaedic literature to address issues with sampling bias and measurement bias by selecting the cases and controls from within an existing cohort study. With the recent development of numerous patient registries in orthopaedics, these nested variations of the case–control study may offer a more cost-effective and rigorous method for determining the associations between risk factors and rare outcomes.

Table 9.2 Univariate and multivariate relative odds of hip fracture for various factors

Factors	Cases	Controls	Univariate relative odds	95% confidence interval	Multivariate relative odds[a]	95% confidence interval
Body mass index per increment of 1 standard deviation (4.3 kg/m^2)	169	485	0.81	0.68–0.97	0.83	0.68–1.01
Education level						
<8 years	140	395	1.00		1.00	
8–12 years	20	64	0.92	0.53–1.60	1.01	0.56–1.85
>12 years	9	26	1.02	0.44–2.35	1.34	0.51–3.55
Physical activity at leisure						
Low	102	221	1.00		1.00	
Moderate	54	217	0.55	0.37–0.81	0.69	0.45–1.05
High	12	47	0.59	0.29–1.17	0.89	0.42–1.87
Smoking						
Never	117	375	1.00		1.00	
Ex-smoker	26	65	1.58	0.86–2.89	1.41	0.72–2.76
Current smoker	26	45	2.51	1.34–4.69	2.17	1.08–4.34
Alcohol intake (grams of ethanol per week)						
0	127	346	1.00		1.00	
1–49	32	118	0.76	0.48 1.21	0.71	0.42–1.20
50–249	3	5	1.72	0.37–8.07	1.05	0.18–6.13
≥249	/	16	1.17	0.43–3.21	1.09	0.34–3.47
Self-rated general health						
Good or fairly good	40	166	1.00		1.00	
Moderate	65	224	1.21	0.78–1.90	1.21	0.75–1.97
Rather poor or poor	63	94	2.67	1.66–4.30	2.70	1.58–4.59
Vertebral fracture						
Grade 0	88	284	1.00		1.00	
Grade 1	41	136	0.93	0.60–1.45	0.96	0.60–1.53
Grade 2	24	60	1.21	0.72–2.04	1.22	0.70–2.15
Grade 3	16	5	10.53	3.46–32.02	12.06	3.80–38.26

Reproduced with permission from Puisto et al.[13]
[a]Adjusted for all the factors listed in this table.

Suggested Reading

Busse JW, Obremskey WT. Principles of designing an orthopaedic case–control study. J Bone Joint Surg Am 2009;91 (Suppl 3):15–20

Morshed S, Tornetta P, Bhandari M. Analysis of observational studies: a guide to understanding statistical methods. J Bone Joint Surg Am 2009;91 (Suppl 3):50–60

Wacholder S, McLaughlin JK, Silverman DT, Mandel JS. Selection of controls in case–control studies. I. Principles. Am J Epidemiol 1992;135:1019–1028

Wacholder S, Silverman DT, McLaughlin JK, Mandel JS. Selection of controls in case–control studies. II. Types of controls. Am J Epidemiol 1992;135:1029–1041

Wacholder S, Silverman DT, McLaughlin JK, Mandel JS. Selection of controls in case–control studies. III. Design options. Am J Epidemiol 1992;135:1042–1050

References

1. Busse JW, Obremskey WT. Principles of designing an orthopaedic case–control study. J Bone Joint Surg Am 2009;91 (Suppl 3):15–20
2. Hulley SB, Cummings SR, Browner WS, et al. Designing Clinical Research. 3rd ed. Philadelphia: Lippincott Williams & Wilkins; 2007
3. Thillemann TM, Pedersen AB, Mehnert F, et al. The risk of revision after primary total hip arthroplasty among statin users: a nationwide population-based nested case–control study. J Bone Joint Surg Am 2010;92:1063–1072
4. Bhandari M, Joensson A. Clinical Research for Surgeons. New York: Thieme; 2009
5. Kelsey JL, Whittmore AS, Evans AS, et al. Methods in Observational Epidemiology. 2nd ed. New York: Oxford University Press; 1996
6. Bhandari M, Tornetta P III, Guyatt GH. Glossary of evidence-based orthopaedic terminology. Clin Orthop Relat Res 2003;158–163
7. Hartz A, Marsh JL. Methodologic issues in observational studies. Clin Orthop Relat Res 2003;33–42
8. Rothman KJ. Epidemiology: An Introduction. New York: Oxford University Press; 2002
9. Wacholder S, Silverman DT, McLaughlin JK, et al. Selection of controls in case–control studies. II. Types of controls. Am J Epidemiol 1992;135:1029–1041
10. Kohatsu ND, Schurman DJ. Risk factors for the development of osteoarthrosis of the knee. Clin Orthop Relat Res 1990;242–246
11. Garcia Mata S, Ardanaz Aicua E, Hidalgo Ovejero A, et al. Legg-Calvé-Perthes disease and passive smoking. J Pediatr Orthop 2000;20:326–330
12. Wacholder S, McLaughlin JK, Silverman DT, et al. Selection of controls in case–control studies. I. Principles. Am J Epidemiol 1992;135:1019–1028
13. Puisto V, Heliovaara M, Impivaara O, et al. Severity of vertebral fracture and risk of hip fracture: a nested case–control study. Osteoporos Int 2011;22:63–68
14. Tabachnick BG, Fidell LS. Using Multivariate Statistics. 5th ed. Boston: Pearson Education Inc.; 2007

10

Cohort Studies

Steven Takemoto, Saam Morshed

"Evidence-based medicine is the conscientious, explicit, and judicious use of current best evidence in making decisions about the care of individual patients."[1]

Summary

The goal of this chapter is to convey the essential concepts one should consider when evaluating, designing, and reporting on studies that involve patient cohorts. The chapter will begin by introducing two pivotal cohort studies to illustrate design challenges and good reporting practices. The key to good study design is prognostication: how well the study informs treatment decisions that improve care of patients. We will provide a historical perspective to illustrate why some methodologists only consider randomized trials when considering medical evidence and provide methodological steps for elevating cohort studies in the hierarchy of evidence. Various cohort methodologies are well suited to address certain questions. We will review methodologies and analytic approaches developed to improve the rigor of cohort studies, as well as checklists that evaluate and improve strength of evidence.

Introduction

What should one consider when evaluating whether new evidence should change how one practices medicine? The study should be of the highest possible quality, provide the best available information, be valid and plausible, and the benefit of change should outweigh the risks of implementation.[2]

What are the elements of a high quality study? What information improves prognostication? How should strength of evidence be rated? Starting in 1992, the *Journal of the American Medical Association* (*JAMA*) published a series of 25 *Users' Guides to Medical Literature,* developed by the Evidence-Based Medicine Working Group at McMaster University. The series succinctly described strategies for gleaning evidence from medical literature to inform treatment decisions.[3] Each guide started with a clinical scenario, criteria to determine whether results are valid, and whether conclusions are applicable to a particular case. We adopted this approach to illustrate strengths and limitations of cohort studies.

The first case examines whether patients with severe limb injuries have comparable outcomes with limb salvage and reconstruction versus amputation and prosthetic replacement. Because of the nature of the injury, blinding and randomization were not possible. Nonetheless, by stratifying by severity of injury, blinding outcome assessors, and selecting informative outcomes, evidence suggests salvage and amputation provide similar outcomes.

At baseline, sociodemographic factors were similar, but patients undergoing amputation had higher rates of contamination and severe bone, soft tissue, neurologic, and skin injury. Patients with reconstruction had higher rates of rehospitalization, but a similar percentage returned to work by 2 years. Functional outcomes, assessed using a 136-item Sickness Impact Profile survey, were similar at 2 years.

Examples from the Literature: Comparison of Outcomes after Amputation versus Reconstruction for Limb-threatening Injuries

Case example 1 is a cohort study comparing complications and patient-reported outcomes for two surgical options for patients with severe leg injury.[4]

Background: Limb salvage for severe trauma has replaced amputation as the primary treatment in many trauma centers. However, long-term outcomes after limb reconstruction as compared to amputation have not been fully evaluated.

Methods: We performed a multicenter, prospective, observational study to determine the functional outcomes of 569 patients with severe leg injuries resulting in reconstruction or amputation. The principal outcome measure was the Sickness Impact Profile, a multidimensional measure of self-reported health status (scores range from 0 to 100; scores for the general population average 2–3, and scores greater than 10 represent severe disability). Secondary outcomes included limb status and the presence or absence of major complications resulting in rehospitalization.

Results: At 2 years, there was no significant difference in scores for the Sickness Impact Profile between the amputation and reconstruction groups (12.6 vs. 11.8, $P = 0.53$). After adjustment for the characteristics of the patients and their injuries, patients who underwent amputation had functional outcomes that were similar to those of patients who underwent reconstruction. Predictors of a poorer score for the Sickness Impact Profile included rehospitalization for a major complication, a low educational level, nonwhite race, poverty, lack of private health insurance, poor social-support network, low self-efficacy (the patient's confidence in being able to resume life activities), smoking, and involvement in disability-compensation litigation. Patients who underwent reconstruction were more likely to be rehospitalized than those who underwent amputation (47.6% vs. 33.9%, P = 0.002). Similar proportions of patients who underwent amputation and patients who underwent reconstruction had returned to work by 2 years (53.0% and 49.4%, respectively).

Conclusions: Patients with limbs at high risk for amputation can be advised that reconstruction typically results in 2-year outcomes equivalent to those of amputation.

The second case example illustrates the challenges of randomizing patients to medical versus surgical treatment. All enrolled patients had leg weakness arising from lumbar spinal stenosis and chose being randomized or opting to select their treatment. This study illustrates problems facing designers of randomized controlled trials (RCTs) in surgery: blinding, and the distinction between "intention-to-treat" and actual treatment.

Primary outcomes were patient reports of bodily pain and physical function using the short-form 36-item General Health Survey (SF-36) and the Oswestry Disability Index. In the randomized cohort, 33% of patients assigned to the surgery declined. Their baseline preference was nonsurgical treatment and their severity of symptoms diminished with time. Conversely, 43% of the patients randomized to the nonsurgical cohort subsequently underwent decompression surgery. These patients not only had an initial preference for surgery, they had greater preoperative pain and disability than others not undergoing surgery. The intention-to-treat analysis of the randomized cohort showed significant improvements in bodily pain (SF-36) after 2 years in the group randomized to surgery, but no difference in physical function or the Oswestry Disability Index. However, the as-treated analysis that attempted to adjust for confounding factors, found significant improvements in all measures of pain and function among those treated operatively versus non-operatively.

> **Examples from the Literature: Comparison of Outcomes after Surgical Versus Nonsurgical Treatment of Lumbar Spinal Stenosis**
> Case example 2 illustrates some of the challenges in implementing and interpreting results of a clinical trial comparing medical and surgical interventions for patients with leg pain due to nerve impingement.[5]
> *Background:* Surgery for spinal stenosis is widely performed, but its effectiveness as compared with nonsurgical treatment has not been shown in controlled trials.
> *Methods:* Surgical candidates with a history of at least 12 weeks of symptoms and spinal stenosis without spondylolisthesis (as confirmed on imaging) were en-

> rolled in either a randomized cohort or an observational cohort at 13 US spine clinics. Treatment was decompressive surgery or usual nonsurgical care. The primary outcomes were measures of bodily pain and physical function on the Medical Outcomes Study 36-item Short-Form General Health Survey (SF-36) and the modified Oswestry Disability Index at 6 weeks, 3 months, 6 months, and 1 and 2 years.
> *Results:* A total of 289 patients were enrolled in the randomized cohort and 365 patients were enrolled in the observational cohort. At 2 years, 67% of patients who were randomly assigned to surgery had undergone surgery, whereas 43% of those who were randomly assigned to receive nonsurgical care had also undergone surgery. Despite the high level of nonadherence, the intention-to-treat analysis of the randomized cohort showed a significant treatment effect favoring surgery on the SF-36 scale for bodily pain, with a mean difference in change from baseline of 7.8 (95% confidence interval 1.5–14.1); however, there was no significant difference in scores on physical function or on the Oswestry Disability Index. The as-treated analysis, which combined both cohorts and was adjusted for potential confounders, showed a significant advantage for surgery by 3 months for all primary outcomes; these changes remained significant at 2 years.
> *Conclusion:* In the combined as-treated analysis, patients who underwent surgery showed significantly more improvement in all primary outcomes than did patients who were treated nonsurgically.

Cohort Studies in the Hierarchy of Evidence

Problems with cohort studies employing historic controls were illustrated in meta-analyses published by Sacks et al. in 1982 comparing outcomes for six therapies in over 100 trials to those achieved with RCTs.[6,7] With cohort studies a significant benefit was noted for 80% of the studies, whereas only 20% of the RCTs indicated these therapies were effective. There are many other examples where conclusions drawn from cohort studies were later invalidated when examined with more stringent study designs. For example, a large multicenter randomized trial dispelled the notion that carotid artery bypass surgery should be performed to treat symptomatic cerebrovascular disease.[8] Guyatt et al. point out other clinical trials that repudiated previous studies. Steroids did not reduce mortality from sepsis or improve facet-joint back pain.[9] Other confounding factors such as severity of illness, comorbid conditions, or a host of other prognostic factors, known or unknown, can confuse the effect of therapy.[10]

Jargon Simplified: Confounder

A confounder must meet two criteria: it must increase or decrease susceptibility or risk of poor outcome, and it must be distributed differently in the groups being compared.[10] Confounder literally means "confuser of effects".[11] By magnifying or canceling measures of the treatment effect, confounders contribute to an inaccurate "causal" association to exposure.

In 1999, Altman and Bland justified the *British Medical Journal*'s position rejecting publication of nonrandomized studies.[12] The simplest cohort design compares outcomes before and after a change in intervention. With historic designs, the effect of unmeasured confounders that have changed over time cannot be measured. Even with contemporary controls, if patients or physicians accept or refuse a particular treatment, unmeasured preferences result in selection bias. Randomization uses probability to reduce bias so that confounders are evenly matched as if one were flipping a coin. If the number of enrolled patients is relatively small, block randomization, where confounders are evenly distributed within smaller sets of cases, can assure the balance of prognostic factors.[13]

Key Concepts: Bias and the Treatment Effect

Selection bias refers to the systematic error in estimation of the association between exposure and outcome due to ascertainment of study subjects. Selection bias is most likely to occur in retrospective study designs (case–control or cohort) because of the presence of disease prior to sample selection, thereby potentially rendering sampling probabilities of different disease-exposure groups to be differential. In prospecitve cohort studies, study participants are (ideally) selected before disease occurs making differential selection based on disease status less likely. Selection bias in prospective cohort studies is more likely to occur secondary to differential loss to follow-up. This is because individuals lost to follow-up may have a different probability of the outcome of interest than those who remain in the cohort for the duration of the study. This will bias estimates of disease incidence, and to the degree that this bias differs between treated and untreated groups, the measures of association (relative risk or rate ratio) as well.

Information bias occurs when completeness or accuracy of measurement of exposure, outcome or covariate data can lead to systematic errors in estimating the association of exposure and outcome.[11] Information bias results from inadequate definitions of study variables or flawed acquisition procedures that can lead to misclassification of exposure and outcome status. In retrospecive cohort and case–control studies, missclassification of exposure can result from inaccuracies in participant **recall** of past exposure or **interviewer** knowledge of outcome altering the way in which exposure information is gathered. In prospective cohort studies, information bias more commonly arises due to errors in outcome ascertainment by **respondents** or **observers**. If misclassification is rendered nondifferential, through such safe-guards as blinding of subjects and assessors, the direction of bias of estimates is typically toward the null, or no effect. However, if misclassification of exposure or outcome is differential, or differs between groups being compared, the direction of bias can either be toward or away from the null effect. To guard against information bias, it is important to thoroughly examine inclusion criteria, each prognostic factor, and outcomes, and to assure that operational definitions are as robust as possible.[16]

The goal of an RCT is to assure internal validity, that is, to make sure that a change in outcome is due to the treatment and not to other factors.[17] With basic science, mice or cultures are used to maximize internal validity by controlling the genetic background to the degree that the only difference between comparators may be a single gene. In a similar way, RCTs seek to control confounders using blinding and randomization so that the only difference between groups is the treatment. Randomization alone may be insufficient. Patients or their clinicians who know they are receiving a new experimental treatment are likely to have an opinion about its efficacy.[18] To eliminate this bias, allocation to treatment groups can be concealed and outcome assessors and patients blinded to treatment. Even with these methodological precautions, RCTs are not immune to information and selection bias.[19]

In 1996, Black argued that clinical experiments in the form of RCTs may be unnecessary, inadequate, or impossible when approaching many clinical questions, and that observational studies are an essential component of the evidence hierarchy.[20] In cases such as the rapamycin trial,[15] where a clear treatment benefit is demonstrated in a well-designed observational trial, further experimentation is unnecessary. RCTs often have inadequate follow-up, small sample size, high cost, and utilize surrogate end points.[21] They are inadequate for assessing the safety of pharmaceuticals. Even with a meta-analysis, it is rare to gain 10 000 person-years of exposure before approval is granted; a single additional death or cardiovascular, kidney, or liver event at this level of exposure is clinically significant.[22] More than half of the drugs approved by the FDA between 1976 and 1985 had at least one adverse reaction that was not detected in initial RCTs,[23] and 10% either received a "black box" warning or were withdrawn from the market.[24]

Issues that potentially limit the external validity of RCTs include the trial setting and physicians; patient eligibility criteria; demographics; severity of disease and co-morbidities; the similarity of protocol and routine care; the clinical relevance and frequency of outcome measures; and the rigor of adverse event ascertainment.[25]

McCulloch et al. expand upon Black's final point, that RCTs in surgery may be impossible.[26] Indeed, it is not possible to blind surgeons to surgical interventions. The variability in technique necessitates precise definition, monitoring of quality, and consideration of learning curves. Case example 1 illustrates the difficulty of randomization when there are rare or life-threatening situations. The low rates of intent-to-treat compliance in case example 2 show how differences in potential risks and benefits for surgical and nonsurgical interventions can affect patient equipoise.

Reality Check: Controlled vs. Observational Studies
The continuum of controlled versus observational methodology can be illustrated by contrasting *efficacy*—the degree of health improvement that can be achieved by an intervention under ideal conditions—and *effectiveness*—improvement achieved by an intervention in the real world.[27] Mice with similar genetic backgrounds provide the optimal setting for assessing the efficacy of a drug to improve bone healing. In a similar manner, prospective trials designed to measure the benefit or "treatment effect" of an intervention minimize confounding through randomization, blinding, and studying homogeneous populations.[17] The goal of a randomized trial is to assure *internal validity*, the extent to which a measured effect is causally associated with an intervention through sound experimental methodology and execution. Cohort studies are often designed to assure *external validity*, the extent that evidence can be applied to a broader patient population. The emergence of electronic health records is enabling multi-institutional HIPAA-compliant research databases (HIPAA: US Health Insurance Portability and Accountability Act).[28] One such database was used to attribute a 25-fold increase in myocardial infarctions to the introduction of Vioxx to the marketplace.[29] Cohort studies can also be derived using administrative claims. Examination of ICD-9 diagnosis codes revealed complication rates for knee arthroplasty procedures in a state-wide hospital discharge database.[30] Similarly, a national registry with over 50 000 hip arthroplasty procedures has been assembled using Medicare claims.[31] Open-label RCT extensions provide additional data alongside standard clinical trials. A re-examination of x-ray images in RCTs for bisphosphonates revealed incidence rates for subtrochanteric fractures.[32] Kidney transplantation is unique in that reporting to the registry is mandatory to be eligible for national sharing of human leukocyte antigen (HLA)-matched organs.[27] Ascertainment of registry outcomes can be expanded by linkage to administrative claims databases.[33] Perhaps the most exciting new development is the blending of RCT and observational methodologies possible with pragmatic clinical trials.[34] With pragmatic trials, patients agree to be randomized to an intervention and data are collected using large-scale cohort methodology.

In 2000, Benson and Hartz[35] and Concato et al.[7] published back-to-back articles in the *New England Journal of Medi-* *cine* revisiting the 1982 analysis by Sacks et al. that compared treatment effects derived by RCTs and cohort studies. Both investigators found treatment effects for a wide array of interventions were remarkably consistent, suggesting that, with modern analytic methods and sufficient sampling, the gap in quality of evidence for these two methodologies has considerably narrowed. When considering whether a study is sufficient to alter the way medicine is practiced, it is often useful to consider a hierarchy of evidence.[36] Efforts to minimize bias and confounding elevate RCTs over cohort studies in this hierarchy. In turn, methodologies employed by cohort studies improve the quality of evidence above that of case series and expert opinion.

Types of Cohort Study Designs

In cohort studies, the investigator does not attempt to control who receives an intervention or exposure, so clinicians are not asked to compromise clinical judgment or perform procedures that they have not mastered.[37] Cohorts are defined on the basis of an exposure and outcomes and are assessed over a period of time. At time zero, a study population of eligible participants is split into cohorts depending on an exposure of interest. The investigator does not intervene in the patient's care, but rather notes what intervention the physician and/or patient choose. These cohorts are then followed with time to determine whether an outcome does or does not occur. Although the implication is that one cohort receives an intervention and the other does not, cohorts can be redistributed into subgroups. In case example 1, the reconstruction cohort was subdivided into dysvascular, tibia, and foot/ankle fracture subgroups, and the amputation cohort into above/through/below the knee and foot subgroups. In case example 2, intent-to-treat cohorts were re-examined "as-treated".

Key Concepts: The Distinction between Cohort, Case–Control, and Nested Case–Control Methods
Cohort studies are selected based on their exposure history, either in the present or the past, and followed forward in time to assess differences in outcome of interest.
Case–control studies consider patients (cases) who experienced an outcome and retrospectively compare their characteristics to a sampling of controls who did not experience the outcome in order to attribute risks to various prognostic factors.
Nested case–control studies use more efficient means of conducting a prospective cohort study by implementing features of case–control design within a well-defined cohort. In such studies, controls are either selected from the baseline cohort or from a pool of candidates at risk at the time that each case arises. Nested case–control, or case–cohort studies as they are often called, are par-

ticularly useful when additional information that was not obtained or measured for the whole cohort is needed, such as when serum samples are collected but not analyzed at baseline.

Case–control studies are cohort studies in reverse. Cases (patients) who experience a particular outcome are matched to controls for whom that outcome was absent.[38] Case–control studies are particularly useful for rare or adverse events requiring a large number of patients and for outcomes such as implant failure that usually occur many years after the index procedure.[20] Case–control studies have traditionally provided a lower level of evidence than cohort studies because the sampling methodology does not provide the information necessary to estimate the total number of patients at risk and also because results are susceptible to information bias.[36]

Although the different conclusions drawn by the 1982 Sacks[6] and 2000 Benson[35]/Concato[7] studies could be attributed to the use of historic or concurrent controls, it does not necessarily follow that prospective designs are superior to retrospective. The strength of prospective cohort studies is that, apart from randomization, many of the safeguards for preventing bias can be implemented. Diagnostic criteria can be standardized, outcome assessors can be blinded when possible, and capture of confounding data can be operationalized and carried forward.[37] But some argue that the most important aspect of a cohort study is not whether data existed at the time of protocol development, but rather whether the research protocol was thoroughly fleshed out before the data were assembled for the study.[39,40] Hospital and multicenter registries are often used to facilitate cohort studies.[41] When establishing a registry, it is important to clearly define outcomes that inform the clinical question and to define parameters that may confound results. Registries generally have high external validity since data are collected in the setting of clinical practice, with large sample sizes and long term follow-up enabling better estimates of outcomes.[21]

With cohort studies, since the total number of patients exposed and experiencing an outcome is known, it is possible to report temporal relationships between exposure and outcome. The effect of exposure to a treatment can be characterized by both relative and absolute risks. Relative risk is the risk of developing an outcome in the exposed divided by the risk or incidence of outcome in the unexposed cohort.[36] In case example 1, outcomes were reported as percentages of patients who experienced an event at 2 years and changes in patient-reported outcome scores at 2 years. Case example 2 compared changes in outcome scores at various times after enrollment. Survival analysis, describing the percentage of patients experiencing treatment failure as a function of time, is another common method for describing outcomes.[27] With case–control studies, it is possible to estimate relative risk using the odds ratio.[36]

Nested case–control is a special type of cohort study where sampling of controls comes from a population of subjects matched on time or other possible confounders, but allows those controls to become cases when followed prospectively.[38] Unlike in case–control studies, estimates of relative risk and relative hazard can be directly produced. Nested case-control studies reduce the labor and cost of performing a prospective observational study while preserving many of the benefits over retrospective designs.

Methods for Reducing Confounding and Assessing Causality

In cohort studies, bias and confounding can be addressed either in the design or analysis phase. Restriction and matching of subjects, based on potentially confounding prognostic factors, are effective design steps to mitigate bias due to such factors. In both of the case examples, exclusion criteria were used to create cohorts that were as uniform as possible, yet broad enough to draw generalizable conclusions. In case example 1, those with transferral more than 24 hours after injury, more than 3 weeks' impaired consciousness, burns, spinal cord deficit, and psychiatric disorders were excluded.[4] In case example 2, patients with less than 12 weeks of symptoms or lumbar instability were excluded.[5]

Both studies used analysis phase steps including stratification and multivariable regression to reduce the impact of confounders and look for differences in treatment effect between subgroups of patients. Stratification allows estimation of treatment effects between subgroups defined by some baseline characteristic. In regression, the outcome of interest is the dependent variable, and baseline measures and the intervention are independent variables.[42] This technique estimates the association of each independent variable with the dependent variable such that the relative contribution of each factor can be weighed. When outcomes are binary, logistic regression can be expressed as an odds ratio which expresses the likelihood of experiencing an outcome such as infection for patients with a certain risk factor compared to those who did not have the risk factor.[43] Linear regression can be used to estimate an effect as a mean difference for continuous outcomes such as range of motion or a functional outcome score such as SF-36. The likelihood of experiencing a time-to-event outcome such as reoperation after total hip replacement can be expressed as a hazard ratio in a multivariable proportional hazards model. Multivariable adjustments for national rates of total joint replacement can be calculated using Poisson regression and expressed as a rate ratio.

A Checklist to Evaluate or Improve the Strength of Evidence

The Strengthening the Reporting of Observational Studies in Epidemiology (STROBE) initiative provides guidelines that make it clear to those evaluating a study what was planned, what was done, what was found, and what conclusions were drawn.[40] The goal is to maximize the strength of evidence for cohort studies by reducing ambiguities and clearly describing potential sources of confounding. For example, they discourage simply calling a study "prospective" or "retrospective" and not providing details regarding how and when data collection took place. Some consider cohort designs "prospective" if data are collected with a plan in place, and reserve "retrospective" for case–control studies. Others define prospective and retrospective in terms of when the idea for the study was developed or whether the outcome occurred prior to when cases were selected.

If we apply the STROBE checklist to our two case examples, we find that both studies describe the setting of the trial, locations and periods of enrollment, but they do not give the date when data collection ended. Variables are clearly defined as well as methods for addressing potential bias. Case example 2 included a flow chart that clearly illustrated the number of potentially eligible patients, and reasons for nonparticipation at every stage of the study.[5] Both studies include tables that show how potential confounders are distributed among groups, and both provide unadjusted and adjusted results, as well as discussing limitations and the generalizability of study results.

Conclusion

In this chapter, we provide a historical perspective that forms the basis for the hierarchy of medical evidence and the position of cohort studies within this framework. As recently as 15 years ago, evidence from cohort studies was not regarded highly. However, randomizing is not always possible to investigate the clinical efficacy of surgical interventions. We have reviewed how robust cohort study designs can be used to measure and report on the effect of confounders and to adjust for them in order to produce less biased estimates of treatment effect. Well-conducted cohort studies can provide high-quality, generalizable evidence when blinding or randomization is not feasible or ethical.

Suggested Reading

Cox E, Martin BC, Van Staa T, Garbe E, Siebert U, Johnson ML. Good research practices for comparative effectiveness research: approaches to mitigate bias and confounding in the design of nonrandomized studies of treatment effects using secondary data sources: The International Society for Pharmacoeconomics and Outcomes Research Good Research Practices for Retrospective Database Analysis Task Force Report—Part II. Value Health 2009;12:1053–1061

Farrokhyar F, Karanicolas PJ, Thoma A, et al. Randomized controlled trials of surgical interventions. Ann Surg 2010; 251:409–416

Hoppe DJ, Schemitsch EH, Morshed S, Tornetta P 3rd, Bhandari M. Hierarchy of evidence: where observational studies fit in and why we need them. J Bone Joint Surg Am 2009;91 (Suppl 3):2–9

Morshed S, Tornetta P 3rd, Bhandari M. Analysis of observational studies: a guide to understanding statistical methods. J Bone Joint Surg Am 2009;91 (Suppl 3):50–60

Vandenbroucke JP, von Elm E, Altman DG, et al. Strengthening the Reporting of Observational Studies in Epidemiology (STROBE): explanation and elaboration. Ann Intern Med 2007;147:W163–194

Weinstein JN, Tosteson TD, Lurie JD, et al. Surgical versus nonsurgical therapy for lumbar spinal stenosis. N Engl J Med 2008;358:794–810

References

1. Sackett DL, Rosenberg WM, Gray JA, Haynes RB, Richardson WS. Evidence based medicine: what it is and what it isn't. BMJ 1996;312:71–72
2. Cone DC, Lewis RJ. Should this study change my practice? Acad Emerg Med 2003;10:417–422
3. Oxman AD, Sackett DL, Guyatt GH. Users' guides to the medical literature. I. How to get started. The Evidence-Based Medicine Working Group. JAMA 1993;270:2093–2095
4. Bosse MJ, MacKenzie EJ, Kellam JF, et al. An analysis of outcomes of reconstruction or amputation after leg-threatening injuries. N Engl J Med 2002;347:1924–1931
5. Weinstein JN, Tosteson TD, Lurie JD, et al. Surgical versus nonsurgical therapy for lumbar spinal stenosis. N Engl J Med 2008;358:794–810
6. Sacks H, Chalmers TC, Smith H, Jr. Randomized versus historical controls for clinical trials. Am J Med 1982;72:233–240
7. Concato J, Shah N, Horwitz RI. Randomized, controlled trials, observational studies, and the hierarchy of research designs. N Engl J Med 2000;342:1887–1892
8. Haynes RB, Mukherjee J, Sackett DL, Taylor DW, Barnett HJ, Peerless SJ. Functional status changes following medical or surgical treatment for cerebral ischemia. Results of the extra-cranial-intracranial bypass study. JAMA 1987;257:2043–2046
9. Guyatt GH, Sackett DL, Cook DJ. Users' guides to the medical literature. II. How to use an article about therapy or prevention. B. What were the results and will they help me in caring for my patients? Evidence-Based Medicine Working Group. JAMA 1994;271:59–63
10. Mamdani M, Sykora K, Li P, et al. Reader's guide to critical appraisal of cohort studies: 2. Assessing potential for confounding. BMJ 2005;330:960–962
11. Vandenbroucke JP, von Elm E, Altman DG, et al. Strengthening the Reporting of Observational Studies in Epidemiology (STROBE): explanation and elaboration. Ann Intern Med 2007;147:W163–194
12. Altman DG, Bland JM. Statistics notes. Treatment allocation in controlled trials: why randomise? BMJ 1999;318:1209
13. Altman DG, Bland JM. How to randomise. BMJ 1999; 319:703–704

14. Deeks JJ, Dinnes J, D'Amico R, et al. Evaluating non-randomised intervention studies. Health Technol Assess 2003; 7:iii–x, 1–173

15. D'Arcy Hart P. A change in scientific approach: from alternation to randomised allocation in clinical trials in the 1940s. BMJ 1999;319:572–573

16. Cox E, Martin BC, Van Staa T, Garbe E, Siebert U, Johnson ML. Good research practices for comparative effectiveness research: approaches to mitigate bias and confounding in the design of nonrandomized studies of treatment effects using secondary data sources: The International Society for Pharmacoeconomics and Outcomes Research Good Research Practices for Retrospective Database Analysis Task Force Report–Part II. Value Health 2009;12:1053–1061

17. Farrokhyar F, Karanicolas PJ, Thoma A, et al. Randomized controlled trials of surgical interventions. Ann Surg 2010; 251:409–416

18. Guyatt GH, Sackett DL, Cook DJ. Users' guides to the medical literature. II. How to use an article about therapy or prevention. A. Are the results of the study valid? Evidence-Based Medicine Working Group. JAMA 1993;270:2598–2601

19. Altman DG, Schulz KF. Statistics notes: Concealing treatment allocation in randomised trials. BMJ 2001;323:446–447

20. Black N. Why we need observational studies to evaluate the effectiveness of health care. BMJ 1996;312:1215–1218

21. Takemoto SK, Arns W, Bunnapradist S, et al. Expanding the evidence base in transplantation: the complementary roles of randomized controlled trials and outcomes research. Transplantation 2008;86:18–25

22. Garrison LP, Jr., Towse A, Bresnahan BW. Assessing a structured, quantitative health outcomes approach to drug risk-benefit analysis. Health Aff (Millwood) 2007;26:684–695

23. Furberg CD, Levin AA, Gross PA, Shapiro RS, Strom BL. The FDA and drug safety: a proposal for sweeping changes. Arch Intern Med 2006;166:1938–1942

24. Lasser KE, Allen PD, Woolhandler SJ, Himmelstein DU, Wolfe SM, Bor DH. Timing of new black box warnings and withdrawals for prescription medications. JAMA 2002;287: 2215–2220

25. Rothwell PM. External validity of randomised controlled trials: "to whom do the results of this trial apply?". Lancet 2005;365:82–93

26. McCulloch P, Taylor I, Sasako M, Lovett B, Griffin D. Randomised trials in surgery: problems and possible solutions. BMJ 2002;324:1448–1451

27. Takemoto SK, Terasaki PI, Gjertson DW, Cecka JM. Twelve years' experience with national sharing of HLA-matched cadaveric kidneys for transplantation. N Engl J Med 2000; 343:1078–1084

28. Weber GM, Murphy SN, McMurry AJ, et al. The Shared Health Research Information Network (SHRINE): a prototype federated query tool for clinical data repositories. J Am Med Inform Assoc 2009;16:624–630

29. Brownstein JS, Sordo M, Kohane IS, Mandl KD. The tell-tale heart: population-based surveillance reveals an association of rofecoxib and celecoxib with myocardial infarction. PLoS One 2007;2:e840

30. SooHoo NF, Lieberman JR, Ko CY, Zingmond DS. Factors predicting complication rates following total knee replacement. J Bone Joint Surg Am 2006;88:480–485

31. Bozic KJ, Kurtz SM, Lau E, Ong K, Vail TP, Berry DJ. The epidemiology of revision total hip arthroplasty in the United States. J Bone Joint Surg Am 2009;91:128–133

32. Black DM, Kelly MP, Genant HK, et al. Bisphosphonates and fractures of the subtrochanteric or diaphyseal femur. N Engl J Med 2010;362:1761–1771

33. Neri L, Rocca Rey LA, Pinsky BW, et al. Increased risk of graft failure in kidney transplant recipients after a diagnosis of dyspepsia or gastroesophageal reflux disease. Transplantation 2008;85:344–352

34. Victora CG, Habicht JP, Bryce J. Evidence-based public health: moving beyond randomized trials. Am J Public Health 2004;94:400–405

35. Benson K, Hartz AJ. A comparison of observational studies and randomized, controlled trials. N Engl J Med 2000; 342:1878–1886

36. Hoppe DJ, Schemitsch EH, Morshed S, Tornetta P 3rd, Bhandari M. Hierarchy of evidence: where observational studies fit in and why we need them. J Bone Joint Surg Am 2009;91(Suppl 3):2–9

37. Bryant DM, Willits K, Hanson BP. Principles of designing a cohort study in orthopaedics. J Bone Joint Surg Am 2009;91 (Suppl 3):10–14

38. Busse JW, Obremskey WT. Principles of designing an orthopaedic case-control study. J Bone Joint Surg Am 2009;91 (Suppl 3):15–20

39. Berger ML, Mamdani M, Atkins D, Johnson ML. Good research practices for comparative effectiveness research: defining, reporting and interpreting nonrandomized studies of treatment effects using secondary data sources: The ISPOR Good Research Practices for Retrospective Database Analysis Task Force Report–Part I. Value Health 2009;12:1044–1052

40. von Elm E, Altman DG, Egger M, Pocock SJ, Gotzsche PC, Vandenbroucke JP. The Strengthening the Reporting of Observational Studies in Epidemiology (STROBE) statement: guidelines for reporting observational studies. Ann Intern Med 2007;147:573–577

41. Ahn H, Court-Brown CM, McQueen MM, Schemitsch EH. The use of hospital registries in orthopaedic surgery. J Bone Joint Surg Am 2009;91(Suppl 3):68–72

42. Normand SL, Sykora K, Li P, Mamdani M, Rochon PA, Anderson GM. Readers guide to critical appraisal of cohort studies: 3. Analytical strategies to reduce confounding. BMJ 2005; 330:1021–1023

43. Morshed S, Tornetta P, 3rd, Bhandari M. Analysis of observational studies: a guide to understanding statistical methods. J Bone Joint Surg Am 2009;91(Suppl 3):50–60

11

Survey Design

Michel Saccone, Susan M. Liew

"The extent to which beliefs are based on evidence is very much less than believers suppose."—Bertrand Russell

Summary

Surveys can be very useful tools for accurately collecting data when they are utilized properly in clinical research. They can be used in a variety of settings and can collect a wide range of data. Various strategies are available for survey design and implementation. Effective survey design requires a balance between simplicity and comprehensiveness. Of utmost importance is ensuring that the survey is valid and that it produces a high response rate.

Introduction

Art into Science—Purpose of a Survey?

Every time we see a patient we are conducting a survey. This "survey" allows us to develop expectations of the ideal management of a specific injury and the subsequent outcomes of the intervention. Surveys also provide us with the opportunity to learn about beliefs, behaviors, knowledge, attitudes, and attributes of our patients. Additionally, it is important to note that these characteristics are not limited to patients; surveys are applicable to a wide spectrum of populations, including surgeons. On its own, a survey will provide a "bare-bones" approach when it comes to levels of evidence; however, when used as a primary component in an attempt to refine a research question for a clinical trial, a survey can be advantageous. An example of this would be using a survey to determine the practice patterns of a target group of surgeons in an attempt to obtain concrete data on a particular intervention. The results of this survey may provide you with the evidence you need to justify your trial, or it may indicate that the intervention controversy you sought to identify was in fact nonexistent. Using a survey in this way is known as a needs assessment.

The Value of a Needs Assessment

In addition to providing evidence for your research question, a needs assessment can identify a wide range of valuable information. When utilized correctly, a needs assessment can determine the optimal strategies for the design and implementation of a study.[1] An example of this is using a survey to select the appropriate target population for a research question you have developed. Optimal strategies will likely vary depending on the target population, so it is important to use a needs assessment rather than relying on the strategies used in previous studies. Your needs assessment should also be paired with a review of the relevant literature. This will allow you to incorporate successful methods of previous surveys and will act as an ideal complement to your needs assessment. Lastly, once you have designed your survey, performing a pilot test is critical to determining if your needs assessment has been successful.

Survey as a Bare-Bones Approach

Despite the general lack of credibility in their evidence, surveys can yield some important findings and should not be overlooked. Due to the absence of the rigorous development process found in more credible research designs, such as prospective cohort studies and randomized controlled trials, a well-designed survey can provide important information in a relatively short time frame.[2] Although the results of these surveys may not be significant enough to instill a change in surgical practice, for example, they may identify a trend that can support the need for additional, more rigorous research studies.[3] Also, in some circumstances, surveys provide the ideal means to answer simple research questions.

> **Examples from the Literature: Fluid Lavage in Patients with Open Fracture Wounds (FLOW): An International Survey of 984 Surgeons**
> Petrisor et al. published the results of their fluid lavage of open wounds survey, which aimed to identify the preferred solution and pressure used for irrigation of open wounds for orthopaedic surgeons.[4] The results identified trends in both the preferred solution and irrigating pressure, but also identified discrepancies in definitions of low pressure. The major finding was that 94.2% of the responding surgeons indicated that they would change

their practice if a randomized controlled trial identified a superior method.[4] This survey not only obtained information on surgeon practice, but also identified gaps in current knowledge and the need for further research.[4]

Identifying a Research Question

As with all research, the key to a good survey-based study is dependent upon having a focused purpose. Clearly defining the objectives of the survey will allow you to focus your research question and subsequently streamline your survey. Dependent on whether you plan to use a survey to identify the need for a clinical trial or whether you intend to use the results of the survey directly, your research question will vary. Generally, surveys used in needs assessments aim to obtain as much relevant information as possible without being so long as to discourage response.[1] Accordingly, research questions used for these purposes tend to be broader in scope.[1] However, if you are using a survey to answer a specific question, it is important to develop a focused research question. The question should be relatively simple, as complex questions will often make it too difficult to create a survey that provides usable results.[2] It is recommended that complex research questions be broken down into multiple simple questions.[2] This also ensures sufficient attention is given to outcomes that may appear less important, such as patient-specific outcomes. Often these "less important" outcomes can prove to be very valuable to your conclusions.

An invaluable resource when developing a research question is an experienced clinical practitioner who is immersed in the area of research you would like to pursue.[2] He or she likely is aware of the controversies that require further investigation and can be very helpful in the development of your survey. Again, this should be combined with a rigorous literature review, and together these steps ensure that the final study question is scientifically sound whilst still being clinically relevant.[1]

Key Concepts: Broad Question or Focused Question?
When a survey is being used as part of a needs assessment, the research question should have a broader scope, while research questions for general surveys for clinical research should have a more focused scope. Along with an extensive literature review, consulting an experienced clinician can be an invaluable resource when developing a research question.

Survey Development

The eminent authority on survey design is Don Dillman.[3] His "tailored design method" should be consulted by the clinical researcher to provide an appreciation of the complexities involved in designing and implementing an effective survey.

Sample Identification

Upon finalizing your research question, the next step is the development of your survey. This process begins with the identification of your sample. In an ideal situation, you should include all eligible individuals from the survey population in order to minimize sampling error.[5] However, this is not always possible. The most important aspect of minimizing sampling error is to ensure the sample size of your survey is large enough to produce reliable conclusions.[5] The sample size will restrict what analyses can be conducted and, accordingly, what questions can be answered.[4,6] Another important factor in sample size calculations is the response rate. Since this value can vary it is important to pilot test your survey to create an expected response rate. It is also recommended to consult the literature, as response rates for similar surveys can be used as an estimate.[6] For surveys, in order to limit biases, response rates of 70% or higher are required. If your pilot test indicates a response rate lower than 70%, it may be worthwhile to review your design and implementation strategies.[7]

Question Development

Now that you have defined your sample, you must determine what questions and how many questions you require to ensure you answer your research question. You must also determine how many questions are needed for each specific topic area. Although this step may at first appear relatively simple, it can be difficult to design a question set that is interpreted in the way that you intend. When a question is able to produce consistent results that are intended, it is termed "valid."[3] Validity is a critical characteristic of a question and a survey as a whole. This will be further discussed later in this chapter. There are a few other key points to consider when developing your question:[3]

- Avoid using open-ended questions.[3,4,6] This applies to questions as a whole and to selections on closed-ended questions that allow answers to vary. Rather, use closed-ended questions, as they are easier to score, enter into a database, and analyze.
- Maximize the versatility of an ordinal scale (or Likert scale). Ensure the appropriate use of unipolar and bipolar formats.
- Avoid asking questions pertaining to nonrecent events; these increase recall bias and reduce the reliability of your data.
- Minimize vague questions and response options.
- Avoid neutral response options.
- Avoid requesting respondents to rank response options.[8]

Wording and phrasing must also be considered when developing your questions. They need to be simple, familiar, and not confusing to the responder.[2,3,6,9,10] If the questions are misunderstood, this can lead to a large variability in your answers which will reduce the quality of your results. If there is any doubt about the suitability of a word or phrase, it is recommended to err conservatively. Dillman's wording recommendations are listed below:[3]

- Avoid using specialized words.
- Use the minimum number of words to ask the question.
- Use complete sentences to ask questions.
- Avoid using the same response options, when more accurate ones are available.
- Use equal numbers of positive and negative response options on ordinal questions.
- Distinguish between neutral responses and undecided options by placing an undecided option at the end of the list.
- Avoid developing response categories that are mutually exclusive.
- Avoid double-barreled questions.

Jargon Simplified: Open-Ended Questions
Questions that offer no specific structure for the respondent's answer are open-ended.[11]

Jargon Simplified: Closed-Ended Questions
Questions that offer fixed answers that cannot be altered by the respondent are closed-ended.[11]

Jargon Simplified: Ordinal Scales
Investigators present ordinal scales to respondents to obtain ratings of their responses.[11] The scales typically have three to nine possible values, which include extremes of attitudes or feelings (such as from "totally disagree" to "totally agree"). Ordinal scales can be unipolar, where the scale is anchored at one end by the "zero point" (e.g., "none of the time" to "all the time") or bipolar, where the "zero point" lies somewhere in the middle (e.g., "totally agree" to "neutral" to "totally disagree").

Key Concepts: Make Sure Your Sample Is Large Enough
Ensure an adequate sample size is available to yield sufficient power to find valid conclusions. Utilize the recommendations described by Dillman[3] when developing the questions in your survey.

Survey Design

Survey Format and Length

Survey format and length can have significant effects on the acceptance of your survey, and subsequently your response rate. Your survey should be formatted in a manner that makes it aesthetically appealing. It should be printed on a single side of the page in portrait layout.[3,9] There should be extra space between questions and consecutive numbering to allow easy navigation from question to question.[3,9] Response options should be a lighter shade than questions and they should be listed vertically, rather than horizontally.[3] Also, specific instructions should be placed directly preceding the question they pertain to, rather than being placed at the beginning of the survey. Your survey should be placed on legal-sized paper rather than letter-sized paper.[3,9] With regard to survey length, the goal is to be as short as possible while still obtaining the required information. Eliminating unnecessary questions is integral to improving response rates and survey acceptance.

Survey Aesthetics

The survey needs to be presented in a way that is visually appealing to the responder.[2,6] Using official letterheads and enlisting the support of your departmental head can help to make your document look professional. Some thought should go into certain visual design concepts as they can help maximize response rates and accuracy of responses. It is particularly important when presenting ordinal variable questions that an even spacing between response categories is used.[2] Not doing this may suggest to some participants that one response may cover a greater section of the response scale than the others, thereby increasing the use of this answer.

Another visual design concept to consider is the font used.[2] The use of consistent font changes can help to differentiate between the question and the response options. Furthermore, the use of consistent font throughout your questions and responses avoids any bias that could incur from answers that look "more appropriate." It is also important to consider your audience demographics when selecting your font size.[10] For example, your response rate from a sample of hip fracture patients may be compromised if you've tried to squeeze your survey into a single page by using 10-point font when a 12-point or larger font might have been appreciated by a group of such patients.

Question Order

Consideration should always be given to the order in which the questions are presented. Questions that are designed to investigate similar topics should be placed together.[3] The introduction and first question need to capture the interest of the respondent and encourage them to complete the survey. The first question should apply to everyone, be easy to read, and emphasize that the survey is relevant to the participant.[3] It should not be a potentially objectionable question as this may prevent the respondent from continuing. Potentially objectionable questions, which may be considered personal or confidential, should be placed toward the end of the survey when the respondent has likely committed to completing the survey.[2] Since the closed-ended format of questions specifies the answer options, it may be appropriate to designate some space at the end of the survey to allow the patient to make any comments about their condition or the survey in general.[3] If your survey is not organized properly, respondents may be able to determine your expectations and may provide answers they think you are expecting, rather than the truthful answers.

> **Key Concepts: Features of a Good Survey**
> Your survey should:
> - Be short but comprehensive;
> - Have an engaging introduction to obtain buy-in;
> - Save controversial and personal questions until the end;
> - Provide opportunity for open-ended comments at the survey's conclusion;
> - Be visually appealing;
> - Use consistent text and formatting to enhance design and avoid bias;
> - Take into consideration special needs of certain demographics (e.g., the need for larger text in older populations);
> - Undergo a pilot test to obtain feedback and ensure that the questions are answered as intended.

Using Existing Surveys

In clinical research, the reality is that few researchers will construct a survey for their study from scratch. Most will take a standardized survey that has already been validated to use in their study and supplement this with additional questions in areas not covered.[4,6] As part of your literature review, you should construct a list of previously published surveys (termed "instruments" in health status/quality of life research) in your topic of interest. A very important resource for clinical researchers is the AO Handbook *Musculoskeletal Outcomes Measures and Instruments*, a publication by the AO Foundation (see Suggested Reading), which describes the instruments for the assessment of both acute and chronic musculoskeletal conditions.[12] It is organized by anatomic region, though some instruments may be applicable to multiple regions of the extremities. The AO Handbook was not intended to provide an exhaustive list, as it only identifies the most commonly used musculoskeletal outcome instruments reported in the literature, lists the populations that the questionnaire has been validated for, and gives the survey a "validity" ranking out of ten.

Survey Validation

Ensuring that your survey is valid for the target population is a critical step in survey development. If validity cannot be established, any results obtained from your survey will be void. This concept also applies to previously validated surveys that have been adjusted, as they must be re-validated for the new target population. From a strictly theoretical point of view, a survey should not be used in a population in which it has not been validated for certain measurement properties.[2] The assessment of measurement properties is necessary to enable reviewers and readers to assess the quality of the methodology of a study, and to help other researchers to determine which instrument would be best for their study. This creates a great conflict between the practical application of survey completion and the theory behind conducting a survey. Validation can be a lengthy, resource-intensive process that tends to be conducted by epidemiologists rather than by surgeons.[6]

The key measurement properties of outcome assessment instruments are reliability, validity, and responsiveness.[3] The evaluation of reliability is undertaken in terms of internal consistency (using Cronbach's alpha, α) and reproducibility (using test–retest reliability).[3] Content and construct validity are the most relevant measures of validity when evaluating questionnaires.[3] Content validity is a qualitative assessment of whether an instrument examines all the important domains and consists of a judgment performed by relevant stakeholders.[3] Construct validity is a type of empirical evidence that shows whether an instrument is measuring what is intended.[4] Construct validity is assessed by investigating logical relationships between an instrument and theoretical concepts (constructs).[3] Responsiveness can be assessed using statistical techniques or where the instrument is proven to detect clinically important change over time.[3] While a number of statistical methods are available to assess responsiveness, the importance of detecting clinically relevant change rather than just statistically significant change must be kept in mind.[3] Moreover, a small improvement in a variable may not be statistically significant but may be considered to be functionally relevant by the patient.[3] To avoid yielding invalid results the instrument should also be specific and sensitive. Key to all this is that whether an instrument displays appropriate measurement properties is not a fixed property: it is dependent upon the context and population being studied.[3]

In addition to directly assessing the validity of your survey, it is important to consider the ability of your tool to avoid response bias. Response bias should be of substantial concern any time the response rate of your survey is less than 100%.[13] Generally, response bias has been presented in the literature by comparing the distribution of measured characteristics of pooled groups of responders and respondents.[13] It is assumed that if the response rate is sufficient and the compared characteristics similar enough, then the results are valid.[13] This represents an appropriate method of validation for single-wave studies; however, for multiwave studies—those which resend surveys to nonrespondents in the hope of increasing response rate—the aforementioned concepts are not sufficient.[13] Each successive wave is obtaining responses from a sample of the nonrespondents, who have increased similarities.[13] Increasing the number of waves results in increasingly similar respondents and nonrespondents, and subsequently a reduced likelihood of response bias.[13] In their assessment of response bias in multiwave studies, Montori et al. found response bias to be negligible and the results to be valid, despite poor response rates.[13] As multiwave studies become increasing popular with the accessibility some of the administration techniques afford (see below), this concept of validation becomes increasingly important.

Jargon Simplified: Reliability
Reliability is a measure of whether an instrument produces reproducible and internally consistent results.[11]

Jargon Simplified: Content Validity
In relation to health-related measures, validity represents the extent to which an instrument is measuring what it is intended to measure.[11]

Jargon Simplified: Construct Validity
A construct is a theoretically derived notion of the domain(s) we wish to measure. An understanding of the construct will lead to expectations about how an instrument should behave if it is valid. Construct validity therefore involves comparisons between measures, and examination of the logical relationships which should exist between a measure and characteristics of patients and patient groups.[11]

Jargon Simplified: Responsiveness
Responsiveness is the ability of a tool to detect a significant difference between two populations that is clinically relevant.

Jargon Simplified: Sensitivity
Sensitivity is measured as the proportion of people who truly have a designated condition who are so identified by the test[11]; in other words, it is a measurement of the ability to avoid false-positives.

Jargon Simplified: Specificity
Specificity is measured as the proportion of people who are truly free of a designated condition who are so identified by the test[11]; in other words, it is a measurement of the ability to avoid false-negatives.

Jargon Simplified: Response Bias
Response bias is the name given to the tendency for a greater response rate to arise from a group of the sample that is bound by a similar characteristic.[11]

Key Concepts: Qualities of a Good Survey
A questionnaire should not be used in a population in which it has not been validated. In order to have an acceptable survey, the survey must be reliable, valid, and responsive. Identifying significant results is irrelevant if the change is not clinically important. Sometimes a result may not be statistically significant, but in the context of the situation the change may be clinically relevant.

Pilot Testing

The last important step before the implementation of your survey is a pilot test or pretest. This should be done in a formal manner, by distributing your survey using the methods you plan to use for your definitive survey.[2,6] The sample for your pilot test should be a subset of your target population. Surgeons, epidemiologists, statisticians, patients, and any other persons with an interest in the study or a research background can all provide useful feedback and advice on your survey. Surgical experts can ensure that they agree with the clinically focused aspects of your survey; methodological experts can provide feedback on the format of your survey; and other people (both eligible patients and members of the public who may not have an injury) are invaluable in ensuring that potential respondents will be able to comprehend the survey's material and that questions are answered as intended for your analysis.[6] Assessing the results from the pilot test will display areas where adjustments need to be made. If the adjustments are relatively small, it is likely that once the changes have been made, the survey will be ready for administration. However, if the adjustments are large, the new survey may require additional pilot testing to ensure the changes made were adequate.

Survey Administration

Best Methods

There are currently four primary methods for survey administration: telephone surveys, mail surveys, fax surveys, and electronic surveys. Each method has its advantages and disadvantages; however, the selection of an appropriate method is ultimately dependent on the study population (**Table 11.1**).

Table 11.1 The four primary methods of survey administration

Method of survey administration	Advantages	Disadvantages
Telephone	Increased accuracy of responses Few missed questions	Difficulty in accessing intended physician Interviewer bias Interviewer distortion
Mail	Increased response rate Convenience Ease of surveying geographically dispersed populations Confidentiality and anonymity Increased validity of answers	Incorrect mailing addresses Ongoing costs Data recording can be inaccurate Longest delay in return time Surgeons may not be able to explain responses as well as in a telephone interview
Fax	Can record data via optical character recognition Fast delivery and return	Can be expensive Largest number of incompletely answered questions
Internet and email	Cost effective Faster responses Ease of sending reminders Reduced labor Smaller number of questions left unanswered Results can be quickly pooled and analyzed	Lower response rate Surgeons may be unfamiliar with Internet or email Easy to delete Out-of-date emailing lists Survey may be viewed as junk mail or computer virus

Telephone Surveys

Telephone surveys represent a primitive form of survey distribution and have limited use because of the poor response rate.[14] This has been further complicated in the past decade with the increasing dependence on cellular phones, which are not listed in general phone books. Telephone surveys also suffer from interviewer bias, interviewer distortion, a lack of confidentiality, difficulty in accessing the intended physician, and requiring a large amount of time and resources.[6] On the other hand, telephone-administered surveys can ensure that all questions are answered with increased accuracy, that the questions are comprehended properly, fewer questions are missed, and that responses are registered properly.[6]

Mail Surveys

Mail surveys, though primitive, remain widely used because of the minimal amount of resources required.[7] This is especially the case when the target population is a group that likely does not have access to or is resistant to the use of electronic mail surveys. They tend to be associated with increased validity and increased response rate because the respondents are able to consult required information.[7] They are superior to telephone surveys when there are questions relating to sensitive or confidential topic areas.[7] They are also particularly useful in situations where there is a large study sample dispersed geographically—mail surveys allow a convenient and easy way to reach these target populations.[6] Although mail surveys are widely used for the above reasons, they can be time consuming and involve ongoing costs due to incorrect

mailing addresses or delays in return time.[6] Additionally, responses may not be as well explained as in a telephone interview.[6]

Facsimile (Fax) Surveys

These surveys are very similar to mail surveys, but they require the respondent to have an available fax number.[6] These permit the use of optical character recognition to record data and ensure a fast delivery and return of the survey.[6] The costs of fax and mail surveying are comparable; however, faxed surveys have the highest number of incompletely answered questions.[6]

Electronic Surveys

The email method of survey has become increasingly popular as the population's dependence on the internet and email has increased over the past few decades.[6] Here, electronic copies of the survey are sent and returned via email or a website link is provided, where the survey is made available to the respondent, thus allowing a faster response and reduced labor.[6] Using a website can provide added security, as it is possible to make access available only to those with a username and password. Websites also introduce the option to use a variety of other techniques in survey administration. An example of these is the ability to control the order of questions respondents can answer.[15] Respondents are only given access to the next question once the previous question has been completed. This decreases the number of questions that are left unanswered and provides a cost-effective way for results to be quickly pooled and analyzed afterwards on a computer.[6]

There are, however, disadvantages associated with this method, of which the low response rate is the most apparent.[15] Surveys may also end up in the junk folder, be viewed as a computer virus, or easily deleted if emailed to participants.[6] For this reason, respondents should be provided with the opportunity to print the survey and return it completed via mail or facsimile.[16] Again, this methodology is not applicable to all populations since some, especially older, surgeons may be unfamiliar with internet or email, but for orthopaedic surgeons, like in the survey conducted by Sprague et al., it can be used effectively.[6]

Mixed-Methods Approach

Since no one survey administration method is superior to all the others, Dillman has suggested using a mixed-methods approach. An example of this approach is using electronic surveys in the first administration and for the second administration using a different method like facsimile. With this approach you are able to better access your population as a whole.[3]

> **Key Concepts: How Best to Administer Your Survey**
> Although there are a variety of methods available for survey administration, if resources permit, the most effective is a mixed-methods approach.

Improving the Response Rate

To maximize response rate it has been shown that a mixed-methods approach of mail-out with telephone or email follow-up works best within the surgical population.[9,10,17–19] Be aware that this does require dedicated staff (paid, student project, or pro bono) and a significant amount of time. Another method of follow-up that can also work well if the patients are still undergoing review is to see them in an outpatient clinic setting. Again, this is tremendously resource intensive. Clinical surgeons likely do not have the time to administer surveys, so they must hire research staff and have clinical space available to provide the survey.

> **Examples from the Literature: Survey Design in Orthopaedic Surgery—Getting Surgeons to Respond**
> Sprague et al. conducted a review of surveys used in orthopaedic surgery to determine which methods of survey administration were most effective in increasing response rate.[6] Cover letters were shown to increase response rate as they allow personalization of the survey to the respondent.[6] The cover letter allows an introduction to the survey so that the respondent understands the importance of his or her response.[6] It should also include contact information. Personalization of the survey can go beyond addressing the cover letter to the respondent;[6] it can include the use of a hand-written signature

on the bottom of the letter, which has been shown to increase response rate by greater than 40%.[20] Contacting the respondent prior to administering the survey to inform them of a forthcoming survey, as well as contacting respondents (multiple times if necessary) after administering as a follow-up, have shown to be beneficial.[6] Providing a stamped return envelope, using professional survey packaging, and knowing the respondent all led to an increased response rate.[6] Some strategies that did not improve response rate included providing a deadline, including incentives, and obtaining the approval of an opinion leader.[6]

> **Key Concepts: Maximizing Response Rate**
> There are a variety of methods that have shown to improve response rate. By incorporating the successful surveying methods outlined above, you will increase the likelihood of obtaining a high response rate.

Ethical Considerations

All surveys require ethics approval prior to implementation. They also should be monitored by an ethics review committee.[8] As part of the ethics process, informed consent is required for all surveys involving patients.[6] All patients should be aware of the role they are playing in the study and be able to have any study-related questions answered by study personnel.[6] Before signing the consent form, the researcher must ensure that the patient completely understands his or her participation.[6] Participants should be provided anonymity and confidentiality, which can be done through coding techniques.[3] When patients are not involved, the ethics process is far less involved. Consent forms are no longer required so a cover letter should be included to explain the purpose of the survey.[6]

Financial Considerations

As mentioned previously, the development of a survey from scratch can be a very resource-intensive process. Unfortunately, an estimate of the finances required to perform this process is dependent on a number of factors, such as the sample size, the number of persons involved, and the target population among others.[6] A good resource for obtaining an estimate would be to contact a surgeon who has performed a survey similar to the one you envision. With regard to the method of administration, internet or email distribution remains the cheapest method because it avoids faxing and postage costs.[6]

Conclusion

The development of a successful survey begins with the identification of a relevant research question. When using a survey as part of a needs assessment, the research question should be broader in nature. When using a survey directly for research purposes, a focused, simple research question will generally produce more effective results. Once a research question has been identified you must determine the target population, what specific questions you are going to ask, and how you are going to ask the questions. Special attention should be paid to the format and aesthetics of the survey and how the questions are organized. While developing your survey, it is important to take patient demographics into account. Often participants will not respond well to long and overly personal questionnaires. To obtain high response rates, use successful strategies established by previous researchers and ensure the proper administration methods are utilized.

After completing the design of your survey, it is integral for it to undergo a pretest or pilot before it is applied to the target population. This enables you to test the validity of your survey to determine whether the results derived will be acceptable. Surveys not only need to be valid, they also must be reliable and responsive. Without a pilot test, there is no way of determining the potential effectiveness of your survey.

Lastly, since the validation process of a newly developed survey is a very time-consuming and resource-intensive endeavor, it is common practice to use previously validated surveys. Many of these, especially instruments used for the assessment of both acute and chronic musculoskeletal conditions, are outlined in the AO Foundation Survey Handbook *Musculoskeletal Outcomes Measures and Instruments* (see Suggested Reading). In order to ensure these previously developed questionnaires are appropriate for your target population, it may be required that you adjust the content of the questionnaire. However, in doing so you must ensure that the adjusted survey is valid in the population you will be testing.

Whether you elect to develop your own survey or decide to alter an existing one, there is a vast amount of knowledge that can be obtained. Surveys are a tool that should not be overlooked when attempting to answer a research question. When performed effectively they can often provide evidence to support the need for more comprehensive clinical trials.

Suggested Reading

Dillman DA. Internet, mail, and mixed-mode surveys: the tailored design method. Hoboken, NJ, USA: Wiley & Sons; 2009

Jepson C, Asch DA, Hershey JC, Ubel PA. In a mailed physician survey, questionnaire length had a threshold effect on response rate. J Clin Epidemiol 2005;58:103–105

Petrisor B, Jeray K, Schemitsch E, et al. Fluid lavage in patients with open fracture wounds (FLOW): an international survey of 984 surgeons. BMC Musculoskelet Disord 2008;9:7

Sprague S, Quigley L, Bhandari M. Survey design in orthopaedic surgery: getting surgeons to respond. J Bone Joint Surg Am 2009;91(Suppl 3):27–34

Suk M, Hanson BP, Norvell DC, Helfet DL. AO Handbook: Musculoskeletal Outcomes Measures and Instruments. Davos: AO Publishing; 2005

References

1. Cavanagh S, Chadwick K. Health needs assessment. National Institute for Clinical Excellence. 2005. Available at www.nice.org.uk. Accessed April 20, 2010

2. Jones D, Story D, Clavisi O, Jones R, Peyton P. An introductory guide to survey research in anaesthesia. Anaesth Intensive Care 2006;34:245–253

3. Dillman DA. Internet, mail, and mixed-mode surveys: the tailored design method. Hoboken, NJ, USA: Wiley & Sons, 2009

4. Petrisor B, Jeray K, Schemitsch E, et al. Fluid lavage in patients with open fracture wounds (FLOW): an international survey of 984 surgeons. BMC Musculoskelet Disord 2008;9:7

5. Asch DA, Christakis NA. Different response rates in a trial of two envelope styles in mail survey research. Epidemiology 1994;5:346–345

6. Sprague S, Quigley L, Bhandari M. Survey design in orthopaedic surgery: getting surgeons to respond. J Bone Joint Surg Am 2009;91(Suppl 3):27–34

7. Zelnio RN. Data collection techniques: mail questionnaires. Am J Hosp Pharm 1980;37:1113–1119

8. Mailey SK. Increasing your response rate for mail survey data collection. SCI Nurs 2002;19:78–79

9. Brehaut JC, Graham ID, Visentin L, Stiell IG. Print format and sender recognition were related to survey completion rate. J Clin Epidemiol 2006;59:635–641

10. Mullner RM, Levy PS, Byre CS, Matthews D. Effects of characteristics of the survey instrument on response rates to a mail survey of community hospitals. Public Health Reports 1982;97:465–469

11. Guyatt G, Rennie D. Users' Guides to the Medical Literature: A Manual for Evidence-Based Clinical Practice. Chicago: American Medical Association Press; 2002

12. Suk M, Hanson BP, Norvell DC, Helfet DL. AO Handbook: Musculoskeletal Outcomes Measures and Instruments. Davos: AO Publishing; 2005

13. Montori VM, Leung TW, Walter SD, Guyatt GH. Procedures that assess inconsistency in meta-analyses can assess the likelihood of response bias in multiwave surveys. J Clin Epidemiol 2005;58:856–858

14. Hocking JS, Lim MS, Read T, Hellard M. Postal surveys of physicians gave superior response rates over telephone interviews in a randomized trial. J Clin Epidemiol 2006;59:521–524

15. Mavis BE, Brocato JJ. Postal surveys versus electronic mail surveys. The tortoise and the hare revisited. Eval Health Prof 1998;21:395–408
16. Braithwaite D. Emery J, De Lusignan S, Sutton S. Using the internet to conduct surveys of health professionals: a valid alternative? Fam Pract 2003;20:545–551
17. Jepson C, Asch DA, Hershey JC, Ubel PA. In a mailed physician survey, questionnaire length had a threshold effect on response rate. J Clin Epidemiol 2005;58:103–105
18. Dillman DA. Why choice of survey mode makes a difference. Public Health Reports 2006;121:11–13
19. Bhandari M, Devereaux PJ, Swiontkowski MF, et al. A randomized trial of opinion leader endorsement in a survey of orthopaedic surgeons: effect on primary response rates. Int J Epidemiol 2003;32:634–636
20. Maheux B, Legault C, Lambert J. Increasing response rates in physicians' mail surveys: an experimental study. Am J Public Health 1989;79:638–639

12

Qualitative Studies

Jennifer Klok

Summary

The place of qualitative methods in surgical research is becoming increasingly apparent. Complex surgical questions related to social behaviors, beliefs, and attitudes are often best addressed using a qualitative approach. The use of descriptive data from observations and interactions can serve as the basis for theory development or as an adjunct to quantitative studies. Quality of life and patient satisfaction are important outcomes in the surgical context, and are initially approached using qualitative means. It is essential that surgeons become familiar with what qualitative research is, when it should be considered for surgical problems, and how to conduct an appropriate qualitative study.

Introduction

As evidence-based medicine (EBM) is being implemented in surgical practice, it is clear that various methodologies are required to address the diversity of research questions faced by clinicians today. One such methodology is qualitative research, which is growing in utilization and acceptance in clinical medicine. While it has been slow to find its position in surgical literature, surgeons are beginning to recognize its role and the additional dimension it adds to more traditional research methods. It is the goal of this chapter to provide surgeons with a general understanding of qualitative methods, an introduction to some of the terms and theories in qualitative research, and practical steps for conducting a qualitative study.

What Is Qualitative Research?

Qualitative research is a method of collecting, analyzing, and reporting information through descriptive and narrative means. It seeks to provide an in-depth understanding of experiences or phenomena with data obtained from natural settings.[1] Qualitative research does not begin with the assumption that there is one underlying truth that must be proven. Rather it is undertaken with the intent of capturing a larger, more diverse picture.[1] It gives insight into the "why" questions and tells a story.[2,3]

In contrast to the deductive methods of quantitative research, qualitative studies are inherently inductive. This means that instead of using data to support a preconceived theory, hypotheses are formulated after the information has been obtained and analyzed.[1,4]

> **Jargon Simplified: Inductive**
> The inductive method uses data, observations, or interactions to generate a theory or hypothesis; this process is inherent to qualitative research.[4]

> **Jargon Simplified: Deductive**
> The deductive method uses data to make conclusions about a predetermined theory or hypothesis; this is the intent of quantitative research.[4]

Essentially, qualitative researchers initiate projects with an open mind and try to understand beliefs and behaviors within a context. As such, it is important that the researcher be aware of his or her own contextual framework and recognize how this influences the way information is gathered and analyzed. This is awareness is known as *reflexivity*.[5]

> **Jargon Simplified: Reflexivity**
> Reflexivity arises from the recognition that a researcher's own contextual framework and worldview influences the collection and analysis of data in qualitative research. In reflexivity, researchers use introspective techniques, such as journaling, to understand their own role in the qualitative process.[1,5]

Qualitative and quantitative methods are often viewed as being in contradiction to each other.[6] The former is perceived as a "soft" science that cannot provide conclusive evidence, while the latter is often thought of as producing definitive, "hard" evidence because of the numerical results it provides. This perception may be especially apparent among surgeons, who desire facts and proof that would allow them to make quick decisions. However it is becoming clear to surgeons that not all questions can be answered with numbers. Qualitative and quantitative research, though inherently distinct, should no longer be seen in opposition to each other. Rather, they are different means of answering surgical questions that can serve to complement each other.[6] **Table 12.1** contrasts the two methods of conducting research.

Table 12.1 Overview of typical distinctions between quantitative and qualitative methodologies

	Quantitative	Qualitative
General aim	How much?	What, how, and why?
Treatment of data	Isolates and defines variables, and tests hypotheses on data	Defines very general concepts and searches for patterns
	Narrow lens (deductive)	Wide lens (inductive)
Toolbox	Surveys	Participant-observation
	Questionnaires	In-depth interviews
	Randomized controlled trials	Focus groups
	Systematic reviews and meta-analyses	Document analysis
Focus	Prediction	Rich description
	Outcomes	Process
	Generalizability	Context

Reproduced with permission from Clark.

Why Is Qualitative Research Important?

The complexity of questions asked in surgery and medicine has increased in recent years.[6] Changes in technology, delivery of patient care, health infrastructure, and patient expectations have made it apparent that not all issues can be understood with quantitative statistics. Additionally, quality of life and patient satisfaction outcomes are becoming imperative subjects of measurement in surgical specialties. These outcomes have significant implications for policy and practice.[3] Qualitative research can provide understanding about patient and healthcare provider behaviors, attitudes and beliefs, information which may have important economic relevance.[7] It can give insight into changing patterns of behavior, aid in the assessment of barriers to the uptake of knowledge, or provide frameworks for describing decision-making processes that quantitative methods cannot adequately reach.

When Should It Be Used in Surgical Research?

Understandably, there continues to be skepticism among surgeons regarding the relevance of qualitative research to the surgical field. When time and resources are so scarce, it may seem like an impractical means to some, particularly when the "end" is not always apparent. Certainly, qualitative research is a time-intensive process that must be approached with a great deal of openness.[2,4] However, as with any research undertaking, qualitative studies need to be conducted with a specific question in mind, with equipoise, and with an end goal that is meaningful to

patients, health care providers, and decision makers. It can add richness to information about an issue and address the complexity of questions in surgical practice.[4,8]

So, which questions in surgery are best addressed using qualitative methods? First, the surgical problem must be related to a social phenomenon. Second, the need for a conceptual understanding of the issue must drive the inquiry.[7] When little is known about an issue in surgery, or when a theory needs to be developed as a step in the initiation of further research, qualitative methods should be undertaken.[4] The guide for the critical appraisal of qualitative research in health care by Guyatt et al. can provide readers with a framework for deciding which questions to explore using this methodology.[7]

More specifically, qualitative methods generate understanding about such issues as why patients do not adhere to prescribed regimens, why certain patients opt not to have surgery despite its proven benefit, or why some patients with good subjective outcomes are dissatisfied with their surgery. Quantitative research can tell surgeons whether or not an intervention was effective from the standpoint of measurable outcomes such as pain or range of motion. However, what it cannot tell clinicians is why patients do not comply with certain therapies, or what barriers exist to communication between patients and surgeons or between residents and staff.[6] These issues not only inhibit patient care, but can decrease efficient and economic practice when not examined or addressed.

The following section provides examples from the literature of the types of questions in surgical specialties that were assessed using qualitative methods.

Examples from the Literature: Orthopaedic Surgery

Kroll et al. conducted eight focus groups in a qualitative study that employed *grounded theory* and *ethnographic* methods to explore the influence of race on decision making in total knee arthroplasty.[9] The intent was to understand why the surgery is under-utilized by certain ethnic groups. Thirty categories emerged from analysis of transcripts. Four main concepts provided important insight into beliefs held by different ethnic groups about total knee arthroplasty. These included perceptions about the disease of osteoarthritis, changes in lifestyle, trust, and paying for surgery. The authors concluded that surgeon–patient communication about total knee arthroplasty needs to be more open and that the varying beliefs about surgery among various ethnic groups must be recognized.

Hudak et al. sought to explore the unexpressed concerns of older patients surrounding orthopaedic surgery.[10] Data were collected using observational qualitative methods (audio-recorded surgical consults) and patient interviews. The triangulation of methods allowed researchers to compare what patients expressed as concerns in interviews with what they communicated to their surgeon. The authors found that the majority of patient concerns were not expressed, and concluded that care would be improved if surgeons encouraged patients to communicate at the close of the visit with a question such as "Is there something else you want to ask me about this surgery?"

Examples from the Literature: Plastic Surgery

Klassen et al. conducted in-depth interviews (n = 48) with women who had undergone breast reconstruction, reduction, or augmentation to explore satisfaction and quality of life among patients following surgery.[3] Interviews were transcribed and coded using grounded theory techniques. A conceptual framework was generated using the six overarching themes that emerged from analysis. Patient emphasis on "process of care" (satisfaction with preoperative information, surgeon, and other members of the care team) presented itself as an important concept. This was an unexpected outcome for the research team and highlighted the relevance of this issue in patient satisfaction with surgery.

The conceptual model and coded items from this research were subsequently used to develop a standardized patient-reported outcomes measure.[11] This is a tangible example of how qualitative data may be utilized, and how it can provide a foundation for future quantitative methods.

How Is Qualitative Research Done?

Now that the relevance of and reasons for conducting qualitative research in surgery have been identified, methodology must be discussed. Practically speaking, how does one actually go about doing a qualitative study? There are a number of theories and methodologies in the qualitative world that are used to guide the research process.[12] The process is quite similar between approaches, though the intentions are slightly different. Information is obtained through field observation, interviews, or document analysis.[7] Grounded theory is one of the most common methods, and of greatest relevance to surgical questions. This will be used to guide the step-by-step approach provided below. The concepts of ethnography and phenomenology, often mentioned in qualitative literature, are presented in the "Jargon Simplified" sections below.

Jargon Simplified: Ethnography

An ethnographic qualitative methodology seeks to understand patterns, beliefs, and behaviors of a group within a social context, such as a culture or team, through observation and interaction.[4]

Jargon Simplified: Phenomenology

A phenomenological qualitative theory seeks to understand how individuals interpret and experience a particular phenomenon from the perspective of their own contextual framework.[1,4,12]

Grounded Theory

Grounded theory uses data from interviews and observations to "ground" the development of a theory. This is an iterative process involving the continuous cycle of data collection and analysis. The following example from the literature provides an example of how grounded theory was used in the surgical context.

Jargon Simplified: Grounded Theory

The grounded theory approach in qualitative methodology uses data from interviews and observations to "ground" the development of a theory; this is an iterative process involving the continuous cycle of data collection and analysis.[1,4,13]

Examples from the Literature: Challenges to the Practice of Evidence-Based Medicine During Residents' Surgical Training—A Qualitative Study Using Grounded Theory

A study by Bhandari et al. used grounded theory to examine the challenges experienced by surgical residents in incorporating EBM into clinical practice.[14] Both semistructured interviews (n = 20) and focus groups (n = 8) were used to collect data.

The study identified the participant population appropriately and provided a rationale for why qualitative methods were used to address the issue. *Purposive sampling* was used to include a wide range of perspectives, and participants included residents from all years and all surgical specialties. *Triangulation* was implemented through the use of both focus groups and interviews. Interviews were semistructured with open-ended questions. Two independent reviewers coded all interviews (open coding), and coding discrepancies were resolved through discussion. A theoretical model reflecting the interrelationships between categories or domains was generated, and this was shown to a group of residents for validation in the final step of the analysis process.

Jargon Simplified: Coding

Coding is the process of assigning labels, called "codes," to data (such as interview phrases or passages) as a means of categorizing concepts and themes that emerge through the qualitative analysis.[4,15]

Jargon Simplified: Purposive (Theoretical) Sampling
Purposive sampling is a method used in qualitative research that seeks to round out concepts and reflect diversity in a population as information is gathered and theory emerges. This process is "responsive to the data"[16]—participants are purposefully selected in each round of sampling with the intent of exploring a concept in greater depth.[5,7,16]

The results showed that barriers to the uptake of EBM exist at several levels, beginning with "causal conditions" (resident barriers; staff surgeon barriers), which were compounded by "intervening factors" (institutional barriers; health care system) that both shaped the "central phenomenon" (powerless and helpless; acceptability of EBM). The interviews provided rich information about resident lack of knowledge about and personal barriers to practicing EBM. It also reflected how staff surgeon characteristics and leadership inhibited EBM implementation.

The use of qualitative methods in this study served to construct theories regarding challenges to EBM among surgical residents. This provides information to surgeons, residents, and policy makers about the barriers surrounding this issue, and what steps should be taken next to address these problems.

Constant Comparison Method

"Constant comparison" is the term used by Glaser and Strauss, the founders of grounded theory, to describe the method of continuous and simultaneous data analysis and theory development.[13,17] In other words, it is not a linear process in which data is first collected, then analyzed, and then synthesized into a conceptual model. Instead it is conducted in a cyclical pattern until *saturation* is achieved and no new information or themes emerge.[5,13,17] The following steps may be considered with the constant comparison method in mind.

Jargon Simplified: Saturation
Saturation is the point at which no new information emerges from the data. It includes the subsequent categorization of meaningful terms, often into domains and subdomains; this often involves development of a conceptual model which illustrates relationships between domains.[1,4,7]

Jargon Simplified: Redundancy
Redundancy occurs when data analysis in qualitative research becomes redundant and no new themes are identified; this may be viewed as an appropriate stopping point for some studies.[7]

Step 1: Develop the Research Question
As with any research undertaking, the question must first be clearly identified. In qualitative research the question is more broadly stated than in quantitative studies.[15] It still has a purpose and population in mind, but allows for flexibility and adaptation. To take an example from the literature, a question may be posed in the following way: Why are some elderly patients with moderate-to-severe arthritis unwilling to consider total joint replacement surgery, and what beliefs influence their decision making regarding surgery?[16] This question, though broad, identifies the population as elderly patients with arthritis who would be appropriately treated with surgery, but for unknown reasons are unwilling to consider this management option.[15]

Step 2: Identify the Patient Population
The next step is to identify the patient population. This has been partly done in establishing the research question. The goal of sampling is to obtain a wide range of perspectives from a diverse group of participants.[15] Unlike quantitative methods, it does not strive for homogeneity within a population. A technique called *"purposive"* or *"theoretical"* sampling is typically used.[7,15] In this process participants are selected purposefully in each round of sampling with the intent of exploring a concept or theme in greater depth. This depends on the topic and the purpose of the study. It may mean selecting the most divergent cases or the most critical cases in a population.[7] The sampling criteria evolve during collection and analysis and are "responsive to the data."[15]

Step 3: Obtain Ethics Approval
Generally, ethics approval must be obtained for any qualitative study.[7] This type of research is often very personal and intimate. The researcher must be aware of the sensitive nature of some of the issues explored in qualitative methods. He or she must make it very clear to participants that all identifying information will be removed from transcripts or other documentation, and that future care will not be impacted whatsoever by participation in the study. It is important that rapport is established between the researcher and participant(s), particularly in the interview and focus group situation. When interviewees feel comfortable, the quantity and quality of information obtained is that much richer in the end.[15]

Step 4: Conduct Patient Interviews and/or Focus Groups
There are multiple forms of data collection in qualitative research, including observation, document review (e.g., medical charts), video, interviews, and focus groups. The use of two or more collection methods is known as *triangulation*.[14,15]

Jargon Simplified: Triangulation
Triangulation appears in several forms: "data triangulation," "investigator triangulation," and "theory triangulation." Generally speaking, triangulation is the use of multiple techniques, investigators, or theories in a qualitative study. Findings are compared between methods, not with the intention of reliability reporting, but with the purpose of producing a more comprehensive set of data.[1,7]

The most commonly employed, and likely most useful, approach in surgery is through in-depth interviews and focus groups.[3,4,14] Interviews are typically semistructured with open-ended questions. This means that participants are encouraged to direct the course of the interview and express their stories openly. The interviewer has a list of topics or probes that may be used to guide the session. This topic list is usually developed from expert opinion and literature review, and is added to as more interviews are conducted.[2] Interviewers should be trained prior to interactions with participants, and be encouraged to carry out this process in a way that allows conversation to flow naturally.

Step 5: Review Transcripts
All interviews should be recorded with a good-quality audio recording device. Some transcription service companies will rent out appropriate audio recorders. Once interviews have been transcribed, they are reviewed, ideally by two or more investigators. Each interview should first be read in its entirety prior to further analysis, to allow researchers to appreciate the overall context and perspective of the interviewee.

Step 6: Carry Out Open Coding
Codes are labels such as "physical mobility," "recovery," "self-confidence," and "fears about surgery" that are used to capture concepts in the phrases and passages of the interview transcripts. Open coding is the process of thoroughly working through an interview transcript, highlighting phrases or passages pertaining to a certain concept or topic, and giving it a label or "code."[2] Certain items may be given multiple codes in this stage. This may be done directly in a word-processing document (e.g., in Microsoft Word, using the "Comments" function).

In this step codes are modifiable, so researchers should not be overly concerned about coding everything "correctly" the first time. Again, this process should be done independently by at least two investigators, who then meet together after an interview has been coded to discuss codes, work out any discrepancies, and start to formulate definitions for the labels chosen to identify certain concepts. Domains, or themes, and subdomains should start to evolve during open coding.

Step 7: Develop a Codebook
After several interviews (approximately 5–10) have been coded in duplicate, a "codebook" with all identified and agreed-upon codes is generated. This is a list of codes with definitions or descriptions for each that explain its meaning and when it should be used to identify a concept. The codes may be organized into themes (or domains) and subthemes (or subdomains) that fall under the broader theme headings. The codebook should be reviewed by and discussed with all members of the research team to ensure comprehensiveness and consensus.[2]

Step 8: Carry Out Focused Coding
The researchers now return to the originally coded transcripts and rework the codes based on themes that have emerged and codes included in the codebook. All future interviews should be coded using the codebook as a guide. However it must be pointed out here that the codebook should be considered adaptable, and when new themes and concepts emerge, it must be adjusted and added to.[2]

In the process of focused coding it is imperative that all coded passages be tracked with an interview, page, and line number.[2] Coded portions can be organized in an ordinary computer spreadsheet, or in more sophisticated programs used for qualitative research such as NVivo, which automatically tracks all coded items.

Step 9: Use and Translate the Information
So how is the data used once it has been collected and coded? One way of looking at the data is to see which codes appear most frequently, in a process known as content analysis.[2,4] This can highlight the importance of certain concepts; however, it should not be used as a means for deciding on the inclusion or exclusion of certain data. All information must be considered as a contextual whole and used to develop a conceptual model. A conceptual model is essentially a representative way of showing the major themes that have emerged and the interrelationships between them.[3,4] It aids in the establishment of theory.

The conceptual model and qualitative data may be used in several ways. The model can exist as a hypothesis and launching point for the exploration of future research questions. It can be used to complement quantitative research in mixed-methods proceedings.[1,6] It may be used in the item generation phase in the development of a new patient reported outcomes measure.[11] When qualitative research stands on its own, it must be presented in a way that is meaningful to its intended audience and takes into consideration the elements presented by Giacomini et al.[7] It is important that reflexivity, "the influence a researcher brings to the research process," be openly addressed in this sort of publication.[5]

Key Concepts: Steps for Conducting a Qualitative Study

Step 1: Develop the Research Question
- The question must be clearly identified! In qualitative research the question is more broadly stated than in quantitative studies.[15]

Step 2: Identify the Patient Population
- The goal of sampling is to obtain a wide range of perspectives from a diverse group of participants.[15]

Step 3: Obtain Ethics Approval
- Generally, ethics approval must be obtained for any qualitative study.[7] This type of research is often very personal and intimate.

Step 4: Conduct Patient Interviews and/or Focus Groups
- Interviews are typically semistructured with open-ended questions. This means that the participants are encouraged to direct the course of the interview and express their story openly.

Step 5: Review Transcripts
- All interviews should be recorded with a good-quality audio recording device. Once interviews have been transcribed, they are reviewed, ideally by two or more investigators.

Step 6: Carry Out Open Coding
- Open coding is the process of thoroughly working through an interview transcript, highlighting phrases or passages pertaining to a certain concept or topic, and giving it a label or "code."[2]

Step 7: Develop a Codebook
- After several interviews (approximately 5–10) have been coded in duplicate, a "codebook" with all identified and agreed-upon codes is generated. This is a list of codes with definitions or descriptions of each that explain its meaning and when it should be used to identify a concept.

Step 8: Carry Out Focused Coding
- The researchers now return to the originally coded transcripts and rework the codes on the basis of themes that have emerged and codes included in the codebook.

Step 9: Use and Translate the Information
- All information must be considered as a contextual whole and used to develop a conceptual model. A conceptual model is essentially a representative way of showing the major themes that have emerged and the interrelationships between them.[3,4]

Conclusion

Qualitative methods are used to address surgical problems that cannot be explained or measured using quantitative means. The open nature of the qualitative approach allows the researcher to explore why certain individuals or particular groups of people behave as they do. In a surgical context, for example, the qualitative approach can help to explain why patients opt not to have surgery when they are perfect candidates for surgery, what factors influence quality of life for a patient following surgery, and what barriers exist in patient–surgeon communication. This chapter has provided the reader with background and examples concerning the relevance of qualitative research in surgery, and has described practical steps for initiating a qualitative study to address a surgical issue.

Key Concepts: The Nature and Uses of Qualitative Research Methods
- Qualitative methods can provide contextual insight into complex surgical issues.
- Qualitative research is an inductive process through which theories emerge.
- Qualitative studies can answer the "why" questions in surgical research.
- The qualitative researcher must approach a study with an open mind while being conscious of the contextual framework that he or she brings to the process of data collection and analysis.

Suggested Reading

Beaton DE, Clark JP. Qualitative research: a review of methods with use of examples from the total knee replacement literature. J Bone Joint Surg Am 2009;91:107–112

Corbin J, Strauss A. Basics of Qualitative Research. Thousand Oaks, CA: Sage Publications; 2008

Giacomini M, Cook D. Qualitative research. In: Guyatt G, Rennie D, Meade M, Cook D, eds. Users' Guides to the Medical Literature: A Manual for Evidence-Based Clinical Practice. 2nd ed. New York, NY: McGraw-Hill Companies; 2008:341–360

Glaser B, Strauss A. The Discovery of Grounded Theory: Strategies for Qualitative Research. Chicago, IL: Aldine; 1967

Kuper A, Lingard L, Levinson W. Critically appraising qualitative research. BMJ 2008;337:a1035

Kuper A, Reeves S, Levinson W. An introduction to reading and appraising qualitative research. BMJ 2008;337:a288

Lingard L, Albert M, Levinson W. Grounded theory, mixed methods, and action research. BMJ 2008;337:a567

Reeves S, Kuper A, Hodges BD. Qualitative research methodologies: ethnography. BMJ 2008;337:a1020

Reeves S, Albert M, Kuper A, Hodges BD. Why use theories in qualitative research? BMJ 2008;337:a949

References

1. Kuper A, Reeves S, Levinson W. An introduction to reading and appraising qualitative research. BMJ 2008;337:a288
2. Shauver MJ, Chung KC. A guide to qualitative research in plastic surgery. Plast Reconstr Surg 2010; 126:1089–1097
3. Klassen AF, Pusic AL, Scott A, Klok J, Cano SJ. Satisfaction and quality of life in women who undergo breast surgery: a qualitative study. BMC Womens Health 2009;9:11
4. Beaton D. Clark J. Qualitative research: a review of methods with use of examples from the total knee replacement literature. J Bone Joint Surg Am 2009;91(Suppl 3):107–112
5. Kuper A, Lingard L, Levinson W. Critically appraising qualitative research. BMJ 2008;337:a1035
6. Pope C, Mays N. Reaching the parts other methods cannot reach: an introduction to qualitative methods in health and health services research. BMJ 1995;311:42–45
7. Giacomini M, Cook D. Qualitative research. In: Guyatt G, Rennie D, Meade M, Cook D, eds. Users' Guides to the Medical Literature: A Manual for Evidence-Based Clinical Practice. 2nd ed. New York, NY: McGraw-Hill Companies; 2008:341–360
8. Rich JA, Grey CM. Qualitative research on trauma surgery: getting beyond the numbers. World J Surg 2003;27:957–961
9. Kroll TL, Richardson M, Sharf BF, Suarez-Almazor ME. "Keep on truckin'" or "It's got you in this little vacuum": race-based perceptions in decision-making for total knee arthroplasty. J Rheumatol 2007;34:1069–1075
10. Hudak PL, Armstrong K, Braddock C 3rd, Frankel RM, Levinson W. Older patients' unexpressed concerns about orthopaedic surgery. J Bone Joint Surg Am 2008;90:1427–1435
11. Pusic AL, Klassen AF, Scott AM, Klok JA, Cordeiro PG, Cano SJ. Development of a new patient-reported outcome measure for breast surgery: the BREAST-Q. Plast Reconstr Surg 2009;124:345–353
12. Reeves S, Albert M, Kuper A, Hodges BD. Why use theories in qualitative research? BMJ 2008;337:a949
13. Lingard L, Albert M, Levinson W. Grounded theory, mixed methods, and action research. BMJ 2008;337:a567
14. Bhandari M, Montori V, Devereaux PJ, Dosanjh S, Sprague S, Guyatt GH. Challenges to the practice of evidence-based medicine during residents' surgical training: a qualitative study using grounded theory. Acad Med 2003;78:1183–1190
15. Clark JP, Hudak PL, Hawker GA, et al. The moving target: a qualitative study of elderly patients' decision-making regarding total joint replacement surgery. J Bone Joint Surg Am 2004;86:1366–1374
16. Corbin J, Strauss A. Basics of Qualitative Research. Thousand Oaks, CA: Sage Publications; 2008:vii–381
17. Glaser B, Strauss A. The Discovery of Grounded Theory: Strategies for Qualitative Research. Chicago, IL: Aldine; 1967
18. Clark JP. Balancing Qualitative and Quantitative Methodology in Health Services Research: How Can Qualitative Research Methods Best Complement Administrative Data Analysis? Newmarket, Ontario: Central East Health Information Partnership; 2000:3

13

Economic Analysis

Volker Alt, Gabor Szalay, Theodoros Pavlidis, Christian Heiss, Reinhard Schnettler

Summary

Due to the tremendous rise of health care costs in the last few decades in the Western world, health economics have become an important part of the assessment of new treatment options. In some countries, such as the UK, Canada, and Australia, new therapies can only enter the public health care system if cost–effectiveness under a certain threshold can be shown. The purpose of this chapter is to give basic information about the field of health economics and to make the reader familiar with basic principles of conducting health economic studies, particularly in the course of prospective clinical trials in orthopaedic trauma surgery.

In most cases a new treatment strategy (e.g., a new implant design, navigation system, or drugs) leads to a medical benefit for the patient at a cost that is higher than the cost for the control group. Certain types of studies in health economics allow us to assess whether this additional cost is "justified" and can be considered as "good value for money". Cost studies, cost–effectiveness, cost-utility, and cost–benefit play major roles in health economics.

Cost studies look purely at the financial costs of compared therapies, without any further focus on the medical effects. In cost–effectiveness, cost-utility, and cost–benefit studies the cost differences between the two therapies are related to the medical improvement achieved by the new therapy.

Cost–effectiveness studies use specific "effectiveness parameters," for example "faster fracture healing time in weeks" or "additional fracture healed," to which the incremental costs are related, leading to what are known as "incremental cost–effectiveness ratios". Cost-utility studies translate different health states into general quality of life parameters, mainly the "quality-adjusted life year" (QALY), which uses defined utilities of health states between 0 (death) and 1 (perfect health). The conclusion of a cost-utility study is given in a cost-utility ratio in incremental costs per QALY. Cost–benefit analyses directly change the medical effects into financial parameters, for example with the so-called "willingness-to-pay" approach.

For practical aspects of the conduct of health care studies in the course of prospective clinical trials, the following key steps should be followed: (1) state the medical benefits of the new technology, (2) define the type of the health economic study, (3) define the methodological approach, (4) define the perspective of the study and the types of costs, (5) discount the costs and benefits, (6) conduct sensitivity analysis, (7) state the measurement of efficiency and the conclusions of the study, and (8) discuss strengths and weaknesses of the study. Rationales and references for the underlying cost data should be given and should be reliable. Approaches to data collection should be conservative and practical in order to make the results as transparent and as relevant as possible to the purpose of the study. Finally, cooperation with a health economist is recommended in the preparation and conduct of trials with health economic aspects.

Introduction

Why Economic Analyses?

During the past few decades there has been a tremendous rise in health care costs in the Western world. In the United States expenditures on health care are estimated to be around $2.3 trillion in 2008. This exceeds more than three times the $714 billion spent in 1990, and over eight times the expenditures of $253 billion in 1980.[1] Aging of the population, new medical technology including new innovative drugs, chronic diseases, and, last but not least, increases in administrative costs are seen as the major cost drivers in this development.

This rise in costs has a strong impact on the various health care systems of all Western countries. Higher expenditures in health care frequently outweigh the financial resources of the system and force the different systems into cost-control measures.

In the context of the introduction of a new therapeutic strategy into the health care system, health economic analysis allows (1) assessment of the "health economic value" of this new technology and (2) helps to optimize the allocation of the limited financial resources of the system. In countries such as Australia, Canada, and the UK, demonstration of a new drug's safety, efficacy, and quality—called the first three "hurdles"—is no longer sufficient for market entry and reimbursement in the public health care system. Manufacturers are also obliged to show cost–effectiveness of the new product, that is, to demonstrate sound health economic data combined with clinical effectiveness by comparing the new product to the currently available standard of care for adoption in the health care system. Thus, each new therapeutic strategy can be characterized by clearly defined health economic figures such as cost–effectiveness ratios that allow one to determine its "health economic value." As those ratios are comparable between different therapies, a "health economic ranking" of different treatment strategies can be generated that helps the available financial resources of the health care system to be allocated in the most useful way.

The UK's National Institute for Health and Clinical Excellence (NICE) allows a new therapy entry to the public health care system (National Health Service, NHS) only if the therapy can demonstrate a cost–effectiveness ratio under a certain threshold, for cost control of the system. If the cost–effectiveness ratio of the new therapy lies above this threshold it will—in general—not be able to enter the NHS.

This form of pressure on manufacturers will also gain more importance in the future for other countries. Therefore, the impact of health economic data and health economic studies will increase in the future, including in the field of orthopaedic trauma surgery, as they will deliver the required information for the decision-making processes of regulatory agencies and health care payers in the context of the adoption of new therapies by the public health care sector.

> **Key Concepts: Health Economics**
> Health economics assesses the "health economic value" of treatment strategies and helps to allocate available resources in the health care system in the best way.

Theoretical Background

General Aspects of Health Economics

Health economics compares different medical treatments in terms of medical and economic consequences. When a new therapy strategy is compared to the standard of care, theoretically, four different situations can result in terms of medical and economic outcome (**Fig. 13.1**). First, the new treatment has a better medical outcome but is more expensive than the standard of care. Second, the new treatment is better from a medical point of view and also less expensive. The third and fourth situations result in a worse medical outcome with the new therapy at a lower cost compared to the standard of care, or a worse medical outcome at a higher cost. Since new therapies should lead to a medical benefit for the patient, these two types of situations should not be pursued from either a medical or a health economic point of view.

If the new therapy is better and cheaper than the standard treatment it can be considered as the *dominant treatment strategy* from a health economic point of view; in reality this is only rarely the case. The first combination—better medical outcome with higher treatment costs com-

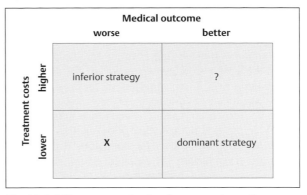

Fig. 13.1 Different scenarios for the comparison of two different treatment strategies from a medical and financial point of view. In most cases new treatment options are better from a medical point of view but also more expensive (upper right box). In these cases a more detailed health economic evaluation is needed.

pared to the standard of care treatment—is the most likely situation for the introduction of new medical strategies nowadays. In this case a more sophisticated evaluation of the health economic value of the new treatment strategy is necessary, and health economics delivers the assessment tools required for this.

The fact that better medical outcomes can be translated into comprehensible economic figures is an essential part of health economic analyses. The ratio between "more expensive" treatment on one hand and "better medical" outcome as expressed in economic figures allows one to draw conclusions as to whether the new medical treatment strategy can be recommended from a health economic point of view.

Types of Studies in Health Economics

The following simple example is intended to facilitate the understanding of the different types of studies in health economics.

> **EXAMPLE**
> A new, growth-factor-coated intramedullary tibial nail is commercially available; its price is $1500 compared to a standard intramedullary nail with a price of $500. A prospective randomized controlled trial could show that the healing rates of closed tibial fractures treated with the new coated nail (group 1) versus the standard uncoated nail (group 2) without secondary intervention were 90% (group 1) versus 80% (group 2) in the first year. Consequently, in the first year 10% of the patients in group 1 and 20% of the patients in the second group had to undergo revision surgery. The cost per revision is $5000 and all other costs are assumed to be equal.

Cost Analysis

This type of economic health study only deals with costs; differences in or consequences of the "medical" outcome of the different treatment strategies are not considered. This means that a cost analysis of the example case would conclude that additional net costs of $500 are associated with the coated nail. The additional initial costs of $1000 are reduced by savings of $500 due to a reduction of 10% for revision surgery for nonunions with costs of $5000 per revision case.

> **Examples from the Literature: A Health Economic Analysis of the Use of rhBMP-2 in Gustilo–Anderson Grade III Open Tibial Fractures for the UK, Germany, and France**
>
> The study, by Alt et al., is a cost analysis of the use of rhBMP-2 in three European countries in open tibial fractures from a societal perspective.[2] In this cost study the authors concluded that from a societal perspective, the overall treatment costs, including the costs of lost productivity, were lower in the study group in which patients were additionally treated with rhBMP-2 than in the group treated with standard soft-tissue management and intramedullary nailing alone. Therefore, the additional rhBMP-2 treatment was concluded to be a net saving strategy for UK, Germany, and France from a societal perspective.

Cost–Effectiveness Analysis

In this form of health economic evaluation the differences in "medical effects" between different treatment strategies in terms of "natural effects" are considered and are related to the cost differences. In our example case an important outcome is "fractures healed after 1 year," for which a difference of 10% exists. The additional cost of $500 per case can be related to the improved fracture healing after 1 year, which is 10%. This means that in ten cases, treatment with the growth-factor-coated nail will lead to the healing of one more fracture than will the control treatment, at an additional total cost of $5000 for the ten cases. This leads to a cost–effectiveness ratio of $5000 per additional fracture healed in one year.

> **Jargon Simplified: Cost–Effectiveness Ratio**
>
> The cost–effectiveness ratio is the ratio of additional costs incurred to achieve a defined better medical outcome for the patient, for example "additional fracture healed."

> **Examples from the Literature: An Economic Evaluation of Early versus Delayed Operative Treatment in Patients with Closed Tibial Shaft Fractures**
>
> Sprague and Bhandari analyzed the cost–effectiveness and cost–utility associated with the adoption of a program of early operative treatment of all closed tibial shaft fractures.[3] The effectiveness parameter was de-

fined as faster fracture healing (measured in weeks). The authors found that fracture healing in the "early surgery" group was faster by 16 weeks, with additional costs of CD$1073 if productivity losses were not included. Thus, the incremental cost–effectiveness ratio in this study was CD$67 per week of faster fracture healing (CD$1073 divided by 16) for the early surgery treatment option—productivity losses not included.

Cost–Utility Analysis

In a cost–utility analysis the medical differences between the two compared treatments are adjusted by utility weights and not expressed as "natural effects" as in cost–effectiveness analysis. Cost–utility studies are nowadays the most important and most frequently conducted form of health economic analysis, as the cost–utility ratio allows comparison not just of two different treatment strategies within one medical discipline, such as orthopaedic trauma surgery, but also between different medical fields, because it quantifies the health care status of a patient by a defined universal and comparable unit.

This unit in cost–utility studies is the "quality-adjusted life year" (QALY), which quantifies a given health state between 0 (death) and 1 (perfect health). It is assumed that all diseases or injuries reduce the health state to a "utility" between $u = 0$ and $u = 1$. For example, the utility value of a patient's health care status after sustaining a closed tibial fracture and before surgery was estimated to be $u = 0.5$.[3] The utility difference between two groups can then be related to differences in QALYs between the two groups, allowing the calculation of a cost/QALY ratio (incremental cost per QALY) as a result of a cost–utility analysis. For example, let us assume that the average utility of one patient treated with a growth-factor-coated (healing rate after 1 year: 90%) nail is $u_1 = 0.8$ versus $u_2 = 0.75$ for a patient treated with an uncoated nail (healing rate after 1 year: 80%) after 1 year, due to the higher fracture healing rates in the groups treated with growth-factor-coated nails. A difference of 0.05 QALY can therefore be assumed in favor of the growth-factor-coated nail group that can be related to the average additional costs per case, resulting in a cost–utility ratio of $500/0.05 QALY = $10 000/QALY. This can be interpreted as follows: at an additional cost of $10 000, 1 year of life in perfect health can be achieved by using a growth-factor-coated nail compared to a standard nail.

> **Jargon Simplified: Utilities**
>
> Utilities help to quantitatively assess the "value" of a certain health state, with utilities between 0 (death) and 1 (perfect health). Utilities can then be transformed into quality-adjusted life years (QALYs).

Decisions from health care institutions on the reimbursement of new therapies are mainly based on incremental cost per QALY ratios from cost–utility studies. For this reason, the researcher in orthopaedic trauma surgery should focus on this type of study unless important reasons advocate another type of study.

Examples from the Literature: Economic Evaluation of Early versus Delayed Operative Treatment in Patients with Closed Tibial Shaft Fractures

The above-mentioned article by Sprague et al. is a good example of a study looking both at cost–effectiveness and cost–utility, and therefore helps to elucidate the differences between the two types of study.[3] As shown before, the cost–effectiveness parameter in this study was "faster fracture healing, in weeks," and the authors found a cost–effectiveness ratio of CD$67 per week of faster fracture healing. For cost–utility analysis, the authors calculated utilities in order to transform the "effectiveness parameter," which showed an acceleration of fracture healing of 16 weeks compared to the delayed group, into a universal and comparable unit of quality of life measurement, the QALY. Utility scores were therefore estimated from expert opinions for the following health states: (1) waiting for an operation ($u = 0.5$), (2) staying in the hospital following surgery ($u = 0.6$); (3) leaving the hospital on crutches with limited activities ($u = 0.7$), (4) experiencing a postoperative complication ($u = 0.5$), (5) delayed union ($u = 0.6$), (6) nonunion that requires reoperation ($u = 0.5$), and (7) returning to normal activities ($u = 0.9$); this allowed calculation of QALYs for each treatment group. From these utility values, an average utility score was estimated for the early surgical group and the delayed surgical group. On the basis of these utilities the authors calculated a mean QALY for the early surgical group of 0.79 and a mean QALY for the delayed group of 0.70. This resulted in a difference of 0.09 QALY in favor of the early surgery group. With additional costs of CD$1073 for the early treatment (see above) there is an incremental cost–utility ratio of $11 922/QALY (excluding productivity losses).

Cost–Benefit Analysis

The cost–effectiveness and cost–utility studies described above measure the "medical difference" between the different treatment strategies either in "physical units" or in utilities (QALYs) but not in monetary terms. Cost–benefit analyses focus on assessment of the medical consequences in monetary terms in order to measure them against the cost difference. However, it is widely accepted that measuring medical consequences in monetary terms is very difficult, which significantly limits the conduct of cost–benefit studies.

There are three possibilities for giving a monetary valuation to medical outcomes: (1) the human capital approach, (2) revealed preferences, and (3) the willingness-to-pay approach. For the human capital approach, for example, average lifetime earnings can be used. In our example, with assumed average annual earnings of $50 000 for a

healed patient versus $0 for an unhealed patient, the "medical difference" due to 10% higher fracture healing in favor of the coated nail group leads to a "monetary difference" of $5000 per case. This results in net savings of $5000 – $500 = $4500 per case for the coated nail group compared with the uncoated-nail group.

Revealed preferences and willingness-to-pay approaches use the relationship between particular medical benefits/risks and the circumstances under which the risk becomes "acceptable" for the patient. This is often done by the so-called bidding game, adapted from O'Brian et al., to estimate patients' willingness to pay in order to have access to the new therapy.[4]

Key Concepts: Cost–Utility or Cost–Benefit Studies are the Most Useful in Orthopaedic Trauma Surgery

Researchers in orthopaedic trauma surgery should focus on cost–utility or cost–benefit studies as health care institutions mainly base their decisions on the ratios produced by these two types of studies.

Examples from the Literature: Treatment of Displaced Femoral Neck Fractures in the Elderly—A Cost–Benefit Analysis

The study by Alolabi et al. looks at willingness to pay in relation to two treatment options for displaced femoral neck fractures (internal fixation versus hemiarthroplasty).[5] The authors calculated that internal fixation of the femoral neck fracture with conservation of the femoral head is a more expensive treatment option than hemiarthroplasty in patients over 60 years in Canada. The medical benefit of internal fixation with conservation of the femoral head is transformed into financial benefit in this study by the bidding game in the willingness-to-pay approach. The conclusion of the study was that the study participants were willing to pay an average of $3.33 per month to have internal fixation available, which shows "good value for money" for this treatment strategy.

Conducting Health Economics Studies

Questions to Ask before Starting the Study

Besides the type of study, as discussed above, there are further important points that should be considered before the start of a health economic evaluation. Several crucial criteria have been identified by Udvarhelyi et al. to assess the quality of health economic studies, and these can be combined with methodological aspects which are essential for the definition of the design of a health economic trial before it is started.[6]

The clinical researcher should address the following aspects, which will help guide the planned health economic study in the right direction:

1. State the medical benefits of the new technology
2. Define the type of the health economic study
3. Define the methodological approach
4. Define the perspective of the study and the types of costs
5. Discount costs and benefits (if costs and benefits occur during different periods)
6. Conduct sensitivity analysis
7. State the measurement of efficiency and conclusion of the study
8. Discuss the strengths and weaknesses of the study

In general, collaboration with a health economist is recommended in order to prevent systematic mistakes and to allow the study to benefit from specialist health economic experience.

1. Medical Benefits of the New Technology

A prerequisite for conducting health economic studies is that the new treatment alternative should show a medical benefit for the patient. This benefit should be clearly stated at the outset, as this is what "justifies" carrying out a health economic study to assess whether the incremental costs for the new therapy can be considered as "good health economic value for money" or not.

In our above example, the statement: "The growth-factor-coated nail leads to a higher rate of fracture healing (90%) compared to the uncoated standard nail (80%) after 1 year" would be an adequate statement in this context.

2. Type of Health Economic Study

The researcher should define whether the health economic study is conducted as a cost, cost–effectiveness, cost–utility, or cost–benefit study.

3. Methodological Approach

In this context the crucial question is whether the health economic evaluation is supposed to be based on medical and financial data collection alongside a particular clinical trial, or whether the study is being conducted using an analytic modeling approach. A third type of methodological approach is retrospective database analysis.

Given the focus of the present book on clinical research, the so-called piggyback evaluation, in which health economic data are collected within a clinical trial, is the most interesting here. The main advantages of piggyback evaluations are the benefits of blinded study design, which reduce bias, in addition to the health economic conclusions. From a practical point of view, the setup of a prospective clinical trial provides the best conditions for data collection as the personnel and processes for data collection are already in place. Another important advantage is that the financial data are generated at the same time as the medical data, so issues of retrospective database analysis can be excluded.

Limitations of piggyback evaluations of which the researcher should be aware are that study patients are often highly selected, and that controlled experimental settings in clinical trials often do not represent actual clinical practice. These limit the conclusions of the health economic data; however, they do still give a reliable case scenario in most cases, and this design is definitely better than retrospective database analysis of clinical trials.[7] For practical aspects of data collection in the course of clinical trials, see below.

Health economic modeling tries to overcome the limitation of piggyback evaluation by including clinical, cost, and health-related quality of life data and information not only from the current clinical trial but also from other studies or relevant literature. It is closely related to statistical decision theory and Bayesian statistics. Key elements of decision analytic models are probabilities and expected values, on which the so-called decision tree or Markov models are based that help to calculate probabilities for certain health states. A Markov model is a tool used when an individual can achieve multiple different health states with different utilities and can move between states according to specific transition probabilities. At the defined end time of the study, with a specific number of time cycles in which transition between the different stages for the patient can occur, the cumulative costs and utilities are calculated and cost–effectiveness and cost–utility ratios can be derived.

Examples from the Literature: Is Prophylactic Fixation a Cost-Effective Method for Preventing a Future Contralateral Fragility Hip Fracture?
The study by Faucett et al. uses a Markov transition-state model to assess costs and utilities for three different, alternative clinical management strategies over the remaining lifetime in women who had sustained either a femoral neck or an intertrochanteric femoral fracture.[8] The alternative management strategies were: (1) surgical treatment of the fractured hip alone, (2) surgical treatment of the fractured plus prophylactic hip fixation of the contralateral side performed at the time of hip fracture surgery, and (3) surgical treatment of the fractured hip with hip pad protection of the contralateral side. The authors had used three health states: "well," "complication," and "dead." In each of the cycles until the study end, the patient could move from the state "well" into the states "well," "complication," or "dead," and from the state "complication" into the states "complication" or "dead." For each transition move there was a specific probability with resulting probabilities for the next health state of that individual. For each cycle the respective costs and utilities were summed. The remaining lifetime of the individual after the first hip fracture was the time horizon of the study. Therefore, all individuals started in the state "well" after surgical treatment of the hip fracture and ended in the state "dead" at the end of the last cycle (**Fig. 13.2**).

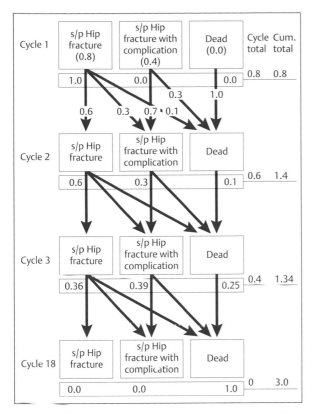

Fig. 13.2 Markov analysis schematic representing a simplified version of a theoretical model with three states. This example shows the model for the health economic analysis of different treatment methods in the prevention of contralateral fragility hip fractures. For each cycle the possible health states and the transition probabilities (arrows) are given. The shaded box gives the fraction of the cohort at each state. Reproduced with permission from Faucett et al.[8]

4. Perspective of the Study and Types of Costs

The perspective from which the study is conducted depends on the following questions: (1) who is paying for the costs? and (2) who is paying for the benefits? Typical perspectives in health economics studies are those of society, insurers, or hospitals. Only costs that have to be covered by the specific "perspective" stakeholder should then be considered in the study. Societal costs most frequently include those for productivity loss in addition to the medical costs of the therapy itself; on the other hand, savings are achieved from averting the disease. An insurance perspective means that only costs that are covered by insurance, such as costs of inpatient and outpatient treatment, medication, etc., are taken into account, and not costs for productivity loss.

The types of costs being studied mainly depend on the perspective that is used. It should be specified which costs are being considered in the study, and they should be documented. In our example case, with the comparison of the two nails, a study can be conducted from the health insurance perspective. In this case the following costs are

considered: the medical costs of the first intervention, the cost of the implant, and medical costs of revision surgery. From this perspective, the cost due to productivity loss is ignored.

In general, health care decision makers are only interested in "direct" medical costs, that is, those that involve direct payments from a stakeholder—payments for inpatient treatment, outpatient treatment, medication, and so on. Less important for these decision makers are indirect costs such as productivity loss, which are more or less theoretical. However, there are some authors, for example in spine surgery, who assert that health economic studies should be done from a societal perspective and include indirect costs such as productivity loss.[9]

The researcher should state his or her rationale for the type of perspective considered for the study and indicate what types of costs will be included. As previously mentioned, the health insurance perspective and hospital perspective are commonly used as both insurance bodies and hospitals are the decision makers in their field and are interested only in costs that affect them directly. However, for each study different arguments have to be balanced, and in certain cases—for example on the impact on society of a road accident prevention program in developing countries—a societal perspective is the best study perspective.

5. Discounting of Costs and Benefits

Frequently, there is a certain time period covering the first occurrence of costs and the last time point with costs and/or benefits that are relevant for the economic calculation. This is mainly related to the time horizon of the study, which should be clearly specified. In addition, the base year (e.g., 2010), should be defined, to which all other financial costs that occur in the next year can be related. The longer the study period, the more important this is in order to adjust future costs and benefits back to their present value. Discounting rates of 3%–5% are recommended if no other rates are announced in the jurisdiction concerned.[10] If the study period is 1 year or shorter, discounting is not necessary.

6. Sensitivity Analysis

Because most health economic studies have to use assumptions for unknown variables, sensitivity analysis should be performed to test the robustness of the results depending on the variability of the underlying assumptions.[6] The uncertain parameters should be identified, possible ranges for the variables should be specified, and an appropriate form of sensitivity testing should be applied.[11] The ranges of uncertain parameters usually lie between 25% and 50%, depending on the uncertainty of the underlying variable. The more unknown and the more uncertain the variable is, the higher the range and the resulting interval for the parameter should be. Forms of sensitivity analysis include one-way analysis, multiway analysis, scenario analysis, and probabilistic analysis. In one-way and multiway analysis, estimates for each critical parameter are made for, respectively, one and several parameters at a time. Scenario analysis is a way of conducting a sensitivity analysis which defines multiple potential outcomes of the underlying variables: for example, base case scenario (best guess), most pessimistic scenario (worst case), and most optimistic scenario (best case). In certain types of health economic studies, such as decision-analytic modeling, that are mainly based on probability concepts of different prognoses that can occur, sensitivity analysis can be performed by probability distributions to the specified ranges of the variables. Randomly drawn samples from these distributions then provide an empirical distribution of the desired efficiency parameter.

7. Measurement of Efficiency and Conclusions of the Study

The results for the respective target parameters, such as cost–effectiveness ratio, cost–utility ratio, and cost–benefit ratio, should be given, including their potential intervals resulting from sensitivity analysis. They should be expressed in incremental costs per parameter such as effectiveness criteria, incremental costs, etc., depending on the type of study performed, unless one treatment alternative is dominant. A clear conclusion should then be derived from the study results.

8. Discussion of Strengths and Weaknesses of the Study

Like other scientific publications, health economic evaluations should undergo a critical appraisal by the authors. Both strengths and weaknesses should be elucidated for the reader. As mentioned before, assumptions about cost data, probabilities, etc., often have to be made in health economic studies; these need clarification and are open for discussion. The more clearly and honestly the weaknesses of the analysis are discussed by the authors themselves, the more transparent and reliable the results will appear. Strengths of the study should also be emphasized to underscore the scientific value of the work.

> **Key Concepts: Items to Address Before Starting a Study**
> 1. State the medical benefits of the new technology
> 2. Define the type of the health economic study
> 3. Define the methodological approach
> 4. Define the perspective of the study and the types of costs
> 5. Discount costs and benefits
> 6. Conduct sensitivity analysis
> 7. State measurement of efficiency and conclusions of the study
> 8. Discuss the strengths and weaknesses of the study

Practical Aspects of Data Collection in Clinical Trials

Referencing of Data and Conservative Approach

Collaboration with a health economist is recommended to optimize planning and physical data collection. Each cost item that is used in the study should be referenced, if possible. In addition, the base case year for each cost item and the currency in which the study is conducted must be stated. For example, if the study includes data on the rate and type of secondary surgical interventions, the relevant financial data for these secondary procedures should be taken from official sources such as diagnosis-related groups (DRGs), Medicare/Medicaid sources, etc., so the calculation can be made transparent to the reader. However, there may be cases in which the researcher is conducting the study from a specific perspective, for example from a specific hospital perspective, for which the respective hospital data are more relevant than official data. In such a case this rationale should be given in the study and the hospital-specific data should be used. If there are differing cost data for which no hard or convincing rationale exists, the more conservative data should be used in order to make the results as reliable and as relevant as possible for decision makers.

> **Key Concepts: Ensuring Reliability of Cost Data**
> Give the rationale and—if possible—references for the underlying cost data. Use reliable, conservative, and practical approaches to data collection.

Calculation of Utilities and Quality-Adjusted Life Years

In cost–utility studies the calculation of utility values and QALYs is of essential importance. Utility values are theoretically determined by the so-called time trade-off (TTO) or standard gamble (SG) technique, which attach a numerical value to a defined health state.

For practical applications in the course of clinical trials, utility value calculation is mainly done by translation of health status data from standard outcome measurement instruments such as the EuroQoL (EQ5D), the Short Form (36) Health Survey (SF36), the Canadian Health Utility Index (UI) III or the Finnish 15D. These questionnaires can be included in the clinical trial and are completed by the patient during the various study visits. The answers to the questions can be used for a description of health care status that can then be translated into utility values, using for example, for SF-36 data, the Brazier index.[12]

Conclusion

Health economics assesses the "value" of medical treatment from an economic perspective. There are four major types of study in health economics: cost studies, cost–effectiveness studies, cost–utility studies, and cost–benefit studies. Cost studies only focus on financial costs, whereas cost–effectiveness, cost–utility, and cost–benefit studies balance the financial costs against treatment outcome. For practical aspects of the conduct of health care studies in the course of prospective clinical trials, the following key concepts should be followed: (1) state the medical benefits of the new technology, (2) define the type of the health economic study, (3) define the methodological approach, (4) define the perspective of the study and the types of costs, (5) discount the costs and benefits, (6) conduct sensitivity analysis, (7) state the measurement of efficiency and conclusions of the study, and (8) discuss strengths and weaknesses of the study. Collaboration with a health economist is recommended when health economic studies are to be included within clinical trials.

Suggested Reading

Brauer CA, Neumann PJ, Rosen AB. Trends in cost effectiveness analyses in orthopaedic surgery. Clin Orthop Relat Res 2007;457:42–48

Drummond MF, Sculpher MJ, Torrance GW, O'Brien BJ, Stoddart GL. Methods for the Economic Evaluation of Health Care Programmes. 3rd ed. Oxford: Oxford University Press; 2005

Neumann PJ. Using Cost-Effectiveness Analysis to Improve Health Care: Opportunities and Barriers. New York: Oxford University Press; 2005

Sprague S, Quigley L, Adili A, Bhandari M. Understanding cost effectiveness: money matters? J Long Term Eff Med Implants 2007;17:145–152

References

1. Centers for Medicare and Medicaid Services, Office of the Actuary, National Health Statistics Group, National Health Care Expenditures Data, January 2010
2. Alt V, Donell ST, Chhabra A, Bentley A, Eicher A, Schnettler R. A health economic analysis of the use of rhBMP-2 in Gustilo-Anderson grade III open tibial fractures for the UK, Germany, and France. Injury 2009;40:1269–1275
3. Sprague S, Bhandari M. An economic evaluation of early versus delayed operative treatment in patients with closed tibial shaft fractures. Arch Orthop Trauma Surg 2002;122:315–323
4. O'Brien BJ, Goeree R, Gafni A, et al. Assessing the value of a new pharmaceutical. A feasibility study of contingent valuation in managed care. Med Care 1998;36:370–384
5. Alolabi B, Bajammal S, Shirali J, Karanicolas PJ, Gafni A, Bhandari M. Treatment of displaced femoral neck fractures in the elderly: a cost-benefit analysis. J Orthop Trauma 2009;23:442–446
6. Udvarhelyi IS, Colditz GA, Rai A, Epstein AM. Cost-effectiveness and cost-benefit analyses in the medical literature. Are the methods being used correctly? Ann Intern Med 1992;116:238–244
7. O'Sullivan AK, Thompson D, Drummond MF. Collection of health-economic data alongside clinical trials: is there a future for piggyback evaluations? Value Health 2005;8:67–79
8. Faucett SC, Genuario JW, Tosteson AN, Koval KJ. Is prophylactic fixation a cost-effective method to prevent a future contralateral fragility hip fracture? J Orthop Trauma 2010;24:65–74
9. Maetzel A, Li L. The economic burden of low back pain: a review of studies published between 1996 and 2001. Best Pract Res Clin Rheumatol 2002;16:23–30
10. Drummond MF, Sculpher MJ, Torrance GW, O'Brien BJ, Stoddart GL. Methods for the Economic Evaluation of Health Care Programmes. 3rd ed. Oxford: Oxford University Press; 2005
11. Briggs A, Sculpher M. Sensitivity analysis in economic evaluation: a review of published studies. Health Econ 1995;4:355–371
12. Brazier J, Usherwood T, Harper R, Thomas K. Deriving a preference-based single index from the UK SF-36 Health Survey. J Clin Epidemiol 1998;51:1115–1128

14

Literature Searches

Laura Quigley

Summary

Systematic literature reviews and meta-analyses require a well-conducted literature search to provide a rigorous review of specific clinical questions. Authors of literature reviews must determine the focus of the review and then conduct the literature search. The literature search in particular requires the following key steps: formulate a research question, identify the most relevant databases, identify the primary search concepts, plan the search strategy, check for the most appropriate vocabulary terms in the selected databases, run the search and create a base set of studies, impose search restrictions, review search strategy as required, and download the search results. The authors then need to identify and select relevant studies, critically appraise relevant studies, collect and synthesize the relevant information, and discuss the findings.

Introduction

A review of the literature can be conducted in many different ways: the most usual are the traditional review, the systematic review, and the meta-analysis.[1] In a traditional (or narrative) review, a senior expert in the field summarizes evidence and recommendations. Usually, these reviews address very broad questions.[1] A traditional review provides an overview of a disease or condition or one or more aspects of its etiology, diagnosis, prognosis, and management. Alternatively, it may summarize an area of scientific inquiry.[2] Traditional reviews typically pose a background-type question to provide a general overview of a topic.[2] An example of a background-type question is: "*What are the clinical presentations, treatment options, and prognosis following femoral shaft fractures in adults?*"[2] Experts are in a good position to provide the review because they know both the pertinent literature and how it should affect actual practice.[1] Authors of traditional reviews typically make little or no attempt to be systematic in formulating the questions that they are addressing, in searching for relevant evidence, or in summarizing the evidence that they consider.[2] The lack of structure of traditional reviews may hide important threats to validity.[1] The literature search may not be clearly outlined (raising the danger that articles may be selectively quoted to support a point of view), and personal experience and conventional wisdom are often included and may be difficult to distinguish from scientific evidence.[1]

> **Jargon Simplified: Validity**
> The degree to which the data measure what they were intended to measure (i.e., the results of a measurement correspond to the true state of the phenomenon being measured). Another word for "validity" is "accuracy."[1]

Systematic reviews are rigorous reviews of specific clinical questions.[1] Systematic reviews typically pose a foreground-type question. Foreground questions are more specific and provide insight into a particular aspect of management.[2] Systematic reviews are "systematic" because they summarize the original research bearing on the question following a scientifically based plan that has been decided in advance and made explicit at every step. Readers are able to see the strength of the evidence and check the validity themselves.[1] Systematic literature reviews are useful for synthesizing the results of multiple primary investigations with the use of strategies to limit bias and random error.[3]

A quantitative systematic review, or meta-analysis, is a review in which statistical methods are used to combine the results of two or more studies. A well-conducted meta-analysis is invaluable for surgeons since it is unusual for single studies to provide definitive answers to clinical questions. Moreover, a well-conducted quantitative review may resolve discrepancies between studies with conflicting results. Guiding principles in the conduct of meta-analyses include use of a specific health care question, use of a comprehensive search strategy, assessment of the reproducibility of study selection, assessment of study validity, evaluation of heterogeneity (differences in effect across studies), inclusion of all relevant and clinically useful measures of treatment effect, and testing of the robustness of the results relative to features of the primary studies (sensitivity analysis).[3]

> **Jargon Simplified: Traditional Review**
> In a traditional review, a senior expert in the field summarizes evidence and recommendations for a broad research question.

> **Jargon Simplified: Systematic Review**
> A systematic review is a rigorous review of specific clinical questions which summarizes the original research following a scientifically based plan that has been decided in advance and made explicit at every step.

> **Jargon Simplified: Meta-analysis**
> A meta-analysis, or quantitative systematic review, is one in which statistical methods are used to combine the results of two or more studies.

All systematic reviews are retrospective and observational. Therefore, they are subject to systematic and random error. The quality of a systematic review, and accordingly its validity, is dependent upon the scientific methods that have been used to minimize error and bias.[3] Explicitly reporting methods for each step of the review enables readers to assess the validity of results.[2] Authors of systematic reviews must make many decisions, including: determining the focus of the review; identifying, selecting, and critically appraising the relevant studies (i.e., the primary studies); collecting and synthesizing (either quantitatively or non-quantitatively) the relevant information; and drawing conclusions.[2]

When to Conduct a Literature Search

The main reason for conducting a literature search is to answer a clinical question. In addition, literature searches are used to form systematic reviews or meta-analyses in order to reconcile previously conducted studies that have inconsistent results. Such a situation may arise when the sample sizes of individual studies are too small to find stable results, or if the results from single studies vary considerably.[4] Other reasons for conducting a meta-analysis or a review are: (1) to assess qualitatively whether a factor has to be considered as a risk factor, (2) to provide more precise effect estimates and increased statistical power, (3) to analyze dose–response relations, (4) to investigate heterogeneity between different studies, (5) to generalize results of single studies, 6) to investigate rare exposures and interactions, and (7) to investigate risks associated with rare diseases.[4]

Clinical decisions are based on the weight of evidence bearing on a question. When a clinician examines an individual study, it is important to question the context of that one piece of evidence by asking whether other good studies exist which examine the same question, and what the studies have shown if they do exist.[1] Systematic reviews are especially useful in addressing a single, focused question.[1] For a systematic review to be useful, strong studies of the question should be available but not so much in agreement with one another that the question is already answered. Also, there should not be so few studies of the question that one could just as well critique the individual studies directly and dispense with the review.[1] The study results should disagree or at least leave the question open; if all the studies agree with one another, there is nothing to reconcile in a review.[1]

How to Conduct a Literature Search

There are nine main steps to conducting a literature search (**Table 14.1**). The *first step* is to formulate a search question.[5,6] A well-built, focused clinical question is based on the clinical problem at hand and is phrased to facilitate searching the literature for a precise answer. Focused clinical questions can be formulated to address problems concerning therapy (or exposure), diagnosis, etiology, and prognosis. Regardless of the type of problem addressed, the components of a well-articulated clinical question include:
- A statement describing the patient *population* or disease process being addressed;
- The *intervention*, or exposure being considered;
- The *comparison* intervention or exposure, when relevant;
- The clinical *outcomes* of interest.[5]

Together these components form the P (patient/problem) I (intervention) C (comparison) O (outcomes) model.[6] Once each applicable component of the PICO model has been identified from the clinical scenario, the research question can be formed.[6] For example, a surgeon who uses both the posterior and direct lateral approach for total hip arthroplasty wonders which approach has shown the best results in terms of dislocations, gait, and sciatic nerve palsy.[7] The review by Jolles and Bogoch provides a good example of a comprehensive literature search for this topic.[7] **Table 14.2** identifies each component of the PICO model present in the clinical scenario studied by Jolles and Bogoch.[7]

Table 14.1 Steps in conducting a literature search

Step 1: Formulate a research question
Step 2: Identify the most relevant databases to search
Step 3: Identify the primary search concepts using your PICO chart
Step 4: Plan your search strategy
Step 5: Check for the most appropriate vocabulary terms in your database
Step 6: Run your search and create your base set
Step 7: Impose restrictions by using the Limit function
Step 8: Revise search strategy as required
Step 9: Print or download or email your search results

PICO, P (patient/problem) I (intervention) C (comparison) O (outcomes).

Table 14.2 Formulating a search question on the basis of the PICO model

Component of PICO model	Clinical scenario
Patient/problem	Adult patients (≥18 years) undergoing total hip arthroplasty for primary osteoarthritis
Intervention	Posterior approach
Comparison	Direct lateral approach
Outcome	Prosthesis dislocation, postoperative Trendelenburg gait, and sciatic nerve palsy

Examples from the Literature: Posterior versus Lateral Surgical Approach for Total Hip Arthroplasty in Adults with Osteoarthritis[7]

In this review by Jolles and Bogoch, the final research question, based on the PICO model in **Table 14.2**, asks: What are "the risks of prosthesis dislocation, postoperative Trendelenburg gait, and sciatic nerve palsy after a posterior approach, compared to a direct lateral approach, for patients aged 18 and older undergoing total hip arthroplasty for primary osteoarthritis?"[7]

The *second step* is to identify the most relevant information sources or database(s) to search.[8,9] MEDLINE, the US National Library of Medicine's comprehensive electronic database of published articles, is a good place to start.[1] The database EMBASE provides strong drug literature coverage.[6] Other approaches to finding studies include reading recent reviews and textbooks, seeking the advice of experts in the content area, considering articles cited in the articles already found through other approaches, consulting databases of articles such as the Cochrane Central Register of Controlled Clinical Trials, and reviewing registries of clinical trials.[1] Unpublished studies and those articles that appear only in conference proceedings or other "gray" literature should be located.[8] Additionally, funding agencies, pharmaceutical companies, personal files, and registries can be searched for relevant literature.[9] Potential information resources that can be used to identify relevant literature include: The Cochrane Library, Bandolier, Best Evidence, MEDLINE, EMBASE, Ovid, HIRU (Health Information Research Unit), the Centre for Evidence-Based Medicine at Oxford, and ACP Journal Club.[2] Once the appropriate databases have been identified, the primary search concepts must be identified by using your PICO chart and adding any related concepts (*Step 3*).

Next, in *Step 4* you plan your search strategy. The search terms can be combined using Boolean operators—"and," "or," and "not"—to create quite complex routines.[8]

Step 5 consists of checking for the most appropriate vocabulary terms in your selected database.[6] Depending on the databases you are searching, these may include Medical Subject Headings (MeSH) terms for MEDLINE, EMBASE terms for EMBASE, the CINAHL thesaurus for CINAHL, the Psychological Abstracts thesaurus for PsycINFO, and textword (keyword) terms for Cochrane.[6] In the databases it is important to read the scope notes for date of entry and previous indexing. It is also important to check the tree structures for related terms and use the Explode function to capture those terms.[6] If the vocabulary terms are inadequate, it may be necessary to simply use text words.

Examples from the Literature: Search Strategy
Jolles and Bogoch clearly outline their search strategy, providing the exact list of search terms and how Boolean operators were used to combine search terms.[7] A trained medical librarian was consulted to develop the optimal search strategy. The authors also clearly state the databases used and the timeframe for each database:
- MEDLINE (1982–2005)
- EMBASE (1982–2005)
- CINAHL (1982–2005)
- Cochrane Musculoskeletal Group Trials Register
- Cochrane Controlled Trials Register (CENTRAL/CCTR)
- Health Technology Assessment database (HTA)
- Database of Abstracts of Reviews of Effectiveness (DARE) (2005)

Step 6 is to run the search and create a base set of studies.[6] At this point you can decide if you need any quality-filtering terms or restrictions to age groups, language, type of study, or publication years.[9] You can then use the Limit function (*Step 7*) to eliminate nonhuman studies and/or non-English articles, to select specific age groups, to limit unpublished data, and determine the time frame from which you want articles.[6,9]

Next, the search strategy should be revised as required (*Step 8*). The focus of the search may need to be broadened or narrowed depending on the results from the base set. Note that very general terms are typically used to formulate the initial clinical question. After the initial question has been stated, the process should be refined by using more specific or alternative terms.[5]

The last step (*Step 9*) is to print, download, or email the search results. References can be downloaded to bibliographic software management packages (e.g., RefWorks or Reference Manager).[6] These reference management tools allow the researcher or clinician to keep track of all references easily.

Study Selection

Following the literature search of many databases and other sources, it is likely that a large number of papers will have been identified. Inclusion and exclusion criteria can now be applied to titles and abstracts.[9] Obtain the full articles for eligible titles and abstracts, and then apply the inclusion and exclusion criteria once again, but this time to the full article, to select the final eligible articles.[9] If more than one reviewer assessed articles for study inclusion, agreement between reviewers should be assessed.[9]

Assessing Methodological Quality of Studies

Having selected the eligible studies, and after deciding which type of study design to include, the reviewers need to assess the methodological quality of the articles.[2,8] It is important to assess whether the results are likely to be misleading due to the study design. The competent reviewer needs a detailed knowledge of study design and the situations in which bias can arise. In brief, studies of effectiveness can be randomized controlled trials (RCTs) or observational studies.[8] The random allocation of patients to intervention and control groups in a RCT should ensure that the two groups are comparable in every way except for the presence of the intervention. In contrast, in observational studies it is possible that any observed difference in outcome between those receiving the intervention and those not may be due to unrecognized differences in the characteristics of the two groups rather than to the effectiveness of the intervention.[8] This may lead to either underestimation or overestimation of the size of any treatment effect.[8] Susceptibility bias has led some to question whether only RCTs should be used as evidence, but others have identified situations in which observational studies may be either preferable or the only possibility.[8] These include where rare side effects are being sought and the trials required to detect them would have to be so large as to be unfeasible, or where the effect of an intervention is so obvious that a trial is not required.[8]

To assess the quality of RCTs in particular, McKee and Britton recommend asking the following questions:[8] Was the population eligible for inclusion representative of the population with which one is concerned? Was the process of randomization rigorous? Were subjects analyzed in terms of the groups to which they were allocated (intention to treat) or according to the treatment they actually received? Did the process of randomization produce similar groups, as far as can be established from available information? Was the follow-up of patients complete? Was assessment of outcome blind to whether the patient was in the intervention or control group? Was the study sufficiently large to be able to show whether any observed effect was statistically significant, or, if no effect was seen, how confident can one be that this was not simply due to a lack of power of the study?[8] McKee and Britton also recommend that similar issues should be considered with observational studies.[8] In particular, questions to ask are: Is there evidence of a systematic difference between the two groups? What is the effect of adjusting for known measures of severity? Were there differences in ascertainment of outcome in the two groups?[8]

Data Extraction and Analysis

Having assessed the quality of the studies and decided which to include, the reviewer should abstract the data if appropriate, or if he or she is conducting a meta-analysis.[2] It is important that the information in abstracts is not relied upon as it has been shown that this will often place disproportionate emphasis on positive results in the paper.[8] In a meta-analysis, results can be pooled and reanalyzed.[8] Statistical pooling of results across studies improves the precision of the final estimates by increasing the sample size.[2] It is most commonly done on the basis of the results published in the papers, but it is also possible to combine individual data supplied by the researchers responsible for the studies included in the review.[8]

Prior to pooling the data statistically, investigators often identify potential sources of differences between studies, or heterogeneity. These a priori hypotheses will be examined if heterogeneity among studies is found.[2] When assessing the data to include in a meta-analysis it is important to consider the risk that studies based on small trials may produce results that differ from those obtained from large trials that have the power, alone, to determine with confidence whether an effect exists.[8] For example, combining studies which were conducted in different patient populations may mask how the effect size varies with factors such as disease severity or age.[8] It is also important to consider publication bias, which can occur as some researchers may be more likely to submit papers that show positive rather than negative effects, or because, after submission, papers showing positive results may be more likely to be accepted by editors.[8]

If heterogeneity among pooled studies is found in the overall meta-analysis, investigators should search for potential differences among these studies by conducting a separate sensitivity analysis. The sensitivity analysis can help identify differences in the magnitude of the effect across patients, interventions, outcomes, and methodology in an attempt to explain within-study and between-study differences in results.[2] Conducting a meta-analysis in orthopaedics is challenging because of the paucity of clinical trials on any single topic. However, to limit bias, investigators must adhere strictly to methodology when performing a systematic review or meta-analysis.[2]

> **Examples from the Literature: Jolles and Bogoch Detail How Data Was Extracted and Analyzed:[7]**
> - Each reviewer extracted data independently using predesigned, standardized data abstraction forms.
> - Extracted data were compared between the two reviewers.
> - Discrepancies were resolved by consensus of the two reviewers.
> - Information was obtained from the primary author when inadequate information was provided in the review.

- Relative risks and 95% confidence limits were calculated for dichotomous outcomes. Weighted mean differences and 95% confidence limits were calculated for continuous outcomes.
- Meta-analyses were conducted with a fixed effects model; however, a random effects model was used when there was statistical evidence of heterogeneity.

Conclusion

Once the data applicable to the systematic review or meta-analysis have been extracted and pooled together, the reviewers need to consider how to summarize the results. A systematic review should provide a critical appraisal of the available literature, and not just a summary of available articles. When summarizing a meta-analysis, the effect sizes with confidence intervals from each of the studies included should be plotted.[8] This will enable readers to determine whether there is consistent evidence of a significant effect or not. It will also draw attention to studies producing apparently aberrant results. These studies can then be examined in more detail to determine whether specific factors can account for the differing results.[8]

Key Concepts: Transparency of the Search Strategy
The search strategy for a literature search should be clearly defined. Readers should be able to replicate the search and produce similar results.

The literature search is an integral part of the systematic review and meta-analysis. If the literature search does not identify all of the articles relevant to a particular research question, the results of the review may be biased. Authors of a systematic review or meta-analysis should clearly define and state the search strategy so that readers who will use the results can judge how comprehensive the review is and update it subsequently if needed.[8] Lastly, the researcher or clinician should ask themselves the following questions:[10]

1. Were the questions and methods clearly stated?
2. Were comprehensive search methods used to locate relevant studies?
3. Were explicit methods used to determine which articles to include in the review?
4. Was the validity of the primary studies assessed?
5. Was the assessment of the primary studies reproducible and free from bias?
6. Was variation in the findings of the relevant studies analyzed?
7. Were the findings of the primary studies combined appropriately?
8. Were the reviewers' conclusions supported by the data cited?

The answers to these questions will indicate whether the systematic review or meta-analysis has been well conducted and provides a valid and critical review of the existing literature.

Suggested Reading

Bhandari M, Devereaux PJ, Montori V, Cinà C, Tandan V, Guyatt GH, for the Evidence-Based Surgery Working Group. Users' guide to the surgical literature: how to use a systematic literature review and meta-analysis. Can J Surg 2004:47:60–67

Bhandari M, Guyatt GH, Montori V, Devereaux PJ, Swiontkowski MF. User's guide to the orthopaedic literature: how to use a systematic literature review. J Bone Joint Surg Am 2002; 84A:1672–1682

Bhandari M, Morrow F, Kulkarni AV, Tornetta P III. Meta-analyses in orthopaedic surgery: a systematic review of their methodologies. J Bone Joint Surg Am 2001;83A:15–24

McKee M, Britton A. How to do (or not to do)... Conducting a literature review on the effectiveness of health care interventions. Health Policy Plan 1997;12:262–267

References

1. Fletcher RH, Fletcher SW. Systematic reviews. In: Sun B, Linkins E, eds. Clinical Epidemiology: The Essentials. 4th ed. Baltimore, MD: Lippincott Williams & Wilkins; 2005: 205–220.
2. Bhandari M, Guyatt GH, Montori V, Devereaux PJ, Swiontkowski MF. User's guide to the orthopaedic literature: how to use a systematic literature review. J Bone Joint Surg Am 2002;84A:1672–1682
3. Bhandari M, Morrow F, Kulkarni AV, Tornetta P III. Meta-analyses in orthopaedic surgery: a systematic review of their methodologies. J Bone Joint Surg Am 2001;83A:15–24
4. Blettner M, Sauerbrei W, Schlehofer B, Scheuchenpflug T, Friedenreich C. Traditional reviews, meta-analyses and pooled analyses in epidemiology. Int J Epidemiol 1999; 28;1–9
5. Doig GS, Simpson F. Efficient literature searching: a core skill for the practice of evidence-based medicine. Intensive Care Med 2003;29:2119–2127
6. Clinical Epidemiology Program, Faculty of Medicine, University of Toronto. Power searching. Health Science Information Consortium of Toronto Power Searching. [Coursebook] Toronto, Ontario: University of Toronto, 2009:1–46
7. Jolles BM, Bogoch ER. Posterior versus lateral surgical approach for total hip arthroplasty in adults with osteoarthritis. Cochrane Database Syst Rev 2006, Issue 3. Art. No.: CD003828. DOI: 10.1002/14651858.CD003828.pub3
8. McKee M, Britton A. How to do (or not to do)... Conducting a literature review on the effectiveness of health care interventions. Health Policy Plan 1997;12:262–267
9. Bhandari M, Devereaux PJ, Montori V, Cinà C, Tandan V, Guyatt GH, for the Evidence-Based Surgery Working Group. Users' guide to the surgical literature: how to use a systematic literature review and meta-analysis. Can J Surg 2004:47: 60–67
10. Oxman AD, Guyatt GH. Guidelines for reading literature reviews. Can Med Assoc J 1988;138:697–703

15

Understanding Effect Sizes

Ivan R. Diamond

Summary

The effect size is a statistic that conveys both the magnitude and direction of the treatment effect. It is a value that provides essential information when applying the results of a clinical trial to patient care and is vital when combining the results of multiple studies in a meta-analysis. This chapter will explain why the P value is inadequate when assessing and comparing the magnitudes of treatment effects and why effect size should be used instead. The chapter will review some of the major types of effect sizes and how to interpret them in the context of both an individual study and a meta-analysis. It will also provide examples and tools to help calculate effect sizes from existing studies—information that can be used in caring for your patients and for performing meta-analysis.

> **Jargon Simplified: Treatment Effect**
> Treatment effect is defined as the impact of a treatment relative to a control: that is, how much better or worse a particular treatment may be relative to the control. Treatment effects are best assessed in randomized controlled clinical trials (RCTs), although they may also be estimated from well-designed nonrandomized comparative studies.

Introduction

The ultimate goal of clinical research is to improve patient care. In order to improve patient care, clinicians need to translate the findings from research into practice. This may be done by critically evaluating individual studies or through meta-analysis that combine results across a series of studies. However, when searching for an answer to a clinically relevant question, it may not be immediately clear how best to interpret or combine findings in a meaningful way.

One key tool in making these interpretations is the effect size. Effect size is an easily interpretable value providing information on the direction and magnitude of a treatment effect. It is a powerful tool in translating the results of studies in a clinically meaningful manner and is essential when combining results across various studies in meta-analysis. Outside of surgery, the American Psychological Association has stated that reporting and interpreting of effect sizes is essential to good research.[1] According to

the CONSORT statement, which is a method for reporting trials and is the format required by most major biomedical journals, the effect size is a key feature that is required when reporting the results of a clinical trial.[2] Despite this, not all researchers and clinicians focus on the effect size when reporting and interpreting research findings. Rather, they focus on P values, which are often misinterpreted as conveying information about the magnitude of an effect.

> **Jargon Simplified: Effect Size**
> The effect size is an easily interpretable value specifying the direction and magnitude of a treatment effect.

The P Value Does Not Assess the Magnitude of a Treatment Effect

We shall first consider why the P value is not an appropriate metric for assessing the magnitude of the impact of a treatment in an individual study or for comparing results across studies. To illustrate this, we shall consider two randomized trials that examined whether antifibrinolytic medications, such as tranexamic acid or aprotinin, reduced the transfusion requirements in patients undergoing spinal surgery. The first of these trials, by Neilipovitz et al., compared tranexamic acid to placebo and concluded that "the total amount of blood transfused in the perioperative period was significantly reduced in the tranexamic group ($P = 0.045$)."[3] The second trial, by Khoshhal et al., compared aprotinin to placebo and reported a P value of 0.021 in favor of aprotinin in terms of reducing transfusion requirements.[4] Since these P values are less than the predefined cut-off of 0.05; the authors correctly concluded that the antifibrinolytic medications resulted in reduced transfusion requirements.

While the P value demonstrates that there is a treatment effect for both medications, the P value does not specify how much more efficacious either antifibrinolytic medication is than the control treatment (saline in both studies). Rather, the P value is merely a quantification of the probability that the results obtained in the study could be due to chance alone. By convention, when the probability of the results being obtained by chance is less than 5%, we conclude that the difference observed is "statistically significant," meaning that there is a difference between the experimental treatment and the control that is unlikely to be explained by chance alone. The question answered by the P value is therefore whether there is any treatment effect at all rather than how large that treatment effect might be.

> **Jargon Simplified: *P* Value**
> The *P* (for probability) value is a statistic that quantifies the probability of the results obtained in a research study (or those more extreme) occurring due to chance alone. By convention, *P* values lower than 0.05 are considered to be "statistically significant," meaning that the results are unlikely to be due to chance alone and may therefore be assumed to derive from the intervention under study.

Although the probability obtained from the *P* value is dependent on the size of the effect, it is also heavily dependent on the sample size. Since it is not possible to separate the contribution of sample size and treatment effect, a *P* value cannot be used to specify how large the difference between treatments may be. For example, a very large study may yield a highly significant difference between two treatments; however, it may be that the real difference between the treatments is small. In other words, the difference may be statistically significant but clinically meaningless. Furthermore, since the magnitude of the *P* value does not specify the magnitude of the treatment effect, it is not correct to use *P* values to draw conclusions as to the relative merits of various treatments. For example, while both aprotinin and tranexamic acid were compared to placebo in the same patient population, the fact that aprotinin had a smaller *P* value (0.021) than tranexamic acid (0.045) does not allow one to conclude that aprotinin is superior to tranexamic acid for preventing transfusion. In contrast to the *P* value, the effect size is a value that conveys information about the magnitude of a treatment effect. It is a key metric that should be used in conjunction with the *P* value in moving beyond the question as to whether there is a difference between treatments, to quantifying that difference in a clinically meaningful manner.

> **Key Concepts: The *P* Value Does Not Specify the Magnitude of a Treatment Effect**
> The *P* value does not specify the magnitude of a treatment effect and is therefore an inappropriate metric for drawing conclusions regarding the magnitude of treatment effect or for making comparisons between treatments. Effect sizes, on the other hand, specify the magnitude of a treatment effect and yield important information when used in conjunction with *P* values.

The Challenge of Comparing Results Across Studies

One of the major challenges in comparing results across studies is that studies may use different measures for similar outcomes. For example, when assessing the efficacy of an analgesic medication on pain in the postoperative period, some studies may make use of a rating scale, such as the visual analogue scale (VAS), whereas others may express the results in terms of dose of analgesic required. This poses a challenge when attempting to make comparisons between various analgesic studies. For example, a 1-point decrease in the VAS rating is not the same as a 1-point reduction in dose of medication. Even when the studies use the same scale, direct comparisons may not always be appropriate since there may be differences in the degree of variability or precision of the ratings between studies. The effect size allows one to overcome this issue by calculating a value that provides the magnitude of the treatment effect that is adjusted for the scale and accuracy of the measurements used across different studies.

> **Key Concepts: Effect Size Enables Comparisons Across Studies**
> Making comparisons across studies can be challenging as studies may use different scales with differing precision to measure similar outcomes. The effect size adjusts for the scale and accuracy of the measurements used in individual studies and therefore allows for comparisons to be made between studies.

Types of Effect Sizes

We shall now consider some of the common types of effect size that can be used when interpreting the results of comparative studies. The specific type of effect size that will be used depends on the type of outcomes reported in the study. Studies examining a treatment effect typically report either continuous or noncontinuous (usually binary) data. Specific effect sizes for each type of data are listed in **Table 15.1**.

Table 15.1 Types of effect sizes commonly reported in studies examining treatment effects

Type of data	Type of effect size	Examples
Continuous	Standardized mean difference	• Cohen's *d* • Hedge's *g* • Glass's *Δ*
Noncontinuous	Effect sizes based on risk	• Absolute risk difference/reduction • Number needed to treat • Relative risk • Relative risk reduction
	Effect sizes based on odds	Odds ratio

Key Concepts: Effect Size Type Depends on the Nature of the Data
The specific type of effect size measure will depend on the nature of the data (continuous/noncontinuous) reported for the outcome of interest.

Effect Sizes for Continuous Outcomes

The first class of effect size that will be considered is the class that is used for continuous outcomes such as the VAS or the dose of analgesic used in the postoperative period. Such effect sizes are known collectively as a standardized mean difference (SMD). Continuous outcomes are generally reported by expressing the mean and standard deviation for both experimental and control groups. While examination of the difference between means provides some understanding as to the treatment effect, the standard deviation allows one to ascertain how much spread there is around the mean response for each group. The SMD as an effect size standardizes the mean difference between the groups on the basis of the degree of variability existing within the sample. The SMD specifies, in standardized units, how much the experimental group mean is greater than the control group mean. The basic form of the equation for the SMD is as follows:

$$\text{Standardized Mean Difference} = \frac{\left[\left(\begin{array}{c}\text{mean of}\\\text{experimental group}\end{array}\right) - \left(\begin{array}{c}\text{mean of}\\\text{control group}\end{array}\right)\right]}{\text{standard deviation}}$$

The SMD can also be calculated from the results of various common comparative statistical tests such as the *t* test or the analysis of variance (ANOVA).

Jargon Simplified: Standardized Mean Difference
The standardized mean difference (SMD) is an effect size statistic that can be used for continuous data. Based on the degree of variability of the outcomes, the SMD specifies in standardized units how much greater the experimental group mean is than the control.

Table 15.1 lists three types of SMD effect sizes. These effect sizes differ in what standard deviation is used to calculate the SMD. *Cohen's d* uses the standard deviation of either the experimental or control group—provided that they are similar. *Hedges' g* uses the pooled standard deviation; this can be thought of as the average standard deviation for the experimental and control groups. *Glass's Δ* uses the standard deviation from the control group. While a detailed discussion of the relative merits of each of these approaches is beyond the scope of this chapter, the basic issues center on whether the treatment affects the degree of variability of the outcomes as this influences the calculation of the effect size. When there is minimal difference in the standard deviation between the experimental and control groups, the SMD will be similar whichever approach is used.

Examples from the Literature: Comparing Effect Sizes for Tranexamic Acid and Aprotinin
In the study comparing tranexamic acid to placebo, the total blood loss was 2453 ± 1526 mL in the experimental group and 2703 ± 1292 mL in the control group. The SMD is therefore:

$$SMD = \frac{[2453 - 2703]}{1292} = -0.19$$

In contrast to this, the SMD for the study comparing aprotinin to placebo can be calculated to be –0.79, suggesting a greater treatment effect for the aprotinin. This notion will be revisited in our in the final example from the literature where we will review the results from a meta-analysis.

For the purposes of understanding possible interpretations of the SMD, we shall consider the Cohen's *d*. When Cohen first developed the statistic, he provided guidance for the interpretation of the effect size, namely that an effect size of 0.2–0.3 might be a small effect, 0.5 a moderate effect, and an effect greater than 0.8 a large effect.[5] However, it is important to note that while this distinction has some merit, the magnitude of effect sizes is related to the context from which they come. The optimal interpretation is relative to other treatments in the same area rather than a somewhat arbitrary classification. For example, effect sizes for the efficacy of antihypertensive medications in reducing cardiovascular mortality would be expected to be much smaller than effect sizes evaluating the efficacy of antibiotics for the treatment of blood stream infection. Comparing the magnitude of effect sizes of various antihypertensives would be valid, whereas comparing the magnitude of an effect size of an antihypertensive to that of an antibiotic would not.

Key Concepts: Interpreting Effect Sizes
Interpretation of effect sizes should be relative to other effect sizes within a particular area.

Effect Sizes for Noncontinuous Outcomes

Many surgical trials report noncontinuous outcomes, the most common being binary outcomes. Results are often reported in terms of the frequency of complications in various treatment groups or as the proportion of subjects in both the experimental and control groups who have a particular outcome. A *P* value is usually reported in conjunction with these results, which answers the question as to whether the frequency of the outcome differed between the groups. To address the magnitude of the difference in outcome between the groups, a number of effect size estimates can also be reported (**Table 15.1**).

Jargon Simplified: Binary Outcome

A binary outcome is one for which there are two mutually exclusive possibilities. Examples of binary outcomes include: alive/dead, recurrence of disease/no evidence of disease recurrence, and occurrence/nonoccurrence of a particular complication.

The first of these effect sizes, known as the *absolute risk difference,* measures the absolute difference between the proportions of outcomes in the experimental and the control group. One of the advantages of reporting the absolute difference in rates of an outcome is that one is able to calculate the number needed to treat, that is, the number of patients that need to be treated in order for a particular outcome to be achieved or prevented in one patient. The difference between the groups can also be expressed in relative terms using either a *relative risk* or an *odds ratio.* The relative risk is typically used in randomized trials and the odds ratio in the setting of case–control studies. The relative risk is more intuitive to interpret and closely matches how clinicians typically think of treatment probabilities. A relative risk of 1 implies that there is no difference in risk between the two groups. A relative risk greater than 1 means that the event is more likely to occur in the experimental group than in the control group. Conversely, a relative risk less than 1 means the event is less likely to occur in the experimental group than in the control group. The final relative measure that can be calculated is the *relative risk reduction*, which examines the extent to which a treatment reduces a risk in comparison to the risk run by patients not receiving the treatment of interest.

The effect size measures for binary outcomes are straightforward to calculate and interpret. Therefore, if not reported in the paper, they can easily be done when attempting to evaluate the results of the studies or when performing a meta-analysis.

Reality Check: Effect Sizes for Binary Outcomes

Consider a hypothetical trial of two antibiotics for prevention of surgical site infection. Drug A is the control drug and Drug B is the newer drug under consideration. The results of this study can be seen in the following 2 × 2 table:

	Drug A	Drug B
Number with infection	100	30
Number in group	1000	1000

The first step is to calculate the event rate for the control and experimental groups. In this example the control event rate (CER) is $100/1000 = 0.1$ and the experimental event rate (EER) is $30/1000 = 0.03$.

The absolute risk reduction (ARR) is calculated as follows:

$$ARR = (EER - CER) = (0.03 - 0.1) = -0.07$$

The number needed to treat (NNT) is calculated as follows:

$$NNT = \frac{1}{ARR} = \frac{1}{0.07} = 14$$

On an absolute scale, there was a 7% decrease in the incidence of infection in the experimental group. Based on the NNT, for every 14 patients who receive drug B instead of drug A, one less infection will be experienced. The relative risk (RR) is calculated as follows:

$$RR = \frac{EER}{CER} = \frac{0.03}{0.1} = 0.3$$

This relative risk implies that the risk of infection with drug B is 30% of that with drug A. The relative risk reduction (RRR) is calculated as follows:

$$RRR = \frac{EER - CER}{CER} = \frac{ARR}{CER} = \frac{0.07}{0.1} = -70\%$$

This relative risk reduction implies that the risk of infection with drug B is reduced by 70%, relative to drug A.

Examples from the Literature: To Continue or Discontinue Aspirin in the Perioperative Period

Surgeons are frequently faced with the question of what to do with preventive treatments that the patient may be on but may have adverse consequences in the perioperative period. One example of this is whether to stop aspirin taken for prevention of adverse cardiac events in the perioperative period, owing to the risk of bleeding. Recently, Oscarsson et al. performed a randomized trial to examine this issue, and an abstract describing the results of their study can be found in **Fig. 15.1.**[6] Overall, they demonstrated a 7.2% absolute risk reduction for the prevention of major adverse cardiac events. This means that the incidence of major adverse cardiac events in the experimental arm (aspirin not stopped) was 7.2% lower than in the control arm. The number needed to treat was 14. Hence, for every 14 patients who received aspirin, one major adverse cardiac event was prevented. Finally, the authors reported a relative risk reduction of 80%, meaning that the continuing aspirin reduced the risk of major adverse cardiac events by 80% relative to those in whom aspirin was stopped. While these results suggest that aspirin should be continued, it is important to note that the trial was underpowered to detect a difference in bleeding complications, and consequently further research is likely indicated in order to draw a firm conclusion as to whether aspirin should be continued.

Background. Major adverse cardiac events (MACEs) are a common cause of death after non-cardiac surgery. Despite evidence for the benefit of aspirin for secondary prevention, it is often discontinued in the perioperative period due to the risk of bleeding.

Methods. We conducted a randomized, double-blind, placebo-controlled trial in order to compare the effect of low-dose aspirin with that of placebo on myocardial damage, cardiovascular, and bleeding complications in high-risk patients undergoing non-cardiac surgery. Aspirin (75 mg) or placebo was given 7 days before surgery and continued until the third postoperative day. Patients were followed up for 30 days after surgery.

Results. A total of 220 patients were enrolled, 109 patients received aspirin and 111 received placebo. Four patients (3.7%) in the aspirin group and 10 patients (9.0%) in the placebo group had elevated troponin T levels in the postoperative period ($P=0.10$). Twelve patients (5.4%) had an MACE during the first 30 postoperative days. Two of these patients (1.8%) were in the aspirin group and 10 patients (9.0%) were in the placebo group ($P=0.02$). Treatment with aspirin resulted in a 7.2% absolute risk reduction [95% confidence interval (CI), 1.3–13%] for postoperative MACE. The relative risk reduction was 80% (95% CI, 9.2–95%). Numbers needed to treat were 14 (95% CI, 7.6–78). No significant differences in bleeding complications were seen between the two groups.

Conclusions. In high-risk patients undergoing non-cardiac surgery, perioperative aspirin reduced the risk of MACE without increasing bleeding complications. However, the study was not powered to evaluate bleeding complications.

Fig. 15.1 Abstract from clinical trial by Oscarsson et al., examining the impact of continuing aspirin in the perioperative period on the risk of major adverse cardiac event (MACE). Reproduced with permission from Oscarsson et al.[6]

Confidence Intervals for Effect Sizes

In addition to calculating a point estimate (single value) for the effect size interval, it is also possible, and highly recommended, to calculate a confidence interval (usually 95% confidence interval) around the point estimate. This can be done for effect sizes for both continuous and noncontinuous outcomes. Although the formulae to achieve these calculations can be complex, confidence intervals are very useful. The value of the confidence interval is that it provides precision for the effect size. A 95% confidence interval provides with 95% certainty the expected range for the effect size should the study be repeated. Therefore, confidence intervals provide an indication of the range for the likely true value of the effect size.

Reality Check: Using Confidence Intervals

Let us compare two SMD effect sizes with the same value: 0.5, which according to Cohen's classification can be considered to be moderate.[5] In one case the effect size has a 95% confidence interval of 0.4 to 0.6, and in the other a 95% confidence interval of 0.1 to 0.8. While the estimate of the effect size is the same in both cases, in the first case you can say with more confidence that it is likely to be a moderate effect, whereas in the second case there is far more uncertainty. In this case, it is possible that the true effect size ranges from small to large, and further study or meta-analysis would likely be indicated.

Confidence intervals also allow one to assess the same question that is addressed by the *P* value, namely whether there is an effect at all. For SMD effect size measures, confidence intervals that include 0 suggest that it is possible that the treatment may not have any effect. Similarly, relative risk confidence intervals including 1 imply a possible lack of treatment response. Confidence intervals that include these critical values (0 for SMD and 1 for relative

risk) suggesting a lack of treatment response are similar to a *P* value greater than 0.05.

In contrast to a *P* value above 0.05, however, these confidence intervals also specify the degree of uncertainty around the effect size estimate and range of possible values for the treatment effect. This is particularly important when examining studies that may be underpowered. A confidence interval that is tightly centered on one of these critical values is more likely to reflect true lack of a treatment effect than a more diffuse confidence interval, which may imply an underpowered study. Also, confidence intervals that include one of the critical values toward the periphery of the confidence interval are more reflective of a sample size issue than they are of the absence of a positive treatment effect.

Key Concepts: Report a Confidence Interval with an Effect Size Measure

Effect size measures should be reported with a confidence interval to specify the degree of uncertainty around the effect size estimate.

Use of Effect Size in Meta-analysis

As mentioned previously, one of the major uses of the effect size is for combining results of many studies in a meta-analysis. This often provides a better understanding of a particular treatment effect than a single study alone. Other chapters in this book will review how to perform a meta-analysis, so we will not focus on this aspect in this chapter. However, it is essential to understand that the data that go into a meta-analysis are a collection of effect sizes from the studies being included. These effect sizes are then entered into the meta-analysis together with a weighting variable. Furthermore, the output from a meta-analysis is generally a pooled (average) estimate of the overall effect size.

Examples from the Literature: The Use of Anti-fibrinolytic Agents in Spine Surgery—A Meta-analysis
Earlier in this chapter, we presented the results and calculated effect sizes from two studies of different antifibrinolytics for the prevention of transfusion in spinal surgery.[3,4] In this final example, we shall review the results of a meta-analysis by Gill et al. that explored this same issue.[7] The authors reviewed studies examining three antifibrinolytics—aprotinin, tranexamic acid, and epsilon-aminocaproic acid—in terms of reducing blood loss and blood transfusions in patients undergoing spine surgery. For each study, the authors computed a SMD (*Hedge's d*) together with a confidence interval. These effect sizes were then plotted for each drug and a pooled estimate of the effect size for each drug was calculated. **Figure 15.2** shows two plots of effect sizes from this meta-analysis. The top panel shows the effect sizes for the impact of aprotinin on blood loss and the bottom panel shows the effect sizes for the impact of tranexamic acid. The lowest line in each panel shows the average ef-

fect size and 95% confidence interval for each drug. The average effect size for aprotinin was –0.691 (95% confidence interval –0.956 to –0.426) and the average effect size for tranexamic acid was –0.668 (95% confidence interval –0.971 to –0.365). On the basis of these results it seems that the effect size for both medications was moderate. Note that, in contrast to our comparison of the effect sizes of the individual studies shown in the first example from the literature, there does not seem to be a meaningful difference between the effect sizes for the two medications. This would need to be studied in "head-to-head" comparisons to draw such a conclusion formally. Nevertheless, the effect size estimates from the meta-analysis provide important implications for the design of this study. Since the effect sizes for the medications were very similar, the difference in the treatment effect of aprotinin relative to that of tranexamic acid would be expected to be quite small. Thus, it is likely that a very large trial would be needed to show any statistically significant difference. The decision to per-

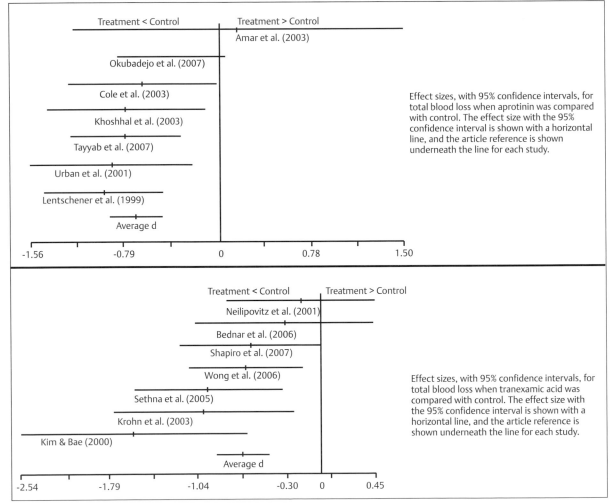

Fig. 15.2 Figures and associated captions from a meta-analysis examining the impact of antifibrinolytics on blood loss in spinal surgery. The top panel shows the effect sizes for the impact of aprotinin on blood loss and the bottom panel the effect sizes for the impact of tranexamic acid. Reproduced with permission from Gill et al.[7]

form such a study should depend on whether the investigators think that the cost of a trial that is anticipated to show a small difference in treatment effects is justified on clinical grounds, including possible differences in the adverse event profile or the cost of aprotinin relative to that of tranexamic acid.

Conclusion

An effect size is a measure of the magnitude of a treatment response. Compared to the *P* value, which simply addresses whether a treatment has any effect at all, an effect size allows one to address the question of how well an intervention works. This facilitates the translation of research findings into a meaningful value, useful for comparisons across studies and for combining studies in meta-analyses.

Suggested Reading

Coe R. It's the effect size, stupid: what effect size is and why it is important. Available at: http://www.leeds.ac.uk/educol/documents/00002182.htm. Accessed April 19, 2012

LeCroy CW, Krysiko J. Understanding and interpreting effect size measures. Social Work Res 2007;31:243–248

Lipsey MW, Wilson DB. Practical Meta-analysis. Thousand Oaks, CA: Sage; 2001

Nakagawa S, Cuthill IC. Effect size, confidence interval and statistical significance: a practical guide for biologists. Biol Rev Camb Philos Soc 2007;82:591–605

Valentine J, Cooper H. Effect size substantive interpretation guidelines: issues in the interpretation of effect sizes. Available at: http://ies.ed.gov/ncee/wwc/pdf/essig.pdf. Accessed April 28, 2010

References

1. Wilkinson, L., APA Task Force on Statistical Inference. Statistical methods in psychology journals: guidelines and explanations. Am Psychol 1999;54:594–604
2. Schulz KF, Altman DG, Moher D; for CONSORT Group. CONSORT 2010 statement: updated guidelines for reporting parallel group randomised trials. BMJ 2010;340:c332
3. Neilipovitz DT, Murto K, Hall L, Barrowman NJ, Splinter WM. A randomized trial of tranexamic acid to reduce blood transfusion for scoliosis surgery. Anesth Analg 2001;93:82–87
4. Khoshhal K, Mukhtar I, Clark P, Jarvis J, Letts M, Splinter W. Efficacy of aprotinin in reducing blood loss in spinal fusion for idiopathic scoliosis. J Pediatr Orthop 2003;23:661–664
5. Cohen, J. Statistical Power Analysis for the Behavioral Sciences. New York: Academic Press; 1969
6. Oscarsson A, Gupta A, Fredrikson M, et al. To continue or discontinue aspirin in the perioperative period: a randomized, controlled clinical trial. Br J Anaesth 2010;104:305–312
7. Gill JB, Chin Y, Levin A, Feng D. The use of antifibrinolytic agents in spine surgery: a meta-analysis. J Bone Joint Surg Am 2008;90:2399–2407

16
Fixed Effects versus Random Effects

Nicole Simunovic, Sheila Sprague, Mohit Bhandari

Summary

The fixed-effects or random-effects model can be used to combine primary study results in a meta-analysis. The impact of the fixed- or random-effects models is dependent on the level of heterogeneity present. It is important to understand the implications associated with the choice of the model to best represent meta-analysis findings. The differences between these models and recommendations for use are presented.

Introduction

A meta-analysis statistically combines treatment effect estimates across similar interventions and outcomes, abstracted from primary studies compiled using a systematic and comprehensive search. A meta-analysis can be useful to increase the statistical power of an effect estimate by combining multiple studies to assemble a larger sample size than that found in an individual trial or observational study, to make sense out of conflicting conclusions, and to answer or propose new and important questions.

The decision to quantitatively pool data may be evaluated at three main stages during the systematic review process. First, at the protocol stage, reviewers should consider whether the research question and eligibility criteria will likely result in a group of studies that may be reasonably combined to form a single study estimate. Second, following data abstraction but before any analysis to prevent data dredging, reviewers can revisit the question of whether it seems reasonable to pool the primary studies for a certain outcome given the available literature. Lastly, at the data analysis stage, reviewers should determine if it is reasonable to present the pooled study estimate based on statistical tests that can quantify the amount of heterogeneity present between individual study estimates.[1]

A reviewer must first be confident that the clinical and methodological diversity is not so great that the primary study data should not be pooled at all. If it is deemed reasonable to pool despite some heterogeneity, reviewers must then determine which statistical model will most plausibly represent these data. Formal tests and considerations for handling heterogeneity are discussed in greater detail in Chapter 17. This chapter will focus on considerations for combining primary study results using either a fixed-effects model or a random-effects model.

Key Concepts: Heterogeneity

- Clinical heterogeneity: Differences between studies in the patient population (old–young, ill–mildly ill, gender, patients who had previous surgery) or treatment under investigation (duration of treatment, intensity, dosage, surgical technique), countries in which the studies were conducted, outcome definitions, and so on
- Statistical heterogeneity: More variation among primary studies than would be expected by chance alone

First, you evaluate possible sources of clinical heterogeneity, then you check with a statistical test to confirm your ideas were correct.[2]

The Data Pool: Fixed Effects versus Random Effects

According to a recent systematic review of orthopaedic meta-analyses, the random-effects model and a combination of both random-effects and fixed-effects models have become significantly more popular over time in the published literature.[3] While we cannot be certain of the reasons for this trend, it is likely that as systematic reviews in orthopaedics improve in methodological quality,[3] authors are considering improved methods for handling within- and between-study heterogeneity.

The fixed-effects model is based on the mathematical assumption that a single common effect underlies every study in the meta-analysis.[4] With fixed effects, "all of the studies you are trying to examine as a whole are considered to have been conducted under similar conditions with similar subjects, the only difference between studies is their power to detect the outcome of interest."[4] Another way to think of the fixed-effects assumption is that if every study was infinitely large, every study would yield an identical result (**Fig. 16.1**). Of course in reality, smaller study pools still demonstrate between-study variability, but under the fixed-effects model, the assumption is that this variability is easily explained by chance.[5]

Rather than assuming that there is one identical true treatment effect common to every study, the random-effects model assumes that the studies included in a meta-analysis are "a random sample of a population of studies."[5] Therefore, each study estimates a different underlying true effect across a normal distribution rather than for a single

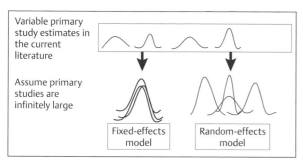

Fig. 16.1 Assumptions underlying the fixed-effects and random-effects models.

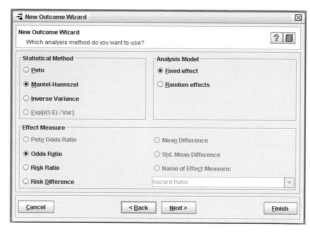

Fig. 16.2 Model and analysis options available in Review Manager.

estimate (**Fig. 16.1**). The meta-analysis estimates the mean and standard deviation of the different effects. Consequently, the random-effects model takes into account both within-study and between-study variability.

Reality Check: Statistical Models Available in Review Manager

There are a variety of statistical models to implement fixed-effects or random-effects methods. A typical application for the fixed-effects model is the Mantel–Haenszel method,[6] and a typical one for the random-effects model is the DerSimonian and Laird method.[7] The inverse variance method combines and weights studies by the inverse of the variance. If the differences within each study are the only sources of variability taken into account, this is a fixed-effects model. When between-study variance is taken into account, this is a random-effects model. These methods are available to pool data using Review Manager (RevMan) software (The Cochrane Collaboration, Copenhagen, Denmark). **Figure 16.2** displays model and analysis options available in Review Manager.

Deciding Which Model to Use

At this point, you have likely gathered the major trade-offs between the fixed-effects and random-effects models. The fixed-effects model is more statistically robust and stable, but based on the overly simplistic and often unreasonable assumption that all primary studies in a meta-analysis are

estimating an identical effect. The random-effects model is based on a more likely assumption, taking into account between-study differences, but is less stable and sometimes unpredictable, while generally resulting in wider, less precise confidence intervals around the pooled estimate (**Table 16.1**). Although neither of two models can be said to be "correct," a substantial difference in the combined effect calculated by the fixed-effects and random-effects models will be seen only if studies are markedly heterogeneous.[9]

If the between-study variance is not beyond that which would be expected by chance, then the fixed-effects and random-effects calculations should give identical results. The Cochrane Collaboration recommends that the primary study data be analyzed in both ways (i.e., select first one option then the other in RevMan) to see how the results vary.[4] If the fixed-effect and random-effect meta-analyses give identical results, "it is unlikely that there is important statistical heterogeneity, and it doesn't matter which one you present."[4]

Examples from the Literature: Impact of the Meta-analysis Model Chosen on the Pooled Estimate of Efficacy (Scenario 1—No Difference in Pooled Estimate)

A recent systematic review comparing Gamma nail and dynamic hip screw fixation found no significant difference in treatment effect on the rates of wound infection

Table 16.1 Respective advantages and disadvantages of the fixed-effects and random-effects approaches to summary point estimation meta-analysis

Model	Principle	Advantages	Disadvantages
Fixed-effects pooling	Common truth	Easy to interpret Applies to whole population	Often simplistic Not applicable with heterogeneity
Random-effects pooling	Range of truth	Allows between-study heterogeneity Realistic	No insight into reasons for heterogeneity Less intuitive

Adapted from Lau et al.[8]

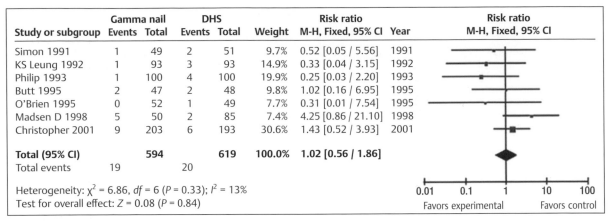

Study or subgroup	Gamma nail Events	Total	DHS Events	Total	Weight	Risk ratio M-H, Fixed, 95% CI	Year	Risk ratio M-H, Fixed, 95% CI
Simon 1991	1	49	2	51	9.7%	0.52 [0.05 / 5.56]	1991	
KS Leung 1992	1	93	3	93	14.9%	0.33 [0.04 / 3.15]	1992	
Philip 1993	1	100	4	100	19.9%	0.25 [0.03 / 2.20]	1993	
Butt 1995	2	47	2	48	9.8%	1.02 [0.16 / 6.95]	1995	
O'Brien 1995	0	52	1	49	7.7%	0.31 [0.01 / 7.54]	1995	
Madsen D 1998	5	50	2	85	7.4%	4.25 [0.86 / 21.10]	1998	
Christopher 2001	9	203	6	193	30.6%	1.43 [0.52 / 3.93]	2001	
Total (95% CI)		**594**		**619**	**100.0%**	**1.02 [0.56 / 1.86]**		
Total events	19		20					

Heterogeneity: $\chi^2 = 6.86$, $df = 6$ ($P = 0.33$); $I^2 = 13\%$
Test for overall effect: $Z = 0.08$ ($P = 0.84$)

Fig. 16.3 Comparison of wound infection rates between the Gamma nail and dynamic hip screw (DHS) using the fixed-effects model. Reprinted from Liu et al.[10]

on the basis of study data pooled using the Mantel–Haenszel fixed-effects method (**Fig. 16.3**).[10] Despite some differences in study results, there was minimal heterogeneity ($I^2 = 13\%$).

We re-evaluated this meta-analysis using the random-effects model (**Fig. 16.4**) and found no significant difference between the final pooled estimates in each model. The only difference is the level of uncertainty surrounding the treatment effect. Because the random-effects model gives smaller studies proportionally greater weight in the pooled estimate, the summary estimates are generally closer to the null with wider confidence intervals (in this case, relative risk 1.02, 95% confidence interval 0.49–2.12), and often provide a more realistic estimate of the range of plausible true values.[5]

If however, the results are heterogeneous (i.e., an I^2 value greater than 20%–50%), you will need to decide which is the better method on which to base your conclusions. Typically, it is best to select the most conservative option.

Examples from the Literature: Impact of the Meta-analysis Model Chosen on the Pooled Estimate of Efficacy (Scenario 2—Difference in Pooled Estimate)

Montori et al. present the example of the effect of magnesium in acute myocardial infarction,[5] in which a series of small trials conducted in the 1980s suggested that magnesium might halve the risk of death.[11] Later, two large trials provided differing estimates. The overall meta-analysis showed significant heterogeneity ($I^2 = 67.9\%$). The fixed-effects summary odds ratio suggests no benefit (i.e., weighted most heavily on the largest trial, ISIS-4), while the random-effects estimate suggests a large benefit from magnesium, driven by the results of the smaller trials. Montori et al. suggest that using fixed effects is not appropriate given that the heterogeneous data clearly violate the assumption of common truth across studies, and recommend presenting the more conservative random-effects estimate.[5]

Study or subgroup	Gamma nail Events	Total	DHS Events	Total	Weight	Risk ratio M-H, Random, 95% CI	Year	Risk ratio M-H, Random, 95% CI
Simon 1991	1	49	2	51	8.8%	0.52 [0.05 / 5.56]	1991	
KS Leung 1992	1	93	3	93	9.7%	0.33 [0.04 / 3.15]	1992	
Philip 1993	1	100	4	100	10.3%	0.25 [0.03 / 2.20]	1993	
O'Brien 1995	0	52	1	49	5.1%	0.31 [0.01 / 7.54]	1995	
Butt 1995	2	47	2	48	12.9%	1.02 [0.15 / 6.95]	1995	
Madsen D 1998	5	50	2	85	17.6%	4.25 [0.86 / 21.10]	1998	
Christopher 2001	9	203	6	193	35.5%	1.43 [0.52 / 3.93]	2001	
Total (95% CI)		**594**		**619**	**100.0%**	**1.02 [0.49 / 2.12]**		
Total events	19		20					

Heterogeneity: $\tau^2 = 0.13$; $\chi^2 = 6.86$, $df = 6$ ($P = 0.33$); $I^2 = 13\%$
Test for overall effect: $Z = 0.05$ ($P = 0.96$)

Fig. 16.4 Comparison of wound infection rates between the Gamma nail and dynamic hip screw (DHS) using the random-effects model. Reprinted from Liu et al.[10]

Conclusion

The impact of using the fixed-effects or the random-effects model is dependent on the level of heterogeneity present in the meta-analysis. Deciding on the most appropriate statistical method for calculating the overall treatment effect will often not matter because both models usually give either identical or similar results.[12] However, when estimates diverge in effect size and/or direction, recommendations specify using the most conservative method (i.e., the random-effects model). This is because it is unlikely that true effects are exactly identical in various populations, which is increasingly clear when there is significant heterogeneity among studies. In general, it is important to understand the implications associated with the choice of the model to best represent the findings of your meta-analysis.

Suggested Reading

Fleiss JL. The statistical basis of meta-analysis. Stat Methods Med Res 1993;2:121–145

Higgins JPT, Green S. Cochrane Handbook for Systematic Reviews of Interventions. Version 5.0.2 [Updated September 2009]. Available at: http://www.cochrane-handbook.org/. Accessed May 1, 2010

Lau J, Ioannidis JPA, Schmid CH. Summing up the evidence: one answer is not always enough. Lancet 1998;351:123–127

Montori V, Ioannidis J, Cook DJ, Guyatt G. In: Guyatt G, Rennie D, Meade MO, Cook DJ, eds. Users' Guides to the Medical Literature: A Manual for Evidence-Based Clinical Practice. 2nd ed. New York, NY: McGraw Hill; 2008:555–562

References

1. Simunovic N, Sprague S, Bhandari M. Methodological issues in systematic reviews and meta-analyses of observational studies in orthopaedic research. J Bone Joint Surg Am 2009;91:87–94
2. Bhandari M, Joensson A. Clinical Research for Surgeons. Stuttgart, Germany: Georg Thieme Verlag; 2009:68–76
3. Dijkman BG, Abouali JAK, Kooistra BW, et al. Twenty years of meta-analyses in orthopaedic surgery: has quality kept up with quantity? J Bone Joint Surg Am 2010;92:48–57
4. Higgins JPT, Green S. Cochrane Handbook for Systematic Reviews of Interventions. Version 5.0.2 [Updated September 2009]. Available at: http://www.cochrane-handbook.org/. Accessed May 1, 2010
5. Montori V, Ioannidis J, Cook DJ, Guyatt G. In: Guyatt G, Rennie D, Meade MO, Cook DJ, eds. Users' Guides to the Medical Literature: A Manual for Evidence-Based Clinical Practice. 2nd ed. New York, NY: McGraw Hill; 2008:555–562
6. Mantel N, Haenszel W. Statistical aspects of the analysis of data from retrospective studies of disease. J Natl Cancer Inst 1959;22:719–748
7. DerSimonian R, Laird N. Meta-analysis in clinical trials. Control Clin Trials 1986;7:177–188
8. Lau J, Ioannidis JPA, Schmid CH. Summing up evidence: one answer is not always enough. Lancet 1998;351:123–127
9. Egger M, Smith GD, Phillips AN. Meta-analysis: principles and procedures. BMJ 1997;315:1533–1537
10. Liu M, Yang Z, Pei F, Huang F, Chen S, Xiang Z. A meta-analysis of the Gamma nail and dynamic hip screw in treating peritrochanteric fractures. Int Orthop 2010;34:323–328
11. Teo KK, Yusuf S. Role of magnesium in reducing mortality in acute myocardial infarction: a review of the evidence. Drugs 1993;46:347–359
12. Engels EA, Schmid CH, Terrin N, Olkin I, Lau J. Heterogeneity and statistical significance in meta-analysis: an empirical study of 125 meta-analyses. Stat Med 2000;19:1707–1728

17

Heterogeneity

S. Samuel Bederman, Anthony Gibson

Summary

Heterogeneity in meta-analyses means the presence of observed study effects that are far more different than what would be expected by chance. Its presence poses a problem for interpreting quantitative summary scores and it can be statistically tested and easily quantified. There are many methods to deal with heterogeneity, from ignoring its presence to incorporating it into the analysis and exploring results using specified factors to explain it.

Introduction

Imagine you are planning a study to look at clinical outcomes following hip fractures. Seems simple enough, right? We will include the 75-year-old woman who slips in her bathtub and sustains a femoral neck fracture. What about the 55-year-old man with multiple myeloma and a pathological subtrochanteric femoral fracture? Do we include the 24-year-old motorcyclist who sustains a femoral head fracture with a hip dislocation? And what about the 13-year-old boy with an acute slipped capital femoral epiphysis? All of these injuries could be considered "hip fractures," but the characteristics of these patients are all distinctly different and would almost certainly account for large differences in outcomes following treatment.

Systematic review is a strategy of collecting the best available evidence with the goal of summarizing what we know in order to answer a relevant clinical question. Once the data have been gathered, the technique of meta-analysis is a statistical method of combining smaller studies by "pooling" the data to effectively increase the sample size. However, proceeding to meta-analysis is only useful if what we are "pooling" is similar or relatively homogeneous. In our planned study above, each different patient is analogous to a different study within a systematic review. Clearly, it would make little sense to combine these patients together to look at outcomes following hip fractures. Similarly, in meta-analyses, it would not make sense to simply combine very different studies only to come up with a statistical value with little clinical meaning.

Heterogeneity Defined

The Cochrane Handbook defines heterogeneity (or statistical heterogeneity) as "the observed intervention effects being more different from each other than one would expect due to random error (chance) alone."[1] This heterogeneity may be due to clinical diversity, methodological diversity, or a combination of the two (**Fig. 17.1**).

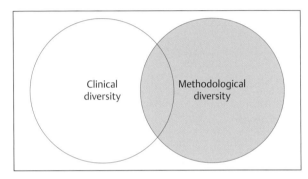

Fig. 17.1 Statistical heterogeneity.

> **Jargon Simplified: Heterogeneity**
> Heterogeneity means differences among individual studies included in a systematic review; typically it refers to study results, but the term can also be applied to other study characteristics.[2]

Clinical heterogeneity includes differences in a study's participants (e.g., inclusion or exclusion criteria), interventions (e.g., type of implant, medication dose), or outcomes studied (e.g., outcome tool used). Methodological heterogeneity includes differences in study design (e.g., prospective, retrospective, randomized), the risk of bias (e.g., concealment of random allocation, blinding), and outcomes (e.g., duration of follow-up).

For example, if we wanted to determine the risk of deep venous thrombosis (DVT) following total knee replacement with low-molecular-weight heparin versus warfarin therapy, we might find some studies that use Doppler ultrasonography for DVT detection while others may use venography. In this circumstance, the different detection methods may suggest that the studies are not all measuring the same thing. However, the presence of significant heterogeneity does not necessarily imply that the effect of different DVT prophylaxis regimens is truly different for each study. Rather, it may signify that the results differ due to variation in detection methods.

> **Key Concepts: Heterogeneity**
> Heterogeneity is the presence of significant variation in treatment effect across studies above what would be expected by chance alone. When significant heterogeneity is present, the interpretation of pooled results is problematic.

Identifying Heterogeneity

Identifying heterogeneity is often as easy as looking at the studies together and applying some common sense. Are the patients, interventions, and outcomes in each of these studies similar enough to combine together in any meaningful way? If we calculate an overall value for the effectiveness of the treatment, does it carry any clinical meaning coming from this varied group of studies? If the answer is "no" then it probably makes little sense to proceed with a meta-analysis once the systematic review is complete. If the studies are sufficiently similar, we can proceed with formal statistical testing for heterogeneity.

As previously mentioned, heterogeneity is the presence of significant variation in treatment effect above what would be expected by chance alone. Statistically, we can see whether there is too great a difference between the overall effect and the sum of each individual effect than what chance alone would predict. The usual statistic for this is Cochran's Q and is computed by summing the squared deviations of each study's estimate from the overall meta-analytic estimate, weighting each study by its overall contribution (sample size or inverse of the variance) and is shown in **Eq. 17.1** where w_i is the study weight, y_i is the study effect for the ith study, and y_w is the weighted overall study effect.[3]

$$Q = \sum_{i=1}^{k} w_i \times (y_i - y_w)^2 \qquad [1]$$

The P value is determined by comparing the statistic with a chi-square (χ^2) distribution with k-1 degrees of freedom where k is the number of studies in the meta-analysis. Typically, if $P < 0.05$ we would assume that there is significant heterogeneity. However, with few studies, the power of Cochran's Q is low and therefore significant heterogeneity might go undetected, which has prompted some to advocate for a less demanding threshold for significance ($P < 0.10$).[4] On the other hand, in meta-analyses where there are many studies, the Q-statistic may be too sensitive and may find significance when the distribution of treatment effects does properly spread over the overall mean.

To better quantify the amount of heterogeneity beyond a P value, the I^2 statistic was developed.[5] The I^2 statistic measures the percentage of variation across studies due to het-

Table 17.1 Interpretation of I^2 values

I^2 value	Interpretation
0–40%	Might not be important
30–60%	May represent moderate heterogeneity
50–90%	May represent substantial heterogeneity
75–100%	Represents considerable heterogeneity

Reproduced with permission from Deeks et al.[1]

erogeneity rather than chance and is shown in **Eq. 17.2**, where Q is Cochran's Q shown above and df is the degrees of freedom.

$$I^2 = \left(\frac{Q - df}{Q}\right) \times 100\% \qquad [2]$$

Values of 0% indicate no heterogeneity while higher values indicate more heterogeneity. The Cochrane Handbook has suggested rough guidelines for its interpretation (**Table 17.1**).[1]

> **Key Concepts: The I^2 Statistic**
> Heterogeneity can be statistically tested and is best quantified by the I^2 statistic. I^2 measures the percentage of variation across studies due to heterogeneity rather than chance.

Dealing with Heterogeneity

Once heterogeneity has been identified the challenge begins—how do we appropriately deal with it? The initial step is to ensure that what we have found is correct. Are the data correct and the statistics properly calculated? Do the effect sizes and their confidence interval widths look different? If so, then we must accept that heterogeneity is present and ask why it exists.

Can we identify sources of heterogeneity? Are there study characteristics that separate out treatment effects? Were these considered in planned subgroup analyses? If so, we may use these factors to better explain the variation observed.

Dealing with heterogeneity can be done in a variety of ways outlined in **Fig. 17.2**. The first and simplest method of dealing with heterogeneity is not to pool the data or perform meta-analysis, but rather to qualitatively describe the findings of the systematic review in light of the variations observed from study to study. This achieves the goal of collecting the best available evidence and allows the reader to make decisions based on it even in the absence of an overall numerical effect size.

The second approach is to ignore the presence of heterogeneity and continue with a "fixed-effects" pooling of the data. Fixed-effects analyses combine the study data with

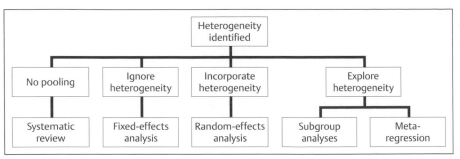

Fig. 17.2 Methods of dealing with heterogeneity.

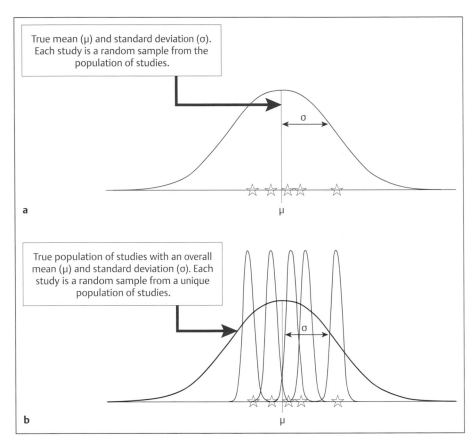

a

b

Fig. 17.3a, b Fixed-effects and random-effects models. **a** Fixed-effects model. It is assumed that each study is a sample from one underlying population with a true effect size. The difference between that study effect and the true effect is simply due to chance alone.
b Random-effects model. It is assumed that no true treatment effect exists, but rather that a distribution of effects exists across different populations. Each study represents a sample from a unique population which estimates that population's true effect with some chance error. The difference between an individual study effect and the mean effect for the true population is the chance difference between the individual study effect and that population's true effect (within-study variation) plus the difference between that population's true effect and the mean effect for all populations (between-study variation).

a weighted average. This approach can provide an estimate of the overall effect size; however, it comes with some difficulty in interpretation. Fixed-effects analyses assume that there is one overall true effect and that each individual study is an estimate of that true effect that varies from the true effect by chance alone (**Fig. 17.3a**). The underlying assumption is that all studies are identical replications from the same population of patients, interventions, and outcome measures. Clearly, these assumptions are rarely valid. However, the pooled estimate gives us some idea of the overall effect size even if no single true effect exists. Furthermore, the confidence interval is artificially narrow because the estimation ignores a large component of the variance—that which exists between studies.

Jargon Simplified: Fixed-Effects Regression

Fixed-effects regression assumes that there is one overall true effect and that each individual study is an estimate of that true effect that varies from the true effect by chance alone. The underlying assumption is that all studies are identical replications from the same population of patients, interventions, and outcome measures.

The third approach involves incorporating the heterogeneity (without necessarily explaining it) by performing a random-effects analysis.[6] In this analysis, we make the assumption that no true effect really exists, but rather that a distribution of effects exists across different populations. Each study represents a sample from a unique population which estimates that population's true effect with some chance error. Each population therefore contributes to an overall distribution of true effect sizes that varies from population to population. In this model, we can estimate the mean effect size and obtain a confidence interval for that distribution of effects with an estimate of the degree of between-study (or between-population) variation. In this way, the difference between the effect in an individual trial and the overall average effect is the difference between the true effect for that trial and the overall averaged effect plus the chance difference between that trial effect and the true effect for that population (**Fig. 17.3b**). Although a random-effects analysis does not explain the heterogeneity, it does incorporate it, and provides a different pooled estimate with a larger confidence interval accounting for both within-study variation (between patients in the same trial) and between-study variation (heterogeneity between trials).

Jargon Simplified: Random-Effects Regression

Random-effects regression assumes that no true treatment effect exists, but rather that a distribution of effects exists across different populations. Each study represents a sample from a unique population which estimates that population's true effect with some chance error. The difference between an individual study effect and the mean effect for the entire population is the chance difference between the individual study effect and that population's true effect (within-study variation) plus the difference between that population's true effect and the mean effect for all populations (between-study variation).

The final method of dealing with heterogeneity is to explain it. This can be done with two main approaches—subgroup analyses or meta-regression. Ideally, characteristics of studies that may contribute to differences in outcomes are specified beforehand (*a priori*), and analyses for each category of the characteristic (subgroup) may be performed to determine whether the overall findings are different for each characteristic.

When the characteristics are prespecified, the conclusions drawn from such subgroup analyses can be reliable. However, in many cases the characteristics are identified after the analysis has been initially performed. When subgroup analyses are performed after the fact (*post hoc*), the results should be interpreted with caution and should only lead to the generation of hypotheses rather than reliable conclusions.

Jargon Simplified: Subgroup Analysis

Subgroup analyses are separate meta-analyses performed for different subsets of studies. The selection of studies for subgroup analysis is specified a priori.

Meta-regression is a technique that goes one step further than separating the analyses. Meta-regression can incorporate the characteristics into the analysis to determine the relationship they have with the outcome. A more detailed explanation is provided in Chapter 21. Briefly, this technique involves performing a meta-analysis using a regression model that includes the characteristics thought to be responsible for heterogeneity as explanatory variables.[7] For example, if we wanted to perform a meta-analysis on outcomes for surgical versus nonsurgical treatment of isthmic spondylolisthesis, we might anticipate that some studies include instrumented posterolateral fusions while some include noninstrumented fusions. In this example, we may plan either a subgroup analysis on the use of instrumentation or include the use of instrumentation as an explanatory variable in the meta-regression.

Jargon Simplified: Meta-regression Analysis

When summarizing patient or design characteristics at the individual trial level, meta-analysts risk failing to detect genuine relationships between these characteristics and the size of the treatment effect. Further, the risk of obtaining a spurious explanation for variable treatment effects is high when the number of trials is small and many patient and design characteristics differ. Meta-regression techniques can be used to explore whether patient characteristics (e.g., younger or older patients) or design characteristics (e.g., studies of low or high quality) are related to the size of the treatment effect.[2]

One additional strategy that may be helpful in rare circumstances is to eliminate outlying studies. This approach is not recommended because it omits valid information and may introduce bias. However, if a clear explanation exists for why one or two studies conflict with the rest of the studies, it may be reasonable to exclude those studies. Ideally, the rationale for exclusion should be prespecified and a sensitivity analysis performed with and without the outlying study.

Key Concepts: Dealing with Heterogeneity

The presence of heterogeneity may be managed in several ways each with unique advantages and disadvantages:

- Qualitative systematic review alone without statistical pooling of studies
- Fixed-effects meta-analysis ignoring the heterogeneity
- Random effects meta-analysis incorporating but not explaining the heterogeneity
- Subgroup analyses or meta-regression to explore causes of heterogeneity

Example from the Literature: Posterolateral Lumbar Spinal Fusion (Heterogeneity from a Single Study)

Gibson and Waddell performed a meta-analysis on surgery for degenerative lumbar spondylosis.[8] In their assessment of radiographic nonunion at 2 years comparing instrumented posterolateral fusion with noninstrumented fusion, the authors identified eight appropriate

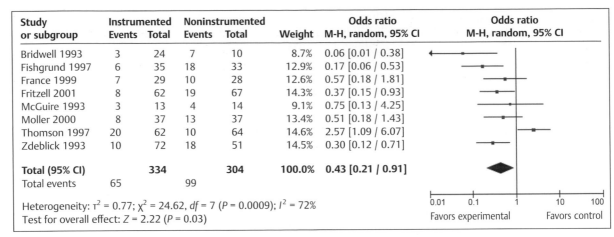

Study or subgroup	Instrumented Events	Total	Noninstrumented Events	Total	Weight	Odds ratio M-H, random, 95% CI	Odds ratio M-H, random, 95% CI
Bridwell 1993	3	24	7	10	8.7%	0.06 [0.01 / 0.38]	
Fishgrund 1997	6	35	18	33	12.9%	0.17 [0.06 / 0.53]	
France 1999	7	29	10	28	12.6%	0.57 [0.18 / 1.81]	
Fritzell 2001	8	62	19	67	14.3%	0.37 [0.15 / 0.93]	
McGuire 1993	3	13	4	14	9.1%	0.75 [0.13 / 4.25]	
Moller 2000	8	37	13	37	13.4%	0.51 [0.18 / 1.43]	
Thomson 1997	20	62	10	64	14.6%	2.57 [1.09 / 6.07]	
Zdeblick 1993	10	72	18	51	14.5%	0.30 [0.12 / 0.71]	
Total (95% CI)		**334**		**304**	**100.0%**	**0.43 [0.21 / 0.91]**	
Total events	65		99				

Heterogeneity: $\tau^2 = 0.77$; $\chi^2 = 24.62$, $df = 7$ ($P = 0.0009$); $I^2 = 72\%$
Test for overall effect: $Z = 2.22$ ($P = 0.03$)

Fig. 17.4a–c Rate of nonunion at 2 years in instrumented vs. noninstrumented posterolateral spinal fusion. M-H, Mantel-Haenzel method. Adapted from Gibson and Waddell.[8]
a Random-effects model.

Study or subgroup	Instrumented Events	Total	Noninstrumented Events	Total	Weight	Odds ratio M-H, fixed, 95% CI	Odds ratio M-H, fixed, 95% CI
Bridwell 1993	3	24	7	10	10.1%	0.06 [0.01 / 0.38]	
Fishgrund 1997	6	35	18	33	17.9%	0.17 [0.06 / 0.53]	
France 1999	7	29	10	28	9.0%	0.57 [0.13 / 1.81]	
Fritzell 2001	8	62	19	67	18.6%	0.37 [0.15 / 0.93]	
McGuire 1993	3	13	4	14	3.5%	0.75 [0.13 / 4.25]	
Moller 2000	8	37	13	37	11.9%	0.51 [0.18 / 1.43]	
Thomsen 1997	20	62	10	64	7.8%	2.57 [1.09 / 6.07]	
Zdeblick 1993	10	72	18	51	21.2%	0.30 [0.12 / 0.71]	
Total (95% CI)		**334**		**304**	**100.0%**	**0.51 [0.36 / 0.73]**	
Total events	65		99				

Heterogeneity: $\chi^2 = 24.62$, $df = 7$ ($P = 0.0009$); $I^2 = 72\%$
Test for overall effect $Z = 3.73$ ($P = 0.0002$)

b Fixed-effects model.

studies with a mix of diagnoses (isthmic spondylolisthesis, degenerative spondylolisthesis, spinal stenosis, and chronic low back pain). Significant heterogeneity was identified in their meta-analysis ($I^2 = 72\%$). Seven of the studies found that instrumentation reduced the rate of nonunion, four of which were statistically significant. Only a single study (Thomsen 1997) favored noninstrumented fusion over instrumentation for the avoidance of nonunion. Because of the heterogeneity, the authors performed a random-effects analysis to account for the significant between-study variation. This analysis found that instrumentation significantly reduced the rate of nonunion [odds ratio (OR) 0.43, 95% confidence interval (CI) 0.21–0.91] (**Fig. 17.4a**). Had the authors ignored the heterogeneity with a fixed-effects regression, they would have come to similar conclusions but with an artificially narrow confidence interval that ignored the between-study variation (OR 0.51, 95% CI 0.36–0.73) (**Fig. 17.4b**).

Reality Check

In this meta-analysis, a single study (Thomsen 1997) has a finding that is inconsistent with the rest. Are there clinical or methodological factors that explain why this study is different? The first step is to check the statistics—is this a true value and are we confident in its interpretation? On the surface, these studies seem similar and no a priori factors for subgroup analysis were considered. However, with further examination, we note that this and one other study (Fritzell 2001) included only patients with chronic low back pain, where all the others included various diagnoses such as isthmic spondylolisthesis, degenerative spondylolisthesis, and spinal stenosis. Fritzell's study also included some patients who underwent circumferential fusion (with anterior or transforaminal interbody fusion). Although we know that all of Thomsen's chronic low back pain patients had a posterior-only instrumented fusion, let's say that in Fritzell's study those who had instru-

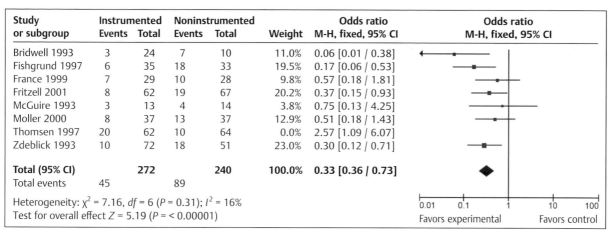

Study or subgroup	Instrumented		Noninstrumented		Weight	Odds ratio M-H, fixed, 95% CI	Odds ratio M-H, fixed, 95% CI
	Events	Total	Events	Total			
Bridwell 1993	3	24	7	10	11.0%	0.06 [0.01 / 0.38]	
Fishgrund 1997	6	35	18	33	19.5%	0.17 [0.06 / 0.53]	
France 1999	7	29	10	28	9.8%	0.57 [0.18 / 1.81]	
Fritzell 2001	8	62	19	67	20.2%	0.37 [0.15 / 0.93]	
McGuire 1993	3	13	4	14	3.8%	0.75 [0.13 / 4.25]	
Moller 2000	8	37	13	37	12.9%	0.51 [0.18 / 1.43]	
Thomsen 1997	20	62	10	64	0.0%	2.57 [1.09 / 6.07]	
Zdeblick 1993	10	72	18	51	23.0%	0.30 [0.12 / 0.71]	
Total (95% CI)		272		240	100.0%	0.33 [0.36 / 0.73]	
Total events	45		89				

Heterogeneity: $\chi^2 = 7.16$, $df = 6$ ($P = 0.31$); $I^2 = 16\%$
Test for overall effect $Z = 5.19$ ($P = < 0.00001$)

Favors experimental — Favors control

c Fixed-effects model, with exclusion of Thomsen 1997.

mentation all had circumferential fusion. One might make the case that in the chronic low back pain population, circumferential fusion with posterior instrumentation is more reliable than posterior-only instrumentation for obtaining a solid fusion. With this in mind, perhaps we have justification to consider removing that study from the analysis and reanalyze the studies to determine if heterogeneity exists and if the results change significantly. In the repeated analysis, we find that no significant heterogeneity persists ($I^2 = 16\%$) and we proceed with a fixed-effects meta-analysis. Our final results demonstrate that the use of instrumentation reduces the risk of nonunion 30% more than in the original analysis (OR 0.33, 95% CI 0.36 to 0.73) (**Fig. 17.4c**).

Example from the Literature: Fixation of Extracapsular Hip Fractures (Heterogeneity across Multiple Studies)
In this meta-analysis by Parker and Handoll, the authors looked at the duration of surgery for short femoral nails versus sliding hip screws in the treatment of extracapsular hip fractures.[9] They identified six relevant studies and found that there was significant heterogeneity

among them ($I^2 = 86\%$). Upon looking at the studies, we see that of the six studies, two favored nails, two favored sliding hip screws, and two were nonsignificant (**Fig. 17.5a**). Here we cannot attribute the heterogeneity to a single study. The authors performed a random-effects meta-analysis to account for the heterogeneity and found that there was no significant difference in operative time between the treatment groups (mean difference 2.48 minutes, 95% CI –3.60 to 8.56). Had they ignored the heterogeneity and proceeded with a fixed-effects analysis, they would have found a similar result but again with a much narrower confidence interval (mean difference 0.34 minutes, 95% CI –1.81 to 2.49) (**Fig. 17.5b**). Although the random-effects model accounts for the heterogeneity, it fails to really explain it.

Reality Check

If we take a closer look at the individual studies, we find that two of them were done by experienced surgeons

Study or subgroup	Short femoral nail			Sliding hip screw			Weight	Mean difference IV, random, 95% CI	Mean difference IV, random, 95% CI
	Mean	SD	Total	Mean	SD	Total			
Adams 2001	55.4	20	203	61.3	22.2	197	18.5%	–5.90 [–10.04 to –1.76]	
Hoffman 1996	56.7	17	31	54.3	16.4	36	15.0%	2.40 [–5.63 to –10.43]	
Kukla 1997	47.1	20.8	60	53.4	6.3	60	17.3%	–6.30 [–11.97 to –0.63]	
O'Brien 1995	59	23.9	53	47	13.3	49	15.6%	12.00 [4.57 to 19.43]	
Ovesen 2006	65	29	73	51	22	73	14.7%	14.00 [5.65 to 22.35]	
Utrilla 2005	46	11	104	44	15	106	19.0%	2.00 [–1.55 to 5.55]	
Total (95% CI)			524			521	100.0%	2.48 [–3.60 to 8.56]	

Heterogeneity: $\tau^2 = 47.36$; $\chi^2 = 34.80$, $df = 5$ ($P = < 0.00001$); $I^2 = 86\%$
Test for overall effect $Z = 0.80$ ($P = 0.42$)

Favors experimental   Favors control

Fig. 17.5a–d Operative time for short femoral nail vs. sliding hip screws for extracapsular hip fracture repair. IV, instrumental variables method. Adapted from Parker and Handoll.[9]
a Random-effects model.

Cont. ▶

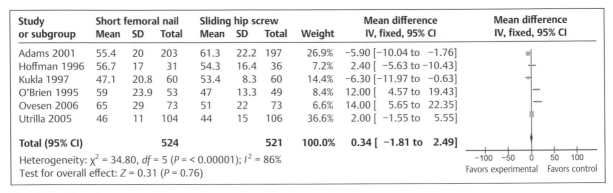

Study or subgroup	Short femoral nail			Sliding hip screw			Weight	Mean difference IV, fixed, 95% CI	Mean difference IV, fixed, 95% CI
	Mean	SD	Total	Mean	SD	Total			
Adams 2001	55.4	20	203	61.3	22.2	197	26.9%	−5.90 [−10.04 to −1.76]	
Hoffman 1996	56.7	17	31	54.3	16.4	36	7.2%	2.40 [−5.63 to −10.43]	
Kukla 1997	47.1	20.8	60	53.4	8.3	60	14.4%	−6.30 [−11.97 to −0.63]	
O'Brien 1995	59	23.9	53	47	13.3	49	8.4%	12.00 [4.57 to 19.43]	
Ovesen 2006	65	29	73	51	22	73	6.6%	14.00 [5.65 to 22.35]	
Utrilla 2005	46	11	104	44	15	106	36.6%	2.00 [−1.55 to 5.55]	
Total (95% CI)			**524**			**521**	**100.0%**	**0.34 [−1.81 to 2.49]**	

Heterogeneity: χ^2 = 34.80, df = 5 (P = < 0.00001); I^2 = 86%
Test for overall effect: Z = 0.31 (P = 0.76)

Fig. 17.5a–d cont.
b Fixed-effects model.

only (Adams 2001, Kukla 1997) while the other four were done by a mix of both experienced surgeons and trainees. If surgeon experience was considered a priori to be a significant factor in accounting for differences in operative time, it could be used to explain any potential heterogeneity in the studies. Subgroup analyses or meta-regression could be performed accounting for surgeon experience. Meta-analysis for mixed surgeons is shown in **Fig. 17.5c** and experienced surgeons in **Fig. 17.5d**. From the four studies of mixed surgeons, we notice that significant heterogeneity remains, although less than in the full analysis (I^2 = 73%). The random-effects analysis of this subgroup found that sliding hip screws were associated with a lower duration of surgery than were short femoral nails (mean difference 7.09 minutes, 95% CI −0.79 to 13.38). In the subgroup of experienced surgeons (two studies), there was no significant heterogeneity and the meta-analysis found that the operative time was lower for the short femoral nail (mean difference −6.04 minutes, 95% CI −9.38 to −2.69). The use of subgroup analyses demonstrates that operative time for nails is much shorter than for screws in the hands of experienced surgeons, but, conversely, in a mixed group of ex-

perienced and trainee surgeons the operative time for screws was lower than that for nails. Failing to explain the heterogeneity would lead to the conclusion that there is no difference in operative time between the implants.

Conclusion

Large differences in group outcomes, or heterogeneity, make the pooling of information difficult to interpret. Clinical diversity, such as the specific population under study, and methodological diversity, such as differences in study design or risk of bias, can both contribute to heterogeneity among studies identified in systematic reviews. Just as pediatric, pathologic, high-energy, and osteoporotic hip fractures should not be combined together to give us any meaningful interpretation of outcome following treatment, studies with significant heterogeneity should not be naively combined together without a careful rationale for dealing with the differences.

Study or subgroup	Short femoral nail			Sliding hip screw			Weight	Mean difference IV, random, 95% CI	Mean difference IV, random, 95% CI
	Mean	SD	Total	Mean	SD	Total			
2.1.1 Experienced and junior surgeons									
Adams 2001	55.4	20	203	61.3	22.2	197	0.0%	−5.90 [−10.04 to −1.76]	
Hoffman 1996	56.7	17	31	54.3	16.4	36	22.5%	2.40 [−5.63 to −10.43]	
Kukla 1997	47.1	20.8	60	53.4	8.3	60	0.0%	−6.30 [−11.97 to −0.63]	
O'Brien 1995	59	23.9	53	47	13.3	49	23.7%	12.00 [4.57 to 19.43]	
Ovesen 2006	65	29	73	51	22	73	21.9%	14.00 [5.65 to 22.35]	
Utrilla 2005	46	11	104	44	15	106	31.9%	2.00 [−1.55 to 5.55]	
Subtotal (95% CI)			**261**			**264**	**100.0%**	**7.09 [−0.79 to 13.38]**	

Heterogeneity: τ^2 = 29.02; χ^2 = 10.99, df = 3 (P = 0.01); I^2 = 73%
Test for overall effect Z = 2.21 (P = 0.03)

Total (95% CI)			**261**			**264**	**100.0%**	**7.09 [−0.79 to 13.38]**	

Heterogeneity: τ^2 = 29.02; χ^2 = 10.99, df = 3 (P = 0.01); I^2 = 73%
Test for overall effect: Z = 2.21 (P = 0.03)
Test for subgroup differences. Not applicable

Fig. 17.5a–d cont.
c Subgroup 1: Experienced and trainee surgeons.

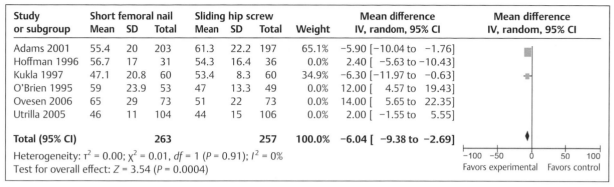

Study or subgroup	Short femoral nail			Sliding hip screw			Weight	Mean difference IV, random, 95% CI	Mean difference IV, random, 95% CI
	Mean	SD	Total	Mean	SD	Total			
Adams 2001	55.4	20	203	61.3	22.2	197	65.1%	−5.90 [−10.04 to −1.76]	
Hoffman 1996	56.7	17	31	54.3	16.4	36	0.0%	2.40 [−5.63 to −10.43]	
Kukla 1997	47.1	20.8	60	53.4	8.3	60	34.9%	−6.30 [−11.97 to −0.63]	
O'Brien 1995	59	23.9	53	47	13.3	49	0.0%	12.00 [4.57 to 19.43]	
Ovesen 2006	65	29	73	51	22	73	0.0%	14.00 [5.65 to 22.35]	
Utrilla 2005	46	11	104	44	15	106	0.0%	2.00 [−1.55 to 5.55]	
Total (95% CI)			**263**			**257**	**100.0%**	**−6.04 [−9.38 to −2.69]**	

Heterogeneity: τ^2 = 0.00; χ^2 = 0.01, df = 1 (P = 0.91); I^2 = 0%
Test for overall effect: Z = 3.54 (P = 0.0004)

−100 −50 0 50 100
Favors experimental   Favors control

d Subgroup 2: Experienced surgeons only.

Heterogeneity is identified by looking at the significance level of Cochran's Q but is better quantified by the I^2 statistic: the P value may underestimate the presence of heterogeneity in a smaller group of studies and may overestimate if the group is larger. High values of I^2 indicate significant heterogeneity, while lower numbers closer to 0% virtually exclude its presence.

Once heterogeneity has been identified, there is no single best method for dealing with it. Avoiding the pooling of data and providing a qualitative interpretation of the systematic review, ignoring the heterogeneity and proceeding with fixed-effects regression, or incorporating it and performing random-effects regression all come with benefits and drawbacks. A fixed-effects analysis answers the question, "What is the most accurate estimate of the true treatment effect?" while the random-effects analysis answers, "What is the average treatment effect across all populations?" While fixed-effects regression is simpler to perform, the confidence interval is artificially narrow and violates many assumptions about the data. On the other hand, random-effects regression accounts for the between-study variation by increasing the width of the confidence intervals but fails properly to explain the heterogeneity.

Subgroup analyses and meta-regression are tools that can explain the differences in effect across different study characteristics. However, these methods are most useful when the individual characteristics are prespecified. When identified after exploring the data, the results can be helpful in generating hypotheses but the conclusions are less reliable.

The identification and management of heterogeneity in meta-analysis requires an approach that balances the clinical relevance of the question with quantitative methods of analysis.

Key Concepts: Crucial Importance of Dealing with Heterogeneity

Identifying and dealing with heterogeneity in meta-analyses is crucial when using systematic reviews of the best available evidence to arrive at recommendations for clinical problems.

Suggested Reading

Deeks JJ, Higgins JPT, Altman DG. Analysing data and undertaking meta-analyses. In: Higgins JPT, Green S, eds. Cochrane Handbook for Systematic Reviews of Interventions. Version 5.0.1. Chichester, England: Wiley-Blackwell; 2008

Higgins JPT, Thompson SG, Deeks JJ, Altman DG. Measuring inconsistency in meta-analysis. BMJ 2003;327:557–560

References

1. Deeks JJ, Higgins JPT, Altman DG. Analysing data and undertaking meta-analyses. In: Higgins JPT, Green S, eds. Cochrane Handbook for Systematic Reviews of Interventions. Version 5.0.1. Chichester, England: Wiley-Blackwell; 2008
2. Guyatt GH, Rennie D, Meade M, Cook D, eds. Users' Guide to the Medical Literature: A Manual for Evidence-Based Clinical Practice. 2nd ed. New York: McGraw-Hill; 2008
3. Hardy RJ, Thompson SG. Detecting and describing heterogeneity in meta-analysis. Stat Med 1998;17:841–856
4. Higgins JPT, Thompson SG, Deeks JJ, Altman DG. Measuring inconsistency in meta-analysis. BMJ 2003;327:557
5. Higgins JPT, Thompson SG. Quantifying heterogeneity in a meta-analysis. Stat Med 2002;21:1539–1558
6. DerSimonian R, Laird N. Meta-analysis in clinical trials. Control Clin Trials 1986;7:177–188
7. Thompson SG, Higgins JPT. How should meta-regression analyses be undertaken and interpreted? Stat Med 2002; 21:1559–1573
8. Gibson JN, Waddell G. Surgery for degenerative lumbar spondylosis: updated Cochrane Review. Spine 2005;30:2312–2320
9. Parker MJ, Handoll HH. Gamma and other cephalocondylic intramedullary nails versus extramedullary implants for extracapsular hip fractures in adults. Cochrane Database Syst Rev 2008;CD000093

18

Uncovering Publication Bias

Vanja Gavranic, Brad A. Petrisor

Summary

Publication bias results from systematic tendencies to publish some types of trials over others. This may result from only publishing positive trials or those trials favoring company products, for example. Publication bias can be detected with statistical tests and may be decreased through the use of trial registries.

Introduction

Systematic reviews and meta-analyses, when conducted with methodological rigor, are considered amongst the highest levels of evidence. However, they lose much of their quality when their validity is compromised. One of the most important ways that validity can be compromised is failure to obtain a representative sample of all the studies that were conducted on a given topic. This is difficult to avoid if *published studies* are systematically different from *all studies* (i.e., both published and unpublished studies)—a problem known as publication bias.

> **Jargon Simplified: Publication Bias**
> Publication bias occurs when the publication of research depends on the direction (positive or negative) of the study results and whether they are statistically significant.[1]

Publication bias results when the strength or direction of results influences whether a study is published. Studies with findings that are statistically significant—*positive studies*—and studies that find in favor of the treatment group are more likely to be published than studies that do not have statistically significant results—*negative studies*—or studies that do not find in favor of the treatment group.[2-6] This bias has been shown in the surgical literature: an analysis of 12 orthopaedic and general surgery journals, which ranged widely in journal rankings and impact factors, found that 91% of published studies were positive or favored the treatment group.[7] Positive studies and studies that find in favor of the treatment group are not only more likely to be published, they also gather more attention: they are cited more frequently, are more likely to be published multiple times, and are also published more frequently in journals with higher impact factors.[2,8] Negative studies and studies that do not find in favor of the treat-

ment group take much longer to be published, giving rise to a type of bias known as time lag bias.[9,10] There may be a delay in publishing these studies, sometimes as high as 1–3 years.[9] It has also been shown that studies conducted in non-English-speaking countries are more likely to be published in English if the results are positive or in favor of the treatment group.[11] Further, studies that are sponsored by pharmaceutical companies are more likely to be published if they find in favor of the company's product.[12] All of this may lead to the preferential publication of positive studies or studies favoring the treatment group.

> **Jargon Simplified: Positive Studies**
> Positive studies are those whose findings are statistically significant.

> **Jargon Simplified: Negative Studies**
> Negative studies are those whose findings are not statistically significant.

> **Key Concepts: Publication Bias**
> Publication bias usually results from a disproportionate contribution to the body of evidence by positive studies and studies that find in favor of the treatment group.

If publication bias exists, it can threaten the validity of any attempts to summarize the evidence. A systematic review will show a disproportionate number of positive studies and studies concluding in favor of the treatment group and can give an overall impression that a treatment is better than it truly is. Indeed, Sutton et al. assessed 48 systematic reviews in the Cochrane Database of Systematic Reviews and estimated that half of all systematic reviews are affected by publication bias, and that 5%–10% of the time the extent of publication bias was large enough to cause results to be misinterpreted.[13] Meta-analyses are also affected when publication bias is present: because there are more positive studies and studies that favor the treatment group, the results of those studies hold more weight in the pooled estimate of treatment effect. This may result in an overestimate of the treatment effect. Publication bias is also a problem in systematic reviews and meta-analyses of observational studies as those studies may, due to their lack of randomization and control group, over or underestimate the truth, with publication bias exacerbating the issue.[2] This is because observational studies are more likely to suffer from other methodological issues such as prognostic differences between treatment groups due to lack of randomization, lack of blinding, and incomplete follow-up.

> **Key Concepts: Distortion Due to Publication Bias**
> Publication bias can result in the impression that a treatment is better than it truly is.

Authors and Publication Bias

Publication bias can occur at any stage of the publication process.[14] There is much evidence to show that publication bias may be caused by investigators most of the time.[2,15–17] Surveys of authors have found that authors have cited negative or unimportant results amongst the main reasons they decided not to publish a study.[2,15–17] This may stem from their perception that the study will be rejected for publication and consequently may not be worth the time or effort to submit. In fact, a survey of investigators revealed that most believe that statistical significance of results is one of the most important factors that journal editors use in determining whether to publish a study.[18] Indeed, this bias has been demonstrated in the editorial review process[2–19]; nevertheless, as discussed, sources of publication bias can be found in both authors and editors.

Detecting and Adjusting for Publication Bias

When conducting a systematic review or meta-analysis, it is important to detect publication bias in order to determine whether the study's validity may be compromised. Publication bias can be detected using a variety of graphical and statistical methods discussed below. All these methods have potential limitations.

Funnel Plot

The funnel plot is a common method used to detect publication bias.[20] Usually, a measure of precision is plotted against a measure of effect size. Standard error can be used to measure precision, and since standard error is correlated with sample size, sample size can also be used. The principle behind funnel plots is that the precision of an estimate of effect (the point estimate) increases with increasing sample size. Therefore, there will be a narrower distribution of point estimates at the top of the graph. Studies with smaller sample sizes are less precise, and the graph will therefore have a wider distribution of estimated effect sizes at the bottom. The graph should take the shape of an inverted funnel if publication bias is not present, and should be symmetrical around the point estimates of the larger studies. Asymmetry in the funnel plot may indicate

the presence of publication bias. Since visual assessment of a funnel plot can be subjective, it is also possible to use statistical tests to determine if publication bias is present.

> **Key Concepts: Statistical Methods to Analyze Funnel Plots**
> ***Egger's linear regression method.*** This method involves calculating a standard normal deviate (defined as the odds ratio divided by standard error) and regressing it against the precision of the estimate (defined as the inverse of standard error). In the presence of publication bias, the regression line will not pass through the origin. The further it is from the origin, the greater the extent of publication bias. This test is limited in that it can provide false-positive results 10% of the time.[21]
> ***Rank correlation test.*** This tests the correlation between standardized effect size estimates and sampling variances.[22] Often, variance is approximately inversely proportional to sample size, so this test can be thought of as determining whether effect size is correlated with sample size. The test is based on the idea that sample size is associated with publication bias, since small studies are more prone to publication bias.[23] Therefore, a correlation should be found between sample size and effect size in the presence of publication bias. A problem with this method is that meta-analyses in surgical research most commonly involve a small number of studies, and in these cases the rank correlation test is not powered to rule out publication bias.

A problem with evaluating funnel plots both visually and statistically is that factors other than publication bias may contribute to asymmetry. Asymmetry in funnel plots can be a result of a variety of different factors: location bias, true heterogeneity, data irregularities, or artifactual factors (e.g., choice of effect measure).[20] Location bias may occur when there is citation bias, English-language bias, or a multiple publication bias—all factors that may influence the symmetry of a funnel plot.[20] True heterogeneity refers to effect size variations that occur as a result of study sample size; here, the intensity of the intervention and differences in underlying risk can substantially influence a funnel plot.[20] Lastly, data irregularities relate to poor methodological designs in small studies, fraud, and inadequate analysis.[20] In addition, the shape of a funnel plot can vary largely depending on the variables chosen for precision and effect size.[24]

Trim and Fill Method

The trim and fill method is based on the funnel plot and involves removing the trials that do not have a counterpart on the other side of what is supposed to be the inverted funnel shape.[25] When those studies are removed, the center of the funnel is estimated. The removed trials are placed back into the graph and their counterparts are reflected upon the calculated center of the funnel. The number of studies that were missing reflects the extent of publication bias. Since this method is based on the funnel plot, it is subject to the same limitations as the latter.

Fail-Safe N

The statistical method known as the fail-safe N calculates how many studies that show no effect would be needed to shift the estimate generated in a meta-analysis from being significant to being nonsignificant.[26] The more studies that that would be needed to change the significance—i.e., the larger the fail-safe N—the more likely it is that publication bias is present. A problem with the fail-safe N method is that it assumes that the missing studies have results that are neutral and does not take into account studies that find in favor of the control group.[27] If the missing studies favor the control group, fewer of these studies would need to be included in order to shift the estimate to being nonsignificant. Thus, fail-safe N can lead to an overestimate of the extent of publication bias. This method also overemphasizes the importance of statistical significance.[27]

Sensitivity Analysis

Sensitivity analysis involves comparing the published trials in a meta-analysis to registered trials to see if the conclusions are different.[28] If there is a difference, publication bias is likely to be present. A problem with this method is that existing trial registers may not be completely comprehensive.[29]

> **Key Concepts: Detecting Publication Bias**
> The presence of publication bias can be detected by graphical and statistical methods, all of which have limitations.

Minimizing the Effect of Publication Bias

Authors of systematic reviews and meta-analyses have a responsibility to reduce the effect of publication bias on their study. They can do this with a thorough search of the literature, to ensure that they have obtained all of the available trials or studies they could. Obtaining all of the published as well as unpublished trials can be difficult; techniques for accomplishing this include looking through any existing registers of published and unpublished trials, searching a variety of databases including the archives of annual meetings, and hand-searching journal indices and the reference lists of relevant trials, as well as speaking to content experts who may be able to identify any unpublished studies. Additionally, since negative studies and stu-

dies that do not favor the treatment group may take longer to be published than positive studies and studies that favor the treatment group, authors may wish to update systematic reviews as more studies become available over time. This works to reduce the effect of time lag bias because negative studies have a chance to "catch up" with the positive studies that were published years earlier.

> **Key Concepts: Possible Measures to Minimize Publication Bias**
> - Looking through trial registers
> - Searching a variety of databases
> - Searching for articles in any language
> - Hand-searching journal indices
> - Looking at reference lists of relevant articles
> - Contacting experts
> - Updating systematic reviews and meta-analyses over time

Although it is important to obtain unpublished data, one should still be careful when using a systematic review or meta-analysis that has collected data from unpublished studies. It should be clear how the data were obtained and analyzed, and the reader should think about the validity of the studies used and whether the data from those studies were chosen selectively.[14] If other investigators are able to access the unpublished data, this makes the review more credible.[14]

A Possible Solution: Trial Registers

Prospective registration of trials has been widely proposed as a solution to publication bias. Registering trials when they are initiated ensures that investigators know of the existence of all trials regardless of their outcome. This removes the potential for publication bias. If a study is not published, then an investigator who is interested in the results would still be aware of the study and would be able to contact those who carried out that study to find the results. A trial registry would need to be inexpensive for users, easy to use, accurate, and comprehensive.[29] ClinicalTrials.gov is one such registry, and in 2007 the US Food and Drug Administration legally required "mandatory registration and results reporting" of some types of trials. Some difficulties with developing a comprehensive trial register are that it is an expensive undertaking, there is no uniform worldwide legislation requiring investigators to register trials, and many are not aware of the importance of trial registration.[29]

Key Concepts: Trial Registers

Trial registers are a potential solution for preventing publication bias. However, there are many challenges in implementing them. ClinicalTrials.gov is a website and trial registry set up by the US National Institutes of Health through the National Library of Medicine in collaboration with the US Food and Drug Administration.

Conclusion

Publication bias may arise from the systematic publication of positive trials or only those trials finding in favor of a particular product. These inherent biases can be detected through a number of statistical tests and accounted for in the analysis of a systematic review. The development of trial registries may help prevent the problem of publication bias in the future; however, strict adherence and compliance with these registries would be necessary for this to occur.

Suggested Reading

Montori VM, Smieja M, Guyatt GH. Publication bias: a brief review for clinicians. Mayo Clin Proc 2000;75:1284–1288

References

1. Guyatt GH, Rennie D, Meade M, Cook D, eds. Users' Guide to the Medical Literature: A Manual for Evidence-Based Clinical Practice. 2nd ed. New York: McGraw-Hill; 2008
2. Easterbrook PJ, Berlin JA, Gopalan R, Matthews DR. Publication bias in clinical research. Lancet 1991;337:867–872
3. Harris IA, Mourad M, Kadir A, Solomon MJ, Young JM. Publication bias in abstracts presented to the annual meeting of the American Academy of Orthopaedic Surgeons. J Orthop Surg (Hong Kong) 2007;15:62–66
4. Hopewell S, Clarke M, Stewart L, Tierney J. Time to publication for results of clinical trials. Cochrane Database Syst Rev 2007;2:MR000011
5. Scherer RW, Langenberg P, von Elm E. Full publication of results initially presented in abstracts. Cochrane Database Syst Rev 2007;2:MR000005
6. Stern JM, Simes RJ. Publication bias: evidence of delayed publication in a cohort study of clinical research projects. BMJ 1997;315:640–645
7. Hasenboehler EA, Choudhry IK, Newman JT, Smith WR, Ziran BH, Stahel PF. Bias towards publishing positive results in orthopedic and general surgery: a patient safety issue? Patient Saf Surg 2007;1:4
8. Gøtzsche PC. Reference bias in reports of drug trials. Br Med J (Clin Res Ed) 1987;295:654–656
9. Hopewell S, Loudon K, Clarke MJ, Oxman AD, Dickersin K. Publication bias in clinical trials due to statistical significance or direction of trial results. Cochrane Database Syst Rev 2009;1:MR000006
10. Krzyzanowska MK, Pintilie M, Tannock IF. Factors associated with failure to publish large randomized trials presented at an oncology meeting. JAMA 2003;290:495–501
11. Egger M, Zellweger-Zähner T, Schneider M, Junker C, Lengeler C, Antes G. Language bias in randomised controlled trials published in English and German. Lancet 1997;350:326–329
12. Lexchin J, Bero LA, Djulbegovic B, Clark O. Pharmaceutical industry sponsorship and research outcome and quality: systematic review. BMJ 2003;326:1167–1170
13. Sutton AJ, Duval SJ, Tweedie RL, Abrams KR, Jones DR. Empirical assessment of effect of publication bias on meta-analyses. BMJ 2000;320:1574–1577
14. Montori VM, Smieja M, Guyatt GH. Publication bias: a brief review for clinicians. Mayo Clin Proc 2000;75:1284–1288
15. Dickersin K, Chan S, Chalmers TC, Sacks HS, Smith H Jr. Publication bias and clinical trials. Control Clin Trials 1987;8:343–353
16. Dickersin K, Min YI. Publication bias: the problem that won't go away. Ann N Y Acad Sci 1993;703:135–146
17. Dickersin K, Min YI, Meinert CL. Factors influencing publication of research results. Follow-up of applications submitted to two institutional review boards. JAMA 1992;267:374–378
18. Shakiba B, Salmasian H, Yousefi-Nooraie R, Rohanizadegan M. Factors influencing editors' decision on acceptance or rejection of manuscripts: the authors' perspective. Arch Iran Med 2008;11:257–262
19. Callaham ML, Wears RL, Weber EJ, Barton C, Young G. Positive-outcome bias and other limitations in the outcome of research abstracts submitted to a scientific meeting. JAMA 1998;280:254–257
20. Egger M, Davey Smith G, Schneider M, Minder C. Bias in meta-analysis detected by a simple, graphical test. BMJ 1997;315:629–634
21. Seagroatt V, Stratton I. Bias in meta analysis detected by a simple, graphical test. Test had 10% false positive rate. BMJ 1998;316:470
22. Begg CB, Mazumdar M. Operating characteristics of a rank correlation test for publication bias. Biometrics 1994; 50:1088–1101
23. Begg CB, Berlin JA. Publication bias: a problem in interpreting medical data. J R Stat Soc A 1988;151:419–463
24. Tang JL, Liu JL. Misleading funnel plot for detection of bias in meta-analysis. J Clin Epidemiol 2000;53:477–484
25. Duval S, Tweedie R. Trim and fill: a simple funnel-plot-based method of testing and adjusting for publication bias in meta-analysis. Biometrics 2000;56:455–463
26. Rosenthal R. The "file drawer problem" and tolerance for null results. Psychol Bull 1979;86:638–641
27. Persaud R. Misleading meta-analysis. "Fail safe N" is a useful mathematical measure of the stability of results. BMJ 1996;312:125
28. Simes RJ. Confronting publication bias: a cohort design for meta-analysis. Stat Med 1987;6:11–29
29. Dickersin K, Rennie D. Registering clinical trials. JAMA 2003;290:516–523

19

Statistical Pooling—Programs and Systems

Michel Saccone, Rudolf W. Poolman, Charles H. Goldsmith

Summary

Statistical pooling is the process whereby data abstracted from individual studies involved in a meta-analysis are combined to calculate an overall effect for an intervention of interest. All conclusions derived from a systematic review and meta-analysis rely on the quality of data produced from the statistical pooling process. As a result, it is imperative to identify the correct statistical pooling program and system to suit your needs. It is even more important to accept that processes which exceed the extent of a basic meta-analysis can be overwhelming for the general clinical researcher. Thus, researchers should look to consult statisticians or researchers with extensive expertise in statistics to minimize errors and improve the quality of research.

This chapter provides you with a brief overview of important concepts of statistical pooling and a review of the available statistical pooling programs and systems.

Introduction

So you have decided to embark on the process of developing a systematic review and meta-analysis. Your goal is to assess the relevant literature in hopes of identifying an overall effect to solidify the evidence present in individual studies on a specific topic. A clinical question has been formulated and eligibility criteria have been developed. Following this, your search strategy is put into effect and identified studies are screened on the basis of eligibility criteria. Once you have selected your studies for review, data abstraction is required to perform the meta-analysis.

What Is Statistical Pooling?

Statistical pooling is the process whereby data abstracted from individual studies involved in a meta-analysis are combined to calculate an overall effect for an intervention of interest.[1] Since all studies are not identical, especially with regard to sample size, it is important to ensure that data abstracted from all studies are not treated as equal. The ability of a study to identify important differences is known as the study's power.[1] Statistical power in a study is largely dependent on the study's sample size. Smaller samples sizes generally provide an inferior ability to detect

differences as they are more susceptible to variability, which is shown in large standard deviations; thus, a smaller sample size can result in reduced validity of any findings produced.[2] This same principle must be taken into account when pooling data. This is done by utilizing weighted averages.[1] Data abstracted from smaller studies are more likely to have greater variability, and accordingly receive less weight than larger studies in an estimate of the overall effect.[1-4] Fortunately, as is shown below, weighting calculations of study results is one of the many analytic techniques performed automatically by statistical pooling programs and systems.

> **Jargon Simplified: Statistical Pooling**
> Statistical pooling is the process by which data abstracted from individual studies are combined into a summary statistic that is produced in a meta-analysis.[5]

Important Concepts in Statistical Pooling

Statistical pooling programs, at least those reviewed in this chapter, provide users with access to virtually all the analytic techniques required to conduct extensive meta-analyses.[6] These programs have been validated, and are constantly monitored and updated.[6]

However, this does not guarantee that any data put into these systems will produce valid results or a technically sound meta-analysis. The quality of a meta-analysis is dependent on the quality of data used.[7] To produce level 1 evidence, a meta-analysis should ideally include data from high-quality primary studies that are homogeneous.[1,2] In reality, the odds of obtaining a group of studies that are completely homogeneous are slim. However, when included studies have heterogeneity, this does not necessarily indicate that the meta-analysis will be of lower quality. Among other techniques, the use of regression models to adjust for heterogeneity is common, and when used properly it can improve the quality of these analyses.[1] A high-quality meta-analysis must also be extensive, in that it identifies not only all relevant published literature, but also the unpublished literature, to avoid publication bias.[8] According to Cucherat et al., the real difficulties associated with meta-analysis are not concerned with arithmetic, but rather lie in the identification of unpublished trials, the selection of trials, data extraction, and in the correct interpretation of results.[8] Fortunately, statistical pooling programs and systems have been developed to guide researchers in their decisions and interpretations. Tools such as funnel plots have been developed to indicate the presence of publication bias, though their effectiveness has been questioned.[1,9–11] The ability to present results in forest plots also enhances interpretability.

Jargon Simplified: Regression Model

A regression model is a statistical model that uses predictor or independent variables to build a statistical model that predicts an individual patient's status with respect to a dependent or target variable.[4]

Jargon Simplified: Publication Bias

Publication bias occurs when the publication of research depends on the direction (positive or negative) of the study results and whether they are statistically significant.[5]

Jargon Simplified: Funnel Plot

A funnel plot is a graphical diagram displaying the treatment effect against a measure of study size; it is used to identify publication bias in a meta-analysis.[9–11]

Jargon Simplified: Forest Plot

A forest plot is a graphical diagram that depicts the relative strength of treatment effects in multiple studies with minimal heterogeneity.[9–11]

One major drawback of statistical pooling systems and software is their inability to dictate the level of heterogeneity in the data identified.[12] This duty is solely the responsibility of the researcher, and the inability to identify the degree of heterogeneity in the data can have serious implications.[1,6,12] The importance of heterogeneity with regard to statistical pooling programs and systems is that the extent of heterogeneity present will determine the model used in the meta-analysis. Most programs and systems developed after the year 2000 have the ability to utilize multiple models, such as fixed-effects and random-effects models.[6,12] However, if more primitive systems are being utilized, it is important to ensure that the correct model is available.[6,12] For more information on these topics, see Chapters 15 and 16.

The uncertainty that is evidently present in the process of statistical pooling is indicative of the need for collaboration between clinicians, researchers trained in methodology, and statisticians. Since accuracy of statistics is of utmost importance to the production of influential conclusions, complex statistical processes should at least involve the consultation of qualified statisticians. This is especially the case in meta-analyses that go beyond the realm of pooling results from well-conducted, good-quality studies.

Examples from the Literature: Evaluating Meta-analyses in the General Surgical Literature—A Critical Appraisal

In their work, Dixon and colleagues identified a number of flaws in the literature using the Overview Quality Assessment Questionnaire.[13] These included improper description or complete lack of appropriate validity criteria, failure to identify selection bias, unexplained search strategies, and improper pooling of data.[13] Furthermore, 22% of studies in journals with impact factors varying from 0.502 to 6.674 did not support their conclusions with the data reported.[13] Among recommendations of increased attention to the QUOROM (Quality of Reporting of Meta-analyses) statement by editors and the need for more rigorous search strategies, Dixon et al. strongly emphasized the need for increased peer review and collaboration between researchers, statisticians, and clinicians.[13]

Why Use Statistical Pooling Programs and Systems?

Statistical pooling programs and systems provide the most comprehensive way to accurately pool, summarize, analyze, and interpret large quantities of data from a variety of sources in a meta-analysis. All high-quality programs are validated with leading statistical software and the programs are consistently monitored and updated.[6,12] Human error is virtually eliminated with the exception of the data input stage, though this is monitored to an extent as most systems have built-in data screening that identify uncharacteristic data entries.[6] All high-quality systems have documentation of the methods users must follow in manual or online form and many provide technical support over the internet or telephone.[6] Most systems also afford the ability to import data from a variety of sources.[6,12] Further, the ability to produce plots, tables, and graphs as part of the system's output enables researchers to present data in easily interpretable and visually appealing formats for publication.[6]

Selecting the Appropriate Programs and Systems: Factors to Consider

As a primary user of a statistical pooling program or system it is essential to ensure that the program or system you have selected is capable of performing all of the analytic techniques and calculations you require. Before determining which program you will use for your meta-analysis, you must be sure to identify all of the major factors that will play a role in determining the program that is best suited to your research.

Study Heterogeneity

As previously mentioned, understanding the level of heterogeneity of the primary studies included in the meta-analysis is critical in determining the model used for analysis. For all programs and systems evaluated, options for fixed- and random-effects models are available.[6,12] Further information on heterogeneity requirements are discussed in Chapter 17.

Outcome Measure Inputted

It is important to know the form of outcome measure or data being inputted into a statistical pooling program. Though all high-quality programs are compatible with binary and continuous data, not all allow for direct input of diagnostic test data.[6]

Required Output

The most practical output of a meta-analysis is the forest plot.[3] Accordingly, this is available in all high-quality statistical programs and systems.[6,12] The funnel plot, used to identify publication bias in meta-analyses, is also available in all programs and systems.[6,12] The receiver-operating characteristic (ROC) provides an indication of the specificity and sensitivity of the overall effect being measured.[3] It can be fitted with a summary ROC curve to enhance interpretation.[3] Hierarchical summary ROC curves can also be determined in the case of bivariate meta-analysis; however, these plots are not available in all programs and systems.[6,12] These outputs are displayed in **Fig. 19.1**.

> **Jargon Simplified:**
> **Receiver-Operating Characteristic (ROC) Curve**
> A figure depicting the power of a diagnostic test. The ROC curve presents the test's true-positive rate (i.e., sensitivity) on the vertical axis and the false-positive rate (i.e., specificity) on the horizontal axis for different cut points dividing a positive from a negative test. An ROC curve for a perfect test has an area under the curve equal to 1.0, while a test that performs no better than by chance has an area under the curve of 0.5.[5]

> **Jargon Simplified: Specificity**
> The specificity (or the compliment of the false-positive rate) of a diagnostic test is a measure of the proportion of people who are truly free of a designated disorder who are so identified by the test. The test may consist of, or include, clinical observations.[5]

> **Jargon Simplified: Sensitivity**
> The sensitivity (or true-positive rate) of a diagnostic test is a measure of the proportion of people who truly have a designated disorder who are so identified by the test. The test may consist of, or include, clinical observations.[5]

Specificity and sensitivity are often multiplied by 100 and expressed as percentages, as the axes labels in **Fig. 19.1c**.

Editing and Programming

All programs and systems reviewed in this chapter allow some form of editing of outputted tables and plots; however, not all allow point-and-click plot editing.[6,12] The capability to program the models used and analyses performed in statistical pooling programs can also be very important. Although this capability is likely only desired by statisticians and researchers familiar with macros and programming languages, it is important to note that its presence is generally reserved to statistical programs.[12]

Review of Programs and Systems

Now that you are familiar with some background knowledge on meta-analysis, the remainder of this chapter will provide a review of available high-quality statistical pooling programs and software. From 1990 to 2010, a variety of programs were developed. Initial programs, developed during the 1990s, utilized DOS-based operating systems and were very primitive in design.[12] They exhibited limited meta-analytic ability and over the years have become obsolete. Since 2000, more advanced Windows-based programs have been developed.[6,12] This chapter focuses solely on the most technologically advanced programs, all of which possess a graphical user interface and allow comprehensive meta-analyses to be conducted.[6,12]

Types of Programs and Systems

Free vs. Commercial Programs and Systems

Before the development of high-quality statistical pooling programs and systems, there was a discrepancy in quality between free programs and commercial programs. Free programs tended to be less user-friendly and they had reduced graphical abilities, reduced output quality, and reduced analytic potential.[3] Furthermore, they lacked the user support available in commercial programs.[3] The discrepancy has dissipated since the year 2000, as free programs and systems are becoming increasingly comprehensive. One point to note is that all high-quality programs

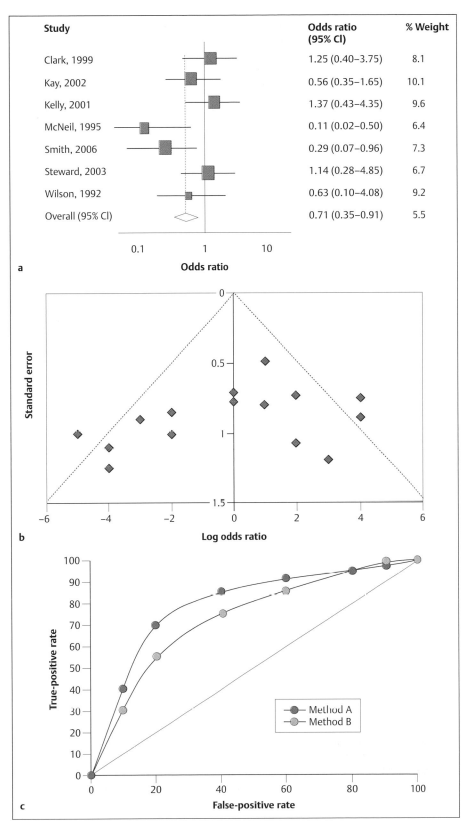

a Forest plot.

b Funnel plot.

c Summary receiver-operating characteristics (SROC) curve.

Fig. 19.1a–c: Examples of outputs from statistical pooling programs and software.
a Forest plot.
b Funnel plot.
c Summary receiver-operating characteristics (SROC) curve.[17]

and systems reviewed in this chapter have been statistically validated with general statistics programs.[6,12]

Meta-analysis-Dedicated Programs vs. Statistical Programs with Meta-analysis Capability

Although most statisticians and some researchers are likely to have a sound background in statistics, a large percentage of clinical researchers do not. They lack the advanced technical skills required to develop macros in statistical programs that are overly command driven. To meet the needs of clinical researchers, menu-driven statistical pooling programs and systems have been developed that are completely dedicated to meta-analysis.[3]

Another focus of the meta-analysis-dedicated programs is on the quality of output.[3] Graphs, tables, and plots are all very important in the publication of findings from meta-analyses, and these programs offer a superior quality to most general statistical programs.

General statistical programs were not initially developed to perform meta-analysis; however, statisticians have created macros in the various command languages to allow basic meta-analyses to be performed by clinical researchers.[6] The benefit of general statistical programs is that they allow capable statisticians to perform virtually any analytical technique available with multiple variations to better suit their needs.[6] Some meta-analysis-dedicated programs have incorporated programming capabilities to increase their analytical sophistication while maintaining the ease of use of the menu-driven format.[6]

Review of High-Quality Statistical Pooling Programs and Systems

The following review of available high-quality statistical pooling programs and systems is derived from a combination of meta-analysis software reviews, program validation literature, and website information. As a result, this review may not be 100% comprehensive, though it should provide sufficient information to aid in your selection of an appropriate program or system. An in-depth comparison of the newest versions of each statistical pooling program is available in **Table 19.1**.

Cochrane Collaboration's Review Manager Version 5.0.24 (RevMan 5.0.24)

The defining feature of RevMan is that it allows its user to complete a full systematic review and meta-analysis in one document once a research question has been determined.[12] RevMan is designed to provide users with extensive features for easy review development that ensures the final product is in the correct format for the Cochrane Collaboration.[12] This format is also applicable to most other journals. However, this feature can also be its downfall if users are looking to conduct a rapid meta-analysis. Rev-

Man requires that individual reviews, along with table types and required comparisons, be completed before data entry and analysis can be performed.[12] Furthermore, RevMan only accepts summary data in two formats (events and sample sizes or means and standard deviations) for effect size calculations, and all data must be entered in the same format.[14] Data in alternative formats must have effect sizes calculated manually. RevMan is also limited in its plotting capabilities and analytical capabilities in comparison to other statistical pooling programs.[14] RevMan is available free of charge at http://www.cc-ims.net/revman and is continually monitored and updated.

Meta-Analyst Version Beta 1.0

Meta-Analyst was reviewed and validated by Wallace et al. in 2009.[6] It was developed with the intent to provide users with the ease of use of dedicated meta-analysis packages and the analytic capabilities offered by general statistical packages. To do this, Meta-Analyst offers a graphical user interface with programming capabilities derived from OpenBUGS statistical software.[6] OpenBUGS also enables Meta-Analyst to perform Bayesian analysis.[6] Furthermore, Wallace et al. realized that there was a void in meta-analysis programs regarding the lack of opportunity to input and perform meta-analysis on diagnostic data.[6] Meta-Analyst does have this capability, but the validation of its ability in this area is limited because of the lack of a suitable reference to compare output results against.[6]

Some distinguishing features of Meta-Analyst include its ability to incorporate multilevel models and perform multivariate analyses, as well as its ability to produce summary receiver-operating characteristics (SROC) curves and bivariate meta-analyses.[6] Meta-Analyst also has multiple options to include covariates and string variables that allow for the introduction of textual descriptions and the ability to specify subgroups for subgroup analyses.[6] Output from Meta-Analyst is highly customizable and able to be exported in a multitude of formats. Another distinguishing feature is Meta-Analyst's lack of tests for publication bias.[6] Although it justifies this omission by citing the lack of reliability in these measures, it is one of the few programs that do not perform this analysis.[6] Meta-Analyst is available free of charge at http://tuftscaes.org/meta_analyst/.

Meta-analysis in Excel (MIX) 2.0

MIX 2.0 is a meta-analysis-dedicated program that was developed as an add-in to Microsoft Excel, gaining access to the calculation and graphics platform of the latter. Its development by Bax et al. in 2006 was spearheaded by a desire to provide an easily accessible and utilizable program for both scientific and learning purposes.[15] The program also incorporates an R/OpenBUGS statistical package to allow for Bayesian analysis and complex meta-analyses without the steep learning curve associated with these programs.[12,15] MIX 2.0 is designed to provide users with the necessary code to input into R or OpenBUGS so that the desired output is achieved.[15] MIX 2.0 also has a data converter which allows it to alter any generic data, such as study estimates with standard errors, into usable data that can be analyzed.[16] From a plotting standpoint, MIX 2.0 in combination with Microsoft Excel produces incomparable vector-based figures that have the highest resolution regardless of size.[16]

MIX 2.0 is available as of May 2010.[16] Two versions will be available for users: MIX 2.0 Lite and MIX 2.0 Pro. The Lite version is currently available at http://www.meta-analysis-made-easy.com/ and is designed solely for teaching purposes.[16] It has most of the features of the Pro version, minus the functionality to create and load data into the program.[16] It will have 30–40 datasets already built in.[16] The Pro version will be available on the same website but will require a licensing fee (see **Table 19.1**). However, it is available free to researchers in developing countries.[16] The MIX website offers a comprehensive learning center with narrated tutorials to guide users through analysis processes. Although it is run through Microsoft Excel, it will not run on current non-Windows Excel programs as they do not have the ribbon interface that is required.[16] MIX 1.7 is free and available online; however, it offers limited meta-analysis capabilities and is no longer being monitored or updated.[16]

Comprehensive Meta-Analysis (CMA) Version 2.0

CMA is a meta-analysis-dedicated program developed by a team of research experts in the United States and the United Kingdom. It allows for over 100 formats of data to be entered and performs most analytical techniques found in general statistical programs.[14] It has multiple functions for assessing publication bias in addition to funnel plots.[14] As of July 2010, it is also in the process of developing advanced support and documentation on the website.[14]

Some notable omissions in its analytic capabilities include Bayesian analysis, multivariate analysis, and the ability to produce SROC curves and bivariate meta-analysis.[14] CMA is available for purchase from its website http://meta-analysis.com/index.html. The cost for licensure varies from US$195 per year for students to US$1295 per year for corporations.[14]

Stata/WinBUGS

Stata is a general statistical program that utilizes programming command language to perform virtually any analysis desired.[6] It is usually paired with WinBUGS to perform Bayesian analysis.[6] Stata is available for purchase at www.stata.com.

Recommendations

The final decision on which statistical pooling program to use for your meta-analysis will ultimately be one of personal preference. As these programs continue to improve, the similarities in their capabilities become uncanny. It is recommended that you consult with colleagues, experienced researchers, and statisticians who have experience with these programs and are able to provide insight on their preferences. Also, an academic institution to which you are affiliated may have a subscription to one of the programs, which may be worth pursuing. Another important factor in determining which program to use is your level of comfort with the graphical user interface the programs provide. It would be worthwhile to try each of the free meta-analysis programs in **Table 19.1**, to find a program that best suits your preferences.

Another factor to consider is that certain journals may have a preference in terms of which formats they require for tables and figures. Since the programs are not identical in their outputs, it is recommended that you consult with the journal you are pursuing for publication. Lastly, your desire to pay for a program and your ability and desire to utilize macros will likely guide your decision making. For the beginning researcher, it is highly recommended that one of the meta-analysis-dedicated programs be used.

Conclusion

Statistical pooling programs and systems allow meta-analyses to be conducted in an organized and timely manner while producing required output tables and figures for publication. Since 1990, statistical pooling programs have progressively developed into complex systems giving users access to a plethora of validated meta-analytic techniques. They allow users to input a variety of data forms, from binary to diagnostic, and subsequently limit the potential human error that exists when these programs are not used. Unfortunately, these systems are not foolproof. They require a substantial level of understanding of meta-analytic concepts, such as study heterogeneity, publication bias, and statistical models. Accordingly, it is recommended that meta-analyses be conducted in collaboration with experienced researchers and statisticians to maintain the integrity of any conclusions.

The five most common statistical pooling programs and systems were reviewed above. Differences amongst them were pointed out, as were the advantages and disadvantages of each. The overwhelming pattern established was the vast similarity in the capabilities of each program. Each program is able to meet a wide variety of meta-analytic requirements and each is suitable for conducting complete meta-analysis. Main points of difference include: free versus non-free programs; dedicated versus general statistical programs; programming capabilities; operating system requirements; output formats; and the list of statistical models the program is capable of utilizing. However, in the end each program is more than capable of fulfilling the requirements of a researcher conducting a meta-analysis. The final decision on which program to utilize is

Table 19.1 Comparison of statistical pooling programs and systems

	RevMan	Meta-Analyst	MIX	CMA	Stata/WinBUGS
Operating system	Windows, Mac, Linux	Windows	Windows	Windows	Windows, Mac, Linux
Version	5.0.24	Beta 1.0	2.0	2	11
Price in USD	Free	Free	155[a]	195[b]	845[c]
Meta-analysis interface	Dedicated	Dedicated	Dedicated	Dedicated	Dedicated
Data characteristics					
Import data	✓	✓	✓	✓	✓
Binary data	✓	✓	✓	✓	✓
Continuous data	✓	✓	✓	✓	✓
Diagnostic data	✓	✓	✓		✓
Multivariate data		✓	✓		✓
Models					
Single-group	✓[d]	✓	✓	✓	✓
Fixed-effects	✓	✓	✓	✓	✓
Random-effects	✓	✓	✓	✓	✓
Multilevel models		✓			✓
Meta-regression		✓	✓	✓	✓
Random-effects meta-regression		✓	✓		✓
Bayesian models		✓	✓		✓
Alternative analyses					
Subgroup analysis	✓	✓	✓	✓	✓
Publication bias tests	✓		✓	✓	✓
Documentation of methods					
Manual	✓	✓		✓	✓
Online assistance		✓	✓	✓	✓
Plotting capabilities					
Forest plot	✓	✓	✓	✓	✓
Funnel plot	✓	✓	✓	✓	✓
SROC	✓				✓
Bivariate meta-analysis		✓			✓
Leave-one-out sensitivity		✓	✓	✓	✓
Additional plots		✓	✓	✓	✓
Exporting abilities	✓	✓	✓	✓	✓
Exporting formats	RevMan	PDF, RTF, Image files	Excel, PowerPoint, PDF	RTF, PowerPoint	RTF
Point-and-click plot editing		✓	✓		✓
Programming capabilities		✓	✓		✓
Up-to-date website	✓	✓	✓	✓	✓

Adapted from Wallace et al.[6] and updated using information from Bax, Bax et al., and Biostat.[12,14,16]

✓, feature is present;, feature is absent; RTF, rich text format (applicable to MS Word); PDF, portable document format; SROC, summary receiver-operating characteristics.

[a] Academic licensure.

[b] Educational licensure of CMA. Rates vary.

[c] Price for standard Stata IC program. Rates vary depending on the model chosen.

[d] Single-group analysis is available for continuous outcomes.

primarily a decision based on preference, familiarity, and the desire to pay for the software.

Suggested Reading

Bax L, Yu LM, Ikeda N, Moons KGM. A systematic comparison of software dedicated to meta-analysis of causal studies. BMC Med Res Methodol 2007;7:40

Hedges LV, Olkin I. Statistical methods for meta-analysis. Orlando, FL: Academic Press; 1985

Sterne JAC, Egger M, Sutton AJ. Meta-analysis software. In: Systematic Reviews in Health Care: Meta-analysis in Context. 2nd ed. BMJ Publishing Group; 2001

Wallace CW, Schmid CH, Lau J, Trikalinos TA. Meta-Analyst: software for meta-analysis of binary, continuous and diagnostic data. BMC Med Res Methodol 2009;9:80

References

1. Hedges LV, Olkin I. Statistical methods for meta-analysis. Orlando, FL: Academic Press; 1985
2. Panesar SS, Bhandari M, Darzi A, Athanasiou T. Meta-analysis: A practical decision making tool for surgeons. Int J Surg 2009;7:291–296
3. Sterne JAC, Egger M, Sutton AJ. Meta-analysis software. In: Systematic Reviews in Health Care: Meta-analysis in Context. 2nd ed. BMJ Publishing Group; 2001
4. Samartzis D, Perera R. Meta-analysis: statistical methods for binary data pooling. Spine J 2009;9:424–425
5. Guyatt G, Rennie D. Glossary. In: Users' Guides to the Medical Literature: A Manual for Evidence-Based Clinical Practice. 2nd ed. (JAMA and Archives Journals.) American Medical Association Press; 2008
6. Wallace CW, Schmid CH, Lau J, Trikalinos TA. Meta-Analyst: software for meta-analysis of binary, continuous and diagnostic data. BMC Med Res Methodol 2009;9:80
7. Simunovic N, Sprague S, Bhandari M. Methodological issues in systematic reviews and meta-analyses of observational studies in orthopaedic research. J Bone Joint Surg Am 2009;91(Suppl 3):87–94.
8. Cucherat M, Boissel JP, Leizorovicz A, Haugh MC. EasyMA: a program for the meta-analysis of clinical trials. Comput Methods Programs Biomed 1997;50:187–190
9. Ionnidis JP, Trikalinos TA. The appropriateness of asymmetry tests for publication bias in meta-analyses: a large survey. Can Med Assoc J 2007;176:1091–1096
10. Lau J, Ioannidis JP, Terrin N, Schmid CH, Olkin I. The case of the misleading funnel plot. BMJ 2006;333:597–600
11. Terrin N, Schmid CH, Lau J. In an empirical evaluation of the funnel plot, researchers could not visually identify publication bias. J Clin Epidemiol 2005;58:894–901
12. Bax L, Yu LM, Ikeda N, Moons KGM. A systematic comparison of software dedicated to meta-analysis of causal studies. BMC Med Res Methodol 2007;7:40
13. Dixon E, Hameed M, Sutherland F, Cook DJ, Doig C. Evaluating meta-analyses in the general surgical literature: a critical appraisal. Ann Surg 2005;241:450–459
14. Biostat. Comprehensive Meta-Analysis. http://www.meta-analysis.com. Accessed April 20, 2010.
15. Bax L, Yu LM, Ikeda N, Tsuruta H, Moons KGM. Development and validation of MIX: comprehensive free software for meta-analysis of causal research data. BMC Med Res Methodol 2006;6:50
16. Bax L. Meta-analysis made easy: MIX 2.0. http://www.meta-analysis-made-easy.com/. Accessed April 20, 2010
17. Krester A, Buntinx F. Meta-analysis of ROC curves. Med Decis Making 2000;20:430–439

20

Meta-analysis of Observational Studies

Nicole Simunovic, Sheila Sprague, Mohit Bhandari

Summary

Meta-analyses of observational studies play an important role in assembling large sample sizes for practical investigation of research questions concerning etiology, prognosis, and estimates of potential risks or harms of treatment. Due to the potential for primary study confounding and bias, reviewers conducting meta-analyses of nonrandomized studies should include the best evidence available for their research question, evaluate whether it is appropriate to combine the resulting study data, and when pooling is deemed appropriate, explore predefined sources of heterogeneity and control for confounding variables whenever possible.

Introduction

Systematic reviews provide comprehensive summaries of studies containing data relevant to a well-defined research question. Compared to narrative reviews, the conduct of systematic reviews requires additional methodological rigor. This allows for the systematic inspection of differences and similarities of the results found in different settings, the formulation of hypotheses, and, ultimately, the identification of the need for future studies.[1]

Every systematic review should start with a protocol written in advance that is centered on a researchable, focused, and clinically relevant question that clearly describes the population, intervention or exposure, comparison group, and outcome(s) of interest.[2] It is important to define the study eligibility criteria prior to a comprehensive search in order to avoid preferential selection of articles. Studies are then selected and data extracted in a reproducible and objective manner. If appropriate, the assembled data may be statistically pooled to derive quantitative estimates of the magnitude of treatment effects and their associated precision using a meta-analysis. Therefore, while every meta-analysis is based on an underlying systematic review, not every systematic review may contingently include a meta-analysis.

Other chapters in this textbook describe the process for conducting systematic reviews of randomized trial data (Chapters 14–19). The methods of assembling systematic review data, including the search for articles, application of the eligibility criteria, and data extraction, are standard irrespective of the design of the included studies. In this section, we address the methods, advantages, and limitations of conducting a meta-analysis of observational studies at the final stage of a systematic review in the context of orthopaedic research.

The Observational Data Dilemma

No Matter How You Slice It, It's Still Baloney

There is nothing you can do to produce good-quality information through a meta-analysis of poor-quality study data. No matter how you extract treatment effect estimates, statistically combine, or explore potential sources of heterogeneity, if the study pool is confounded, biased, and/or incomplete, the meta-analysis results will remain just that—baloney. The meta-analysis of randomized trials is based on the assumption that each trial provides an unbiased estimate of treatment effect, "with the variability of the results between studies being attributed to random variation."[1] The overall effect calculated from a group of sensibly combined and representative randomized trials will provide an unbiased estimate of the treatment effect with adequate precision.[1] In the case of observational studies, however, estimates of association may deviate from true underlying relationships beyond that expected by chance, and therefore, beyond the reach of the meta-analytic method. This may be due to the effects of confounding, bias, or both.[1]

> ### Jargon Simplified: Confounding Bias
> A confounding factor is one that is associated with the outcome of interest and is differentially distributed in patients exposed and those who are unexposed to the outcome of interest.[3]

While it is necessary to use the best available evidence for any systematic review in order to avoid biased estimates of effect, in some cases, for ethical, feasibility, and applicability reasons, observational studies may represent the highest form of evidence in the literature.[2] In fact, many important questions cannot be answered by a randomized trial. For example, etiologic research, where patients do or do not have a particular condition—for example, in a study on the effect of bone mineral density on fracture risk or the incidence of falls—is not amenable to randomization. Incidence studies, such as one determining the rate of meniscal tears associated with tibial plateau fractures, may best be pursued using a prospective cohort study.[4]

Thus, a comprehensive summary and analysis of this literature can help to inform clinical practice and, in some cases, define the need for further research to definitively answer the research question. However, given the potential for bias and confounding, meta-analyses of observational studies require rigorous and systematic compilation, analysis, and interpretation.

Meta-analysis of Observational Data: Process and Recommendations

As has been previously mentioned, the summary of information contained in a systematic review may or may not be quantitative. The advantage of implementing a meta-analysis is that, compared with the results of individual studies, pooled results can increase statistical power and lead to a more precise estimate of treatment effect.[2,5] Data are generally pooled using a forest plot under one of two common statistical models: (1) the fixed-effects model, and (2) the random-effects model. Both models are described in greater detail in Chapter 16. Briefly, the fixed-effects model assumes that the true effect of a treatment is the same for every eligible study.[5,6] The random-effects model assumes that an effect may in fact vary across studies due to differences between studies.[6] Due to the increased potential for unknown or unmeasured variability among observational studies, the random-effects model is the most conservative and therefore the preferable choice for observational data pooling.[2]

> **Jargon Simplified: Forest Plot**
> A forest plot is a graphical diagram depicting the relative strength of treatment effects in multiple studies with minimal heterogeneity. An example of a forest plot is shown in **Fig. 20.1**.

The decision to actually pool study data (Chapter 19) must be considered at three stages in the review process. First and foremost at the protocol development stage, reviewers should consider whether the research question and eligibility criteria will likely result in a group of studies that may be reasonably combined to form a single summary estimate. For example, in a review examining osteoporosis prevention, combining education, policy, and drug-related interventions would result in a meaningless and convoluted pooled estimate because each method is expected to have a differential effect on the prevalence of the disease.[2] However, a reviewer could plan to perform more than one meta-analysis for this question and group study data related to the same intervention and outcome.

Second, reviewers should evaluate if it is likely that the results can be pooled following data extraction before any analysis. Given that it is difficult to predict the available studies and how they were conducted for a particular

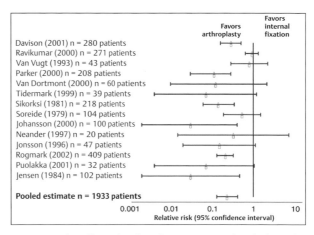

Fig. 20.1 The effect of arthroplasty compared with that of internal fixation on revision rates associated with displaced fractures of the femoral neck. Reproduced with permission from Bhandari et al., p. 1678.[12]

research question, by first examining the treatment or exposure patient groups and outcomes that it was possible to extract, reviewers prevent data-driven analyses. This means that the decision to pool study data is based only on a reviewer's decision that it is reasonable and meaningful to do so, and not because of an observed pattern of effect, likely due to chance. Montori et al. note that as long as the reviewer is "determining the best estimate of the same underlying truth that all of the studies being pooled are trying to measure," there should be no hesitation to pool the study results.[7]

Lastly, at the data-analysis stage, reviewers should determine if it is reasonable to present the pooled study estimate based on statistical tests that can quantify the amount of heterogeneity between individual study estimates. Formal tests of heterogeneity include the Cochran chi-square test (Cochran Q) and the I^2 statistic. While the Cochran Q statistic tests for heterogeneity at a predefined threshold of significance, the I^2 shows the proportion of variability across studies that can be attributed to heterogeneity rather than to sampling error or chance.[2,8,9] Any test for heterogeneity is generally underpowered, meaning that it is more likely to show statistically significant heterogeneity when none exists. Some argue that clinical and methodological diversity will occur in any meta-analysis,[10] especially with observational study data, due to the increased chance of confounding and selection bias. Therefore, testing for the presence or absence of between-study variability based on a statistically significant or nonsignificant P value for a given threshold of significance, such as Cochran's Q, may not be relevant. Instead, the I^2 statistic can quantify inconsistency across studies. Rough guidelines state that an I^2 greater than 25% is considered to indicate low heterogeneity, 50% moderate heterogeneity, and 75% high heterogeneity.[6] The importance of the observed value of I^2 depends on (1) the magnitude and direction (positive or negative) of the effects, and (2) the strength of evidence for heterogeneity (i.e., how wide or narrow the confidence intervals are for a given pooled final estimate).[10]

Key Concepts: Heterogeneity

- Clinical heterogeneity: Differences between studies in the patient population (old–young, ill–mildly ill, gender, patients who have had previous surgery) or treatment under investigation (duration of treatment, intensity, dosage, surgical technique), countries in which the studies were conducted, outcome definitions, and so on
- Statistical heterogeneity: More variation among primary studies expected than by chance alone
- First, you evaluate possible sources of clinical heterogeneity and then you check with a statistical test to confirm your ideas were correct.[11]

Jargon Simplified: Selection Bias

Selection bias occurs when the study and control group subjects differ in the distribution of factors that might affect a given outcome of interest. These factors may be unknown or unmeasurable (e.g., motivation). Selection bias can only be controlled by random allocation into treatment groups such that each subject (with known and unknown characteristics) has an equal chance of being in either treatment group.

Reality Check: Forest Plot

Take the example of a meta-analysis conducted by Bhandari et al. which compares internal fixation and arthroplasty for the treatment of femoral neck fractures.[12] The forest plots (**Figs. 20.1, 20.2**) show the point estimates of the individual primary studies and the pooled overall effect size described as a relative risk. In the case of the revision surgery outcome (**Fig. 20.1**), note that the confidence intervals of the primary studies generally overlap and each point estimate lies to the same side of the null (i.e., favoring arthroplasty). Although

the confidence intervals of the final pooled estimate are somewhat wide, moderate heterogeneity may not preclude combining the study data here. For the mortality outcome (**Fig. 20.2**), the primary study point estimates lie on either side of the null with no clear direction, but the confidence intervals of the primary studies are not as wide as those for the revision surgery outcome. In this case, the confidence intervals of the pooled estimate are narrow and likely precise in showing no statistically significant effect of the surgical treatments on mortality rates. Both plots demonstrate conditions where it is reasonable and likely accurate to present pooled study data with low to moderate heterogeneity. Of course, reviewers should still explore potential sources of heterogeneity as per the original protocol.

Again, to prevent unsystematic data dredging, reviewers should present all potential sources of heterogeneity and maintain their plan to evaluate these subgroups of patients, interventions, exposures, and/or outcomes from the initial protocol. Further, if heterogeneity remains unexplained, reviewers should alert readers to these inconsistencies in order to prevent misleading conclusions.

A Hierarchy within a Hierarchy: Types of Observational Data

Although some studies have shown that well-done observational studies produce estimates of effect similar to those of randomized controlled trials,[13–15] many argue that poorly done observational studies can systematically overestimate the magnitude of the treatment effect and are therefore less valid than randomized controlled trials.[1] However, high-quality observational studies make sense when the outcome is rare, it is unethical to randomize patients, technical expertise is highly varied across groups, and prognostic factors are under study.

In the hierarchy of observational studies, prospective cohort studies remain generally less biased than retrospective studies or case series. Cohort studies deal with two or more cohorts (i.e., a group of individuals identified as having a particular common exposure, risk factor, or treatment) which are followed prospectively and compared for the outcome(s) of interest.[16] By measuring the common exposure, risk factor, or treatment before the outcome, investigators establish a time sequence of events, which prevents investigator influence due to knowledge of the outcome(s) under study. This is especially true for subjective outcomes such as time to fracture healing. The prospective approach also allows investigators to measure multiple exposures and events more completely and accurately than is possible retrospectively.[17]

A retrospective case–control study compares a group of individuals who have already experienced a particular outcome with a matched group of control patients who are similar to the study patients with respect to important

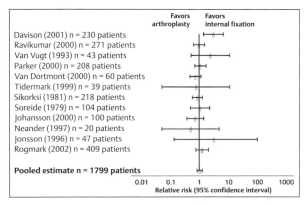

Fig. 20.2 The effect of arthroplasty compared with that of internal fixation on mortality associated with displaced fractures of the femoral neck. Reproduced with permission from Bhandari et al., p. 1678.[12]

known risk factors, but have not experienced the study outcome.[16] Both groups are then examined for any associations between the unmatched variable and the outcome. The retrospective design prevents one from estimating the incidence or prevalence of the outcome and the attributable or excess risk. Further, bias is more likely because such studies usually employ medical records or patient recall, leading to incomplete or incorrect data. An example of recall bias is shown in a study evaluating spinal fusion to treat low back pain.[18] Pellisé et al. found significant differences in patient self-evaluation scale scores when the same patients were asked to recall their preoperative clinical status compared to when they completed the self-evaluation prospectively (prior to treatment).[18]

Case series present clinical observations about a set of patients undergoing the same treatment or experiencing similar outcomes. These studies are retrospective and do not include control groups. Therefore, it is not possible to ascribe the outcomes to a particular treatment that was administered, and in the absence of a control group it is impossible to pool treatment estimates statistically.

Because only the best designed studies may achieve enough safeguards to protect against bias and provide the most reasonable estimate of the true association between exposure and outcome, it is necessary to use the best available evidence for any systematic review.[2] The importance of study design in a meta-analysis of observational studies was shown in a systematic review evaluating in-hospital patient fall risk assessment tools.[19] Simulated application of these tools to retrospective patient chart data was shown to "provide biased and overly optimistic results" compared to prospectively collected data.[19]

On the other hand, an association may be strengthened if the results of high-quality observational studies with differing study designs consistently support the superiority of one treatment over the other.[13] For example, a recent systematic review evaluating the effect of surgical delay on patient mortality found similar benefits of early surgery across both prospective and retrospective studies.[20]

Perhaps the most important consideration when including observational studies in a meta-analysis is whether the estimates of effect are adjusted or unadjusted. As previously stated, observational studies are subject to confounding, bias, or both. Confounding occurs when patients exposed to the factor under investigation differ in other aspects that are relevant to the risk of developing the disease or condition in question.[1] Using the previous example, when examining the effect of surgical delay on elderly patient mortality, a likely contributing factor would be that patients whose surgery is delayed tend to be sicker on admission and are therefore more likely to die than those who undergo immediate surgery. Other factors such as age, gender, and American Society of Anesthesiologists (ASA) classification are also likely to influence mortality risk. It is therefore best to pool studies only after these and other important confounding variables have been controlled or "adjusted" using multivariate logistic regression or proportional hazards models. This would require identifying all key confounders prior to the systematic review and then carefully assessing whether or not these variables were controlled for in the design and/or analysis of the individual included studies. Usually only adjusted effect estimates are then pooled, given the high risk of confounding in unadjusted observational data.

Examples from the Literature:
Adjusted versus Unadjusted Meta-analysis

Indeed, it is not surprising that the results of our adjusted meta-analysis comparing early versus delayed hip fracture surgery were more conservative (relative risk 0.81; 95% confidence interval, 0.68 to 0.96; **Fig. 20.3**) than the unadjusted estimates at 1 year (relative risk 0.55; 95% confidence interval 0.40 to 0.75; **Fig. 20.4**).[21]

Study or subgroup	Log [risk ratio]	SE	Early surgery Total	Delayed surgery Total	Weight	Risk ratio IV, random, 95% CI	Risk ratio IV, random, 95% CI
Zuckerman, 1995^^	−0.42722	0.271849	267	100	10.2%	0.65 [0.38 – 1.11]	
Beringer, 1996	−0.406	0.220283	133	70	15.5%	0.67 [0.43 – 1.03]	
Smektala, 2007	−0.0747	0.127	609	1629	46.7%	0.93 [0.72 – 1.19]	
Orosz, 2004	−0.264	0.173	398	780	25.2%	0.77 [0.55 – 1.08]	
Rae, 2007^	−0.16651	0.569231	137	85	2.3%	0.85 [0.28 – 2.58]	
Total (95% CI)			1544	2664	100.0%	0.81 [0.68 – 0.96]	

Heterogeneity: $\tau^2 = 0.00$; $\chi^2 = 2.67$, $df = 4$ ($P = 0.61$); $I^2 = 0\%$
Test for overall effect: $Z = 2.44$ ($P = 0.01$)

0.1 0.2   0.5   1   2   5   10
Favors early surgery   Favors delayed surgery

Fig. 20.3 Forest plot of adjusted relative risks for the impact of early vs. delayed surgery on all-cause mortality. At a minimum, estimates were adjusted for patient age and pre-existing medical conditions. ^ indicates that the study used a cutoff of 48 hours for delay, and ^^ indicates that the study used a cutoff of 72 hours for delay. For all other studies, a cutoff for delay of 24 hours was used. Diamonds indicate the pooled relative risk estimates. Squares represent point estimates around which 95% confidence intervals are denoted by a horizontal line. CI: confidence interval; "Random": a random-effects model was used to pool the data. Reproduced with permission from Simunovic et al.[21]

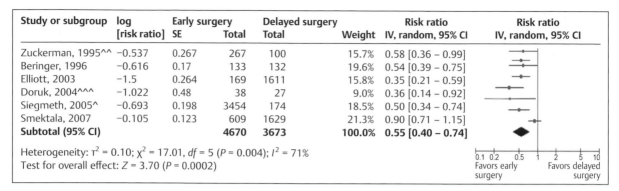

Study or subgroup	log [risk ratio]	Early surgery SE	Total	Delayed surgery Total	Weight	Risk ratio IV, random, 95% CI	Risk ratio IV, random, 95% CI
Zuckerman, 1995^^	−0.537	0.267	267	100	15.7%	0.58 [0.36 – 0.99]	
Beringer, 1996	−0.616	0.17	133	132	19.6%	0.54 [0.39 – 0.75]	
Elliott, 2003	−1.5	0.264	169	1611	15.8%	0.35 [0.21 – 0.59]	
Doruk, 2004^^^	−1.022	0.48	38	27	9.0%	0.36 [0.14 – 0.92]	
Siegmeth, 2005^	−0.693	0.198	3454	174	18.5%	0.50 [0.34 – 0.74]	
Smektala, 2007	−0.105	0.123	609	1629	21.3%	0.90 [0.71 – 1.15]	
Subtotal (95% CI)			**4670**	**3673**	**100.0%**	**0.55 [0.40 – 0.74]**	

Heterogeneity: $\tau^2 = 0.10$; $\chi^2 = 17.01$, $df = 5$ ($P = 0.004$); $I^2 = 71\%$
Test for overall effect: $Z = 3.70$ ($P = 0.0002$)

Fig. 20.4 Forest plot of unadjusted relative risks for the effect of early compared with delayed hip fracture surgery on all-cause mortality. ^ indicates that the study used a cutoff of 48 hours for delay, ^^ indicates that the study used a cutoff of 72 hours for delay, and ^^^ indicates that the study used a cutoff of 5 days for delay. For all other studies, a cutoff for delay of 24 hours was used. Diamonds indicate the pooled relative risk estimates. Squares represent point estimates around which 95% confidence intervals are denoted by a horizontal line. CI: confidence interval; "Random": a random-effects model was used to pool the data. Reproduced with permission from Simunovic et al.[21]

It is also important to note that even with adjustment, residual confounding may still threaten study validity. Therefore, the results of meta-analyses of observational studies must be interpreted cautiously.

> **Jargon Simplified: Residual Confounding**
> Residual confounding arises when a confounding factor cannot be measured with sufficient precision to be quantified for the purposes of statistical adjustment.

Conclusion

Meta-analyses of observational studies play an important role in assembling large sample sizes for practical investigation of research questions concerning etiology, prognosis, and estimates of potential risks or harms of treatment. In fact, in recognition of the importance of systematic reviews of observational studies and the need to improve the quality of reporting in such studies, a checklist was developed by the Meta-analysis Of Observational Studies in Epidemiology (MOOSE) Group.[22] Special care must continue to be exercised for meta-analyses of nonrandomized studies. In particular, reviewers must consider the best evidence available, evaluate whether it is appropriate to combine the resulting study data, and, when pooling is deemed appropriate, explore predefined sources of heterogeneity and control for confounding variables whenever possible.

Suggested Reading

Higgins JPT, Green S. Cochrane Handbook for Systematic Reviews of Interventions. Version 5.0.2 [Updated September 2009]. Available at: http://www.cochrane-handbook.org/. Accessed April 12, 2010

Higgins JP, Thompson SG, Deeks JJ, Altman DG. Measuring inconsistency in meta-analyses. BMJ 2003;327:557–560

Hoppe DJ, Schemitsch EH, Morshed S, Tornetta P III, Bhandari M. Hierarchy of evidence: where observational studies fit in and why we need them. J Bone Joint Surg Am 2009;91:2–9

Simunovic N, Sprague S, Bhandari M. Methodological issues in systematic reviews and meta-analyses of observational studies in orthopaedic research. J Bone Joint Surg Am 2009;91:87–94

Stroup DF, Berlin JA, Morton SC, et al. Meta-analysis of observational studies in epidemiology: a proposal for reporting. Meta-analysis Of Observational Studies in Epidemiology (MOOSE) group. JAMA 2000;283:2008–2012

References

1. Egger M, Schneider M, Davey Smith G. Spurious precision? Meta-analysis of observational studies. BMJ 1998;316:140–144

2. Simunovic N, Sprague S, Bhandari M. Methodological issues in systematic reviews and meta-analyses of observational studies in orthopaedic research. J Bone Joint Surg Am 2009;91:87–94

3. Guyatt GH, Rennie D, Meade M, Cook D, eds. Users' Guide to the Medical Literature: A Manual for Evidence-Based Clinical Practice. 2nd ed. New York: McGraw-Hill; 2008

4. Schemitsch EH, Bhandari M, McKee MD, et al. Orthopaedic surgeons: artists or scientists? J Bone Joint Surg Am 2009;91:1264–1273

5. Lau J, Ioannidis JP, Schmid CH. Quantitative synthesis in systematic reviews. Ann Intern Med 1997;127:820–826

6. Zlowodzki M, Poolman RW, Kerkhoffs GM, Tornetta P 3rd, Bhandari M; International Evidence-Based Orthopedic Surgery Working Group. How to interpret a meta-analysis and judge its value as a guide for clinical practice. Acta Orthop 2007;78:598–609

7. Montori VM, Swiontkowski MF, Cook DJ. Methodologic issues in systematic reviews and meta-analyses. Clin Orthop Relat Res 2003;413:43–54

8. Devereaux PJ, Beattie WS, Choi PTL, et al. How strong is the evidence for the use of perioperative β blockers in non-cardiac surgery? Systematic review and meta-analysis of randomised controlled trials. BMJ 2005;331:313–321

9. Higgins JP, Thompson SG, Deeks JJ, Altman DG. Measuring inconsistency in meta-analyses. BMJ 2003;327:557–560

10. Higgins JPT, Green S. Cochrane Handbook for Systematic Reviews of Interventions. Version 5.0.2 [Updated September 2009]. Available at: http://www.cochrane-handbook.org/. Accessed April 12, 2010

11. Bhandari M, Joensson A. Clinical Research for Surgeons. Stuttgart, Germany: Georg Thieme Verlag; 2009:68–76

12. Bhandari M, Devereaux PJ, Swiontkowski MF, et al. Internal fixation compared with arthroplasty for displaced fractures of the femoral neck: a meta-analysis. J Bone Joint Surg Am 2003;85:1673–1681

13. Shrier I, Boivin JF, Steele RJ, et al. Should meta-analyses of interventions include observational studies in addition to randomized controlled trials? A critical examination of underlying principles. Am J Epidemiol 2007;166:1203–1209

14. Concato J, Shah N, Horwitz RI. Randomized, controlled trials, observational studies, and the hierarchy of research designs. N Engl J Med 2000;342:1887–1892

15. Ferriter M, Huband N. Does the non-randomized controlled study have a place in the systematic review? A pilot study. Crim Behav Ment Health 2005;15:111–120

16. Hoppe DJ, Schemitsch EH, Morshed S, Tornetta P III, Bhandari M. Hierarchy of evidence: where observational studies fit in and why we need them. J Bone Joint Surg Am 2009;91:2–9

17. Hulley SB, Cummings SR, Browner WS, Grady DG, Newman TB. Designing Clinical Research. 3rd ed. Philadelphia, PA: Lippincott Williams and Wilkins; 2007

18. Pellisé F, Vidal X, Hernández A, Cedraschi C, Bagó J, Villanueva C. Reliability of retrospective clinical data to evaluate the effectiveness of lumbar fusion in chronic low back pain. Spine 2005;30:365–368

19. Haines TP, Hill K, Walsh W, Osborne R. Design-related bias in hospital fall risk screening tool predictive accuracy evaluations: systematic review and meta-analysis. J Gerontol 2007;62:664–672

20. Shiga T, Wajima Z, Ohe Y. Is operative delay associated with increased mortality of hip fracture patients? Systematic review, meta-analysis, and meta-regression. Can J Anaesth 2008;55:146–154.

21. Simunovic N, Devereaux PJ, Sprague S, et al. Effect of early surgery following hip fractures reduces mortality and complications: a systematic review and meta-analysis. CMAJ 2010;19;182:1609–1616

22. Stroup DF, Berlin JA, Morton SC, et al. Meta-analysis of observational studies in epidemiology: a proposal for reporting. Meta-analysis Of Observational Studies in Epidemiology (MOOSE) group. JAMA 2000;283:2008–2012

21

Meta-regression

Eleanor M Pullenayegum

Summary

Meta-regression is a tool used in a meta-analysis to investigate factors that are associated with the effectiveness of an intervention, or, equivalently, to investigate sources of between-study heterogeneity. This chapter will provide an overview of the role of meta-regression in exploring heterogeneity, and the basics of how meta-regression is undertaken, looking specifically at descriptive analyses and study weighting. As with all study designs and analytic techniques, meta-regression has important limitations. Findings from a meta-regression are observational rather than causal, and since there is limited scope for including more than one or two variables in a regression model, it is difficult to account adequately for confounding. Unless carefully planned and interpreted, meta-regression can be liable to flag spurious associations due to the temptation to data dredge. However, when used well, meta-regression can help to identify factors associated with increased or decreased effectiveness of an intervention.

Introduction

Meta-regression is a regression analysis of a meta-analysis. Specifically, the effect sizes in each trial are regressed onto some attribute of the trial, for example year of publication, mean age of participants, or drug dose. Meta-regression is thus concerned with explaining between-study variation in effect sizes, that is, with exploring potential effect modifiers. At the simplest level, a meta-regression can formalize a subgroup analysis: instead of simply analyzing the results separately in each subgroup, we could instead ask whether subgroup is an important predictor of effect size. By entering subgroup as a predictor into a regression model, we can test whether there is a statistical difference between the pooled effects in each subgroup.

Jargon Simplified: Meta-regression

When summarizing patient or design characteristics at the individual trial level, meta-analysts risk failing to detect genuine relationships between these characteristics and the size of the treatment effect. Further, the risk of obtaining a spurious explanation for variable treatment effects is high when the number of trials is small and many patient and design characteristics differ. Meta-regression techniques can be used to explore whether patient characteristics (e.g., younger or older patients) or design characteristics (e.g., studies of low or high quality) are related to the size of the treatment effect.[1]

Examples from the Literature:
Examining Heterogeneity in Meta-analysis

Furlan et al. explore the sources of heterogeneity in a meta-analysis of interventions for low back pain.[2] In a comparison of surgery versus conservative treatments, they found an overall odds ratio of 2.18 (95% CI 1.52–3.12) in favor of surgery. Important predictors of the strength of the effect were study type [ratio of odds ratios (ROR) 3.93; 95% CI 2.14–7.24; $P < 0.001$, for randomized versus nonrandomized studies] and the percentage of patients with worker's compensation (ratio of odds ratios 0.27; 95% CI 0.15–0.50; $P < 0.001$); diagnosis was not statistically significantly associated with effect size (ROR 1.00; 95% CI 0.48–2.07; $P = 0.994$ for disc herniation versus degenerative disease).

There are several questions we might ask at this point. How, amongst the many possible factors that could be considered, were these three chosen? How does one go about fitting a meta-regression? What is a ratio of odds ratios? Is this a direct output of the meta-regression, or must it be calculated? How should these results be interpreted?

This chapter provides an overview of answers to these questions in the general scenario, drawing on specific examples when needed. We shall first look further at heterogeneity and discuss how it is measured, then turn to how a meta-regression might be carried out in practice, consider what the limitations of a meta-regression are, and, finally, turn to how to interpret the findings of a meta-regression.

Heterogeneity and Meta-regression

Meta-regression can serve a number of purposes. Underlying all of them is an exploration of heterogeneity. Heterogeneity can be present as clinical heterogeneity (e.g., differences between study populations, study types, implementation of interventions, or measurement of outcome), or as statistical heterogeneity (i.e., variation in the effectiveness of the intervention across studies). Since clinical heterogeneity will usually lead to statistical heterogeneity, and conversely the presence of statistical heterogeneity is often an indicator of clinical heterogeneity, it has been argued that sources of clinical heterogeneity should be investigated as sources of statistical heterogeneity. This can, for example, help to identify subgroups of patients in whom the intervention is more or less effective.[3]

There are various measures of statistical heterogeneity, the most popular of which is the I^2, which quantifies the proportion of variation in the study-level effect sizes that can be attributed to between-study variation rather than to within-study variation.[4] Part of the I^2's popularity is due to its ease of interpretation. The drawback, however, is that the I^2 is related to study size; in fact, as the sizes of the included studies increase whilst the between-study variability remains the same, the I^2 will increase.[5] For this reason, it has recently been observed that the I^2 should not be interpreted in isolation, but should rather be presented alongside an estimate of the between-study variation itself (usually denoted τ^2). There are also tests of heterogeneity, which test the null hypothesis that the between-study variability (τ^2) is equal to zero; however, these should be interpreted with caution because, as with all hypothesis tests, the P value is as much a function of the amount of data as it is of any genuine effect.[6] In many circumstances, a test of heterogeneity will lack power and hence return a nonsignificant P value even when important heterogeneity is present; in contrast, in meta-analyses including many studies the test for heterogeneity may have excessive power and hence return a highly significant P value even when the degree of heterogeneity is unimportant.

Jargon Simplified: Heterogeneity
Heterogeneity means differences among individual studies included in a systematic review. Typically it refers to study results, but the term can also be applied to other study characteristics.[1]

Jargon Simplified: I^2
The I^2 statistic is a measure of heterogeneity. Specifically, the I^2 measures the proportion of variability in the observed effect sizes that is due to variability between studies.

There are thus two main purposes that meta-regression can serve. It may be an exploratory hypothesis-generating analysis of heterogeneity in the data, or it may be an attempt to answer an existing question about effect modifiers. For example, Furlan et al. ask a priori whether randomized and nonrandomized studies of interventions for low back pain give different estimates of treatment efficacy.[2]

Meta-regression Mechanics

At the simplest level, meta-regression involves a regression of the study-specific treatment effects onto one or more study-level covariates. This can be done both for continuous outcomes and for binary outcomes; however, since the latter are by far the most common, we shall restrict our discussion to these. For simplicity, we shall focus on odds ratios, although the methods described can also be used for relative risks. The unit of analysis in a meta-regression is the study: thus, if the meta-analysis includes ten studies, we would have ten rows in our meta-regression dataset. The dependent variable in the meta-regressions we shall discuss is the log odds ratio.

As in most statistical analyses, it is usually wise to begin with some graphs to gain an understanding of the data. The relationship between the effect size and the covariate should ideally be presented visually. For a categorical covariate this can be done through the forest plot, as seen in **Fig. 21.1**. With a continuous covariate the forest plot does not easily capture the nature of any association, and it is instead recommended that the effect size be plotted versus the covariate value for each study, with the size of

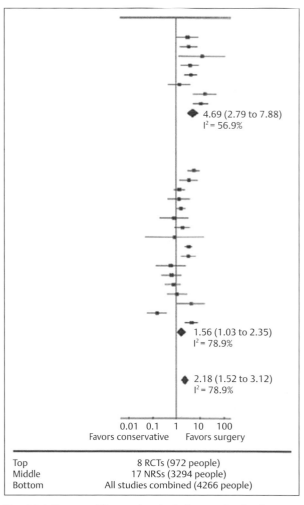

	4.69 (2.79 to 7.88) I^2 = 56.9%
	1.56 (1.03 to 2.35) I^2 = 78.9%
	2.18 (1.52 to 3.12) I^2 = 78.9%

0.01 0.1   1   10   100
Favors conservative   Favors surgery

Top	8 RCTs (972 people)
Middle	17 NRSs (3294 people)
Bottom	All studies combined (4266 people)

Fig. 21.1 Extract of forest plot depicting randomized controlled studies (RCTs) versus nonrandomized studies (NRSs) investigating surgery versus conservative treatment for the management of low back pain. Reproduced with permission from Furlan et al.[2]

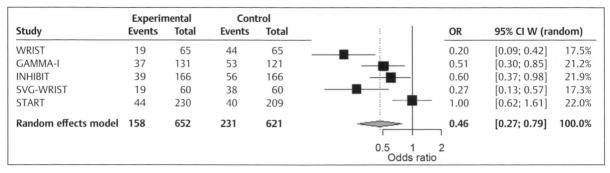

Fig. 21.2 Forest plot of meta-analysis of Uchida et al.[7] CI, confidence interval; W, weight.

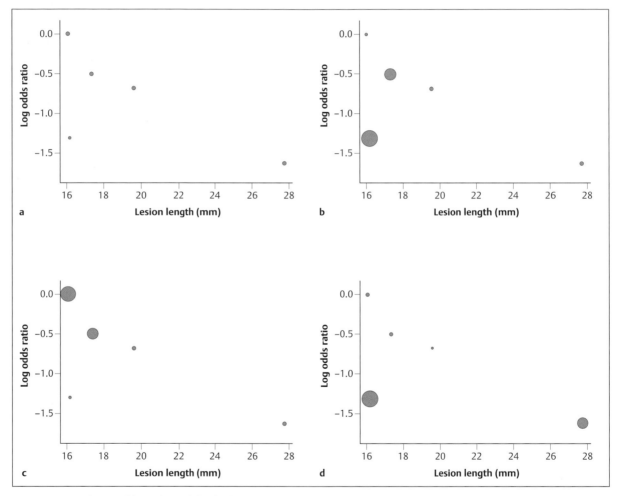

Fig. 21.3 Actual (**a**) and hypothetical (**b–d**) plots of effect size (log odds ratio) vs. lesion length in the meta-analysis of Uchida et al.[7] The size of the points is proportional to the weight the study receives in the meta-regression. Notice how the weight received by each study impacts the visual impression of the relationship between effect size and lesion length.

the plotting character proportional to the weight of the study in the meta-regression. This type of plot, known as a L'Abbé plot, gives a much clearer presentation of which studies are influential than a plot without information on weighting. Consider, for example, a meta-analysis by Uchida et al. on intracoronary beta- and gamma-radiation therapy for in-stent restenosis,[7] a forest plot of which ap-

pears in **Fig. 21.2**. Here the primary outcome is the occurrence of a major adverse cardiac event, and this is compared amongst five studies for brachytherapy versus placebo. **Figure 21.3** shows a plot of the study-specific estimate of the log odds ratio versus the lesion length, using the actual study weights, which in this case are very similar to one another. Compare, however, the different messages that would be implied had the study weights been different, in **Fig. 21.3b–d**. For this reason, visual presentation of the results should include information on the study weights in order to give a clear impression of the underlying associations.

> **Examples from the Literature:**
> **A Meta-analysis of Randomized Controlled Trials of Intracoronary Gamma- and Beta-Radiation Therapy for In-Stent Restenosis**
> Uchida et al. report a meta-analysis of the effects of beta- and gamma-radiation therapy for in-stent restenosis.[7] In a meta-regression, they regress effectiveness onto lesion length. For an illustration of the importance of accounting for study size, see **Fig. 21.3**.

> **Jargon Simplified: L'Abbé Plot**
> The L'Abbé plot is a plot of study-level effect size versus a continuous study-level covariate, in which the size of the plotting symbol is proportional to the weight received by the study in the analysis.

After some initial data exploration, formal analysis can begin. One of the important mechanics of implementing a meta-regression is the need to weight studies. That is, it would be a mistake simply to regress the log odds ratios from each study onto the covariates, since this would not account for study size. In such an unweighted analysis, a study of 10 000 patients would carry the same weight as a study of 100 patients—clearly not a desirable feature. The weights used in a meta-regression should be the inverse of the within trial plus the residual between-trial variance. The residual between-trial variance is the variability between trials after accounting for the between-trial covariates, and acknowledges that the meta-regression may not explain all the heterogeneity. Including this residual variance in the meta-regression weights amounts to conducting a random-effects meta-regression as opposed to a fixed-effects meta-regression; a similar concept to random- versus fixed-effects meta-analysis. Random-effects meta-regression is preferred over fixed-effects meta-regression as it better controls the type I error rate.

> **Jargon Simplified: Random-Effects Analysis**
> Random-effects analysis is a method of pooling or meta-regression that allows for unexplained variability in effect sizes among studies.

> **Jargon Simplified: Fixed-Effects Analysis**
> Fixed-effects analysis is a method of pooling or meta-regression that assumes that all the variability in effect sizes among studies has been accounted for.

Although meta-regression is an exploration of between-study heterogeneity, it is still meaningful when Cochran's Q test is not significant, or if the I^2 is zero. Cochran's Q test may be nonsignificant due to lack of power, and the point estimate for the I^2 is just that: an estimate. Just because it is zero does not exclude the possibility of important heterogeneity amongst the studies. Moreover, even in the event of an I^2 estimate of zero or a nonsignificant test result for heterogeneity, the random-effect weights should still be used in the meta-regression.[8]

Meta-regression can handle many different types of covariates. Binary study-level covariates, for example study type or blinding, can be incorporated through the use of dummy variables as in a linear regression. Continuous study-level covariates, for example year of publication, can be incorporated just as they are. Covariates that are binary at the individual patient level, for example gender, are usually incorporated as the study-specific percentages. Thus, if a study population was 55% male, the gender covariate for that study would be 0.55. Similarly, covariates that are continuous at the individual patient level are usually incorporated as study-level means, or as medians in the case of very skew covariates. For example, age would typically be incorporated as the mean age of patients in each study. Meta-regression will tend to work best when the characteristic of interest has a lot of variability between trials, specifically when the variability between trials is large compared to the variability within trials. If the characteristic of interest does not vary much between trials, then there is little scope for meta-regression to explain between-trial heterogeneity.

One type of covariate that must be handled with caution is control group event rates, i.e., the prevalence of the outcome in the control group. The issue with control group event rates is that the sampling error in the dependent variable in the regression (the log odds ratio) is correlated with the sampling error in the covariate (control event rate), and this association must be correctly accounted for in the analysis. Traditional meta-regression methods ignore the sampling error in the covariate, resulting in misleading results in the case where the two sampling errors are correlated. The most common method for exploring the relationship between treatment effect and event rates is through a Bayesian analysis, an example of which is given in Talati et al.[9]

Interpreting a Meta-regression

The output of a meta-regression is a statement about the extent to which the covariate of interest modifies the treatment efficacy. Thus, the most helpful way to report the association when the outcome of interest is binary will be a ratio of odds ratios (ROR), or, less commonly, a ratio of relative risks (RRR). For example, Furlan et al. report an ROR of 3.93 (95% CI 2.14–7.24) for randomized versus nonrandomized studies comparing the effectiveness of surgery versus conservative treatments for low back pain.[2] This means that the odds ratio is almost four times as high for randomized studies as compared to nonrandomized studies. Note, however, that there is a wide confidence interval, ranging from two to seven, as will be typical of such interaction terms. Many meta-regressions will, however, simply be reported as a regression coefficient, often unhelpfully referred to as a β-coefficient (simply because this is how statisticians choose to write down their equations). Provided that the summary measure is an odds ratio, this can be translated into an ROR by exponentiating (to base e). For example, Furlan et al. would have had a regression coefficient of 1.37 for study type, which can be exponentiated to derive the ROR: $e^{1.37}$ = 3.93. Importantly, confidence intervals for the ROR need to be derived first for the regression coefficient, and then exponentiated. In our example, the regression coefficient of 1.37 would have had an associated standard error of 0.31. A 95% CI for the regression coefficient is then given by 1.37–1.96 × 0.31 to 1.37+1.96 × 0.31, i.e., 0.76 to 1.98. On taking exponentials, we have the confidence interval for the ROR: $e^{0.76}$ = 2.14 and $e^{1.98}$ = 7.24. Note that this is not the same thing as exponentiating the coefficient, exponentiating the standard error, and then taking the exponentiated coefficient ±1.96 times the exponentiated standard error, a procedure which would give a flawed, and possibly nonsensical, confidence interval.

Reality Check

Furlan et al. report an ROR of 3.93 (95% CI 2.14–7.24) for randomized as compared to nonrandomized studies in their study of surgical versus conservative management of low back pain. This means that randomized studies have odds ratios that are roughly four times as large as the odds ratios from nonrandomized studies, and that we can be fairly confident that this ratio is no smaller than 2 and no larger than 7. Since in this case an odds ratio that is greater than 1 favors surgery, this means that randomized studies are showing more favorable results than nonrandomized studies.

One explanation for this finding is that observational studies are more susceptible to bias. For example, it may be the case that in observational studies it was the patients with most severe pain who received surgery, and that the confounding variables adjusted for in the study-level analyses did not adequately capture this selection effect.

There are, however, alternative explanations, for example that surgical interventions were implemented better, with better follow-up, in the randomized trials, or that the inclusion/exclusion criteria in the trials were such that the population studied was a selected group who were most likely to do well with surgery.

The meta-regression does not tell us which of these explanations for the association is correct; it simply tells us that the association exists.

There are two vital points to keep in mind when interpreting the findings of a meta-regression. Firstly, meta-regression yields information about observational associations rather than causal relationships, even if the component studies are randomized trials. This is because randomized trials provide causal inference only with respect to the factor that is randomized, which will be the treatment or intervention; all the other associations remain observational.

Key Concepts: Association Not Causation

The regression coefficients from a meta-regression represent observational associations, not causal relationships!

Secondly, any meta-regression associations represent between-trial associations rather than within-trial associations, a point that is particularly important for meta-regression covariates that are patient averages. To illustrate the difference, consider **Fig. 21.4**. The within-trial associations in the left-hand panel suggest effect modification, but this is masked once the mean effect sizes are compared to

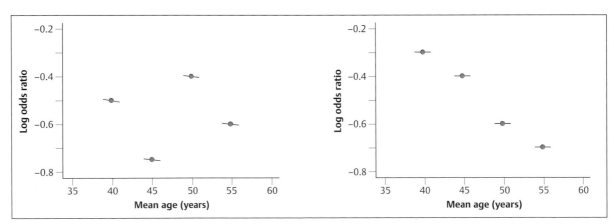

Fig. 21.4 Hypothetical relationships between effect size and mean age in a meta-regression. Each point represents one study, and the line through each point represents the relationship between effect size and age within each study. Thus in the left-hand panel there is a relationship between age and effect size within each study, which would be missed in a meta-regression, whereas in the right-hand panel a meta-regression would reveal a relationship between effect size and mean age where no genuine relationship was present.

the mean covariate value. Conversely, there may be little within-trial association, but once averages are compared, an association emerges.

The ideal method for assessing this type of relationship is of course a meta-regression based on individual-level patient data. In this analysis, patient-level data including treatment assignment, the outcome of interest, and any relevant covariates are retrieved from the authors of each included study and then pooled, typically using a hierarchical model to account for study-level variation. The advantages of this approach are numerous: it allows for investigation of within-trial associations whilst allowing for between-trial variability; there is greater power to detect effect modifiers, which individual studies are usually too small to detect (studies are usually powered on the basis of between-group comparison on the primary outcome only); and the number of observational units will often be in the thousands, allowing for far more extensive and robust regression analysis as compared to using study-level summaries, which will typically include 10 or fewer studies. See Simmonds et al. for a review of methods for individual patient data meta-analysis.[10]

Limitations of Meta-regression

Conceptually, meta-regression can be problematic. Ideally, the covariates to be included in a meta-regression should be specified a priori to avoid the possibility of bias or data dredging. The reason is as follows: suppose we have just two studies in our meta-analysis and substantial heterogeneity. Then any covariate that differs substantially between the two studies will be an important predictor of effect size. Similarly, suppose we have five studies, four of which are relatively homogeneous and one which shows quite different results. Then as long as we can find one covariate that differs substantially between the four homogeneous studies and the one outlying study, we will have a good chance of a significant meta-regression, irrespective of whether that covariate was important or not. However, prespecification is very rarely done.[11] Moreover, in many cases the choice of covariates to be included will be prompted by associations noticed amongst existing trials, i.e., in the data to be included in the meta-analysis, which does not avoid the problem of bias.

One counterargument to the call for prespecification of meta-regression covariates is that the results of the meta-regression are intended to be exploratory and hence hypothesis-generating. However, by the time a meta-analysis has been done, often the totality of the evidence will already have been gathered—there will often be no intent to do further trials—and hence no occasion to verify the exploratory hypotheses.

Furlan et al. describe an example of successful prespecification.[2] They first conducted a literature review to identify potential effect modifiers, and through the published literature identified 44 experts. The resulting list of 55 factors was then sent to the 44 experts, who were asked to identify the ten most important factors in explaining variability in intervention efficacy. The number of experts choosing each factor was then used to rank the factors. Since the number of studies included in the meta-analysis was limited, the top three factors were included in the meta-regression.

> **Key Concepts: Number of Covariates**
> Because most meta-analyses include relatively few studies (often ten or fewer), there will be limited scope to include more than one or two factors in a meta-regression model.

Some practical considerations of meta-regression also deserve attention. Associations between the log effect size and the covariate are usually assumed to be linear, without any verification. For example, why would it be a good assumption that the log odds ratio increases linearly for each additional year of mean age? Moreover, there is usually limited ability to include more than one covariate in the regression. Typically a meta-analysis contains between 5 and 10 studies; analyses with more than 30 studies are rare. Using a rule of thumb of at least 10 observations per covariate, this means that it will usually not be possible to include more than one covariate and still achieve stable estimates.

A particular point of concern is empirical evidence, derived through simulation studies,[12] that the P values for meta-regression coefficients from meta-regressions derived from standard meta-analysis software are often too small (that is, standard statistical tests used in meta-regression often have inflated, anticonservative, type I error rates). Whilst this is a general concern, settings where this is a particular danger include cases where there are few studies included in the analysis, settings where several covariates are tested without adjusting for multiplicity, and the use of fixed-effects meta-regression when residual heterogeneity is present. Permutation tests, whilst computationally more complex, can lead to more reliable P values[12]; however, they do not provide the associated confidence intervals.

Conclusion

Meta-regression is a useful tool in investigating between-study heterogeneity in meta-analyses, and in exploring potential effect modifiers. Its use is becoming more widespread; however, findings should be interpreted in the light of the observational nature of the associations, the difficulty in prespecifying covariates of interest, and the tendency for analytic techniques to give anticonservative, inflated P values.

Suggested Reading

Higgins JP, Thompson SG. Controlling the risk of spurious findings from meta-regression. Stat Med 2004;23:1663–1682

Sutton AJ, Abrams KR, Jones DR, Sheldon TA, Song F. Methods for Meta-analysis in Medical Research. Wiley Series in Probability and Statistics—Applied Probability and Statistics Section. Chichester, UK: Wiley; 2000

Thompson SG, Higgins JP. How should meta-regression analyses be undertaken and interpreted? Stat Med 2002;21:1559–1573

References

1. Guyatt GH, Rennie D, Meade M, Cook D, eds. Users' Guide to the Medical Literature: A Manual for Evidence-Based Clinical Practice. 2nd ed. New York: McGraw-Hill; 2008
2. Furlan AD, Tomlinson G, Jadad AA, Bombardier C. Examining heterogeneity in meta-analysis: comparing results of randomized trials and nonrandomized studies of interventions for low back pain. Spine (Phila Pa 1976) 2008;33:339–348
3. Thompson SG. Why sources of heterogeneity in meta-analysis should be investigated. BMJ 1994;309:1351–1355
4. Higgins JP, Thompson SG, Deeks JJ, Altman DG. Measuring inconsistency in meta-analyses. BMJ 2003;327:557–560
5. Rucker G, Schwarzer G, Carpenter JR, Schumacher M. Undue reliance on I(2) in assessing heterogeneity may mislead. BMC Med Res Methodol 2008;8:79
6. Altman DG, Bland JM. Absence of evidence is not evidence of absence. BMJ 1995;311:485
7. Uchida T, Bakhai A, Almonacid A, Shibata T, Cox B, Kuntz RE. A meta-analysis of randomized controlled trials of intra-coronary gamma- and beta-radiation therapy for in-stent restenosis. Heart Vessels 2006;21:368–374
8. Thompson SG, Higgins JP. How should meta-regression analyses be undertaken and interpreted? Stat Med 2002; 21:1559–1573
9. Talati R, Reinhart KM, White CM, et al. Outcomes of perioperative beta-blockade in patients undergoing noncardiac surgery: a meta-analysis. Ann Pharmacother 2009; 43:1181–1188
10. Simmonds MC, Higgins JP, Stewart LA, Tierney JF, Clarke MJ, Thompson SG. Meta-analysis of individual patient data from randomized trials: a review of methods used in practice. Clin Trials 2005;2:209–217
11. Higgins J, Thompson S, Deeks J, Altman D. Statistical heterogeneity in systematic reviews of clinical trials: a critical appraisal of guidelines and practice. J Health Serv Res Policy 2002;7:51–61
12. Higgins JP, Thompson SG. Controlling the risk of spurious findings from meta-regression. Stat Med 2004;23:1663–1682

22

Preparing a Statistical Analysis Plan

Charles H. Goldsmith

Summary

Suppose you have worked all day seeing many patients in the operating room and the recovery room, you attended two study meetings, and you got home late at 7:30 pm for dinner to be greeted by your spouse who mentions that you made the headlines in the local paper today. The headline reads: "Local Surgeon Misleads Journal Readers." The article goes on to name you as the culprit. You are one of the Canadian Institutes of Health Research (CIHR) grant holders that Chan et al. meant when they quoted that CIHR grant holders do not always report the primary outcome measure that they had put into their CIHR grant application.[1] This chapter shows how you might minimize the opportunity for the headline to apply to your studies by creating a statistical analysis plan (SAP) which should increase the transparency and credibility for your funded research project.

Not following the protocol and the corresponding SAP as planned may compromise your ability to publish in some top line journals. This chapter provides an overview on how to develop an SAP.

Introduction

Once a project has been designed and the grant has been submitted, it is time to think carefully of all the things that should be considered around the details of how the study should be managed, analyzed, and reported. This plan is often called a statistical analysis plan or SAP. The SAP is usually an appendix to many protocols; however, since few protocols were published until recently, the existence of the SAP is often not obvious to those who peruse the literature. On one research ethics board of which the author of this chapter was a member, few of the protocols submitted for approval had SAPs. SAPs are especially important as protocols are being published before a trial is initiated and many funding agencies and regulatory bodies require that trials be registered before patients are enrolled. These procedures are in place to help ensure that the proposed protocol and corresponding SAP are followed.

> **Reality Check: Purpose of a Statistical Analysis Plan**
> A statistical analysis plan should guide you during the study to be clear about all those technical procedures that keep you honest as a credible scientist when you are reporting the results of your study.

Data Management

Data entry and how the data will be cleaned need to be documented in detail. This includes copies of data forms, particularly if they are entered in a computer-oriented way with TeleForm or DataFax. The levels of cleaning to be used before any data analyses are done should be specified.

> **Jargon Simplified: Data Management**
> Data management is the list of things one does for data entry into a database, data cleaning, and file construction in preparation for statistical analysis.

Statistical Procedures

There should be a database dictionary of all variables and definitions for everything at an operational definition level, including missing data indicators and units. Examples include: height (m), weight (kg), with body mass index (BMI) computed.

Those who read this chapter and are rusty on the interpretation of basic statistical principles may want to refer to Bhandari and Joensson, *Clinical Research for Surgeons*, Section III C: Practical Guide to Statistical Analysis.[2]

Specify statistical procedures that are used to describe the data, check assumptions for statistical testing and what will happen if there are missing data: imputation strategies should be outlined.

Data listings for eyeball checking and other data integrity checks should be specified.

It is okay to not mention a reference for a two-sample Student's t test or χ^2 (chi-square) test for a 2×2 contingency table; however, more specialized or less common procedures such as multiple imputation methods for missing data or a Cox proportional hazard model to handle time-dependent covariates should be referenced.

Outline what is the backup plan for the raw data as well as all intermediate and final analyses.

If multiple comparisons are to be used, specify the method and references with a rationale for their usage. This should include the family of hypothesis tests that are the justification for the multiple comparison procedure.

Draft statistical text to be used in manuscripts might also be included, sometimes called boiler-plate text.

"Whatever statistical task is defined, it is inappropriate, and indeed unethical, to try several methods and report only those results that suit the investigator."[3]

What is the plan for detection and handling of outliers? What will be done about violated assumptions?

Stratification and blocking should be described and should be taken into account in the analyses since these are restrictions on the randomization.

Details of the randomization should be described, including details of blocking using Meinert's principles.[3] The details of the blocking in randomization should be concealed from any investigators or staff who are recruiting patients or are checking the patients for inclusion and exclusion criteria, to prevent selection bias.

The use of multivariate analysis should be considered to draw inferences when the primary and secondary analyses may give conflicting answers, or when the multiple outcomes may be integrated into some index of success.

Data Safety and Monitoring Board

Committee structure for various study types is outlined in Bhandari and Joensson, *Clinical Research for Surgeons*, Section III B: Conducting a Research Study,[2] and also in Chapters 6 and 8 of this book.

What data and interim findings such as adverse reactions, lost patients, rates of missing data, etc., will be made available to the Data Safety and Monitoring Board (DSMB)?

The SAP should specify how all analyses are related to the committee structure of the study: for example, preparing regular reports to the DSMB for their monitoring and meetings. It might also include reports on the recruiting progress of the study for the investigators and funders of the research. The time lines and due dates for such reports should be visible to those who need to prepare such reports.

Sample Size

The sample size justification for a study is a function of eight items; $n = f(\alpha, \beta, \delta, \sigma,$ tails, test, outcome, design); these items are referred to as the Four Greeks and the Four Others. The Four Greeks are:
1. α, the type I error rate;
2. β, the type II error rate (and its complement called power, $1-\beta$, often expressed as a percentage);

3. δ, the size of the minimum clinically important difference (MCID) that the investigators wish to detect for the primary outcome in their study (it is okay to specify MCIDs for all outcome measures);
4. σ, the size of the standard deviation that the proposed study design is likely to have.

The Four Others are:

Tails—whether the type I error will be distributed into one or two tails of distribution of the test statistic;

Test—the type of statistical tests that will be used to detect whether the data suggest rejection or acceptance of the null hypothesis;

Outcome—the primary outcome variable that will be used to judge the success or failure of the study;

Design—the type of statistical design to be conducted.

Sample size may be computed for all other outcomes too, with details in the SAP. Details of software used to compute the sample size and for a variety of different values of the eight items are commonly detailed in the SAP, even if they are not placed in the protocol. This allows readers and investigators to see whether the study has a possibility of detecting secondary outcomes and functions as a reference for manuscript writing at the end of the study.

"It is also critical that authors specify how and when they developed each null hypothesis in relation to their consideration of the data. Statistical theory and acceptable clinical research practice require that null hypotheses be fully developed before the data are examined—indeed, before even the briefest view of preliminary results. Otherwise the *P* values cannot be interpreted as meaningful probabilities."[4] Dates of SAP development and revisions help to clarify credibility under this concept.

"Authors should always specify whether they are using two-tail or one-tail tests; one-tail tests should be vanishingly rare."[3]

Interim Analysis

An interim analysis looks at the data accrued so far in the study to demonstrate futility of the study, possible early large clinically important results that challenge the ethics of withholding the new therapy from patients, and seeing whether the evidence is sufficient to stop the study early for either safety or efficacy reasons. Whether there will be any interim analyses and, if so, whether the interim analyses will be used for decisions about the trial, such as early stopping, should be outlined for decision making. If the protocol does not contain any interim analysis statements, consider approaching the research ethics board with a strategy that will be a protocol amendment. The writing of an interim analysis may lead to the creation of an α-spending function that attributes some of the set α to the interim analysis and the remainder to the end of study analysis. Please refer to Chapter 25 for more details on interim analysis.

Reports to Investigators

What reports will be made available for the investigators, such as on recruiting progress or balance of the stratification factors, types of patients being recruited, and progress by center if relevant, etc?

Control charts should be kept on recruiting: usually a c-chart if counts are used, with the four tests that are used to measure being "in control." For example, in Minitab 16, they are: (1) points beyond 3 standard deviations from the center line, (2) 9 points in a row on the same side of the center line, (3) 6 points in a row that are all increasing or decreasing, (4) 14 points in a row that are alternating up and down like saw teeth. Predictions for the future can then be made for "in control" recruiting processes. Graphical displays should be created with the target sample size and study completion date, with a cumulative graph done weekly to show progress. Have the recruiting graph visible to all personnel associated with the study.

Sensitivity Analysis

Outline which variables will be used for sensitivity analysis and whether a factorial design will be used or not.

> ### Jargon Simplified: Sensitivity Analysis
> Sensitivity analysis is a term referring to any test of the stability of the conclusions of a health care evaluation over a range of probability estimates, value judgements, and assumptions about the structure of the decisions to be made. This may involve the repeated evaluation of a decision model in which one or more of the parameters of interest are varied.[5]

Tables for Presentation and Publication

Mock data tables for manuscripts and reports to agencies, companies, and archives should be constructed. Along with these mock tables, the number of decimal places to be used to record each variable should be specified. Units for each variable should be in the SI (Système International) format, if possible.

Document whether the analyses will be rerun at time of abstract/paper submission to check that all table entries come from an identified set of computer output. Timelines to accommodate these extra analyses should be built into the submitting times for abstracts and papers.

Policies on rounding of data output for reports, presentations, and manuscripts should be in the SAP. If the target meeting or journal has guidelines for reporting, then copies of these should be referenced and available to those who need to prepare tables, graphs, and materials specific to the meeting and journal.

Possible Presentations and Publications

Possible publications include a meta-analysis of previous literature,[6,7] protocol and statistical analysis plan, primary trial outcomes, secondary trial outcomes, and implications for clinical practice.

Some problems to avoid are outlined in various chapters of Bhandari et al., *Writing Your Research Paper for Publication*,[8] such as Chapter 4: Common Pitfalls in the Reporting of Surgical Results, which includes a detailed explanation of CLEAR NPT[9] for surgery studies with examples of models of good and bad text.

Possible presentations (with abstract deadlines): Canadian Orthopaedic Association Annual Meeting (October), American Academy of Orthopaedic Surgeons (June).

Graphical Displays

Graphical displays will need to be created for presentations and publications, including descriptive as well as inference graphs. They should be displayed in mock form with suitable computer code to make them simple to produce when they are needed. References for graphic principles include van Belle, Robbins, Lang and Secic as well as Chapter 23 in *Writing Your Research Paper for Publication*.[8,10-12]

Software

List available software and version numbers with computers available for computation, such as Minitab 16, SAS 9.0.1, StatXact 9, SPSS 18, R, Splus. If other statistical software such as PASS is used for sample size calculation, it should also be documented. Sap Maker 2.0 from ClinTrialStat and other packages for study management might be considered to manage the study.

Document any special software written specifically for the project, and how it was validated.

Reporting Guidelines

CONSORT and other guidelines should be specific to the study design. A good source for these checklists is the Equator network, which is regularly kept up to date and is a source of documents for reporting different types of studies.[13] CLEAR NPT should also be cited, particularly for surgical trials where experience may play a central role and blinding of the treatment provider may not be feasible.[9] Please refer to Chapter 28 for more details on reporting guidelines.

General Policies

A policy should be established on who has access to raw data; whether the database will be locked after cleaning is completed; and whether there will be any future changes allowed.

There should be a written policy on data disclosure by staff, with contravention leading to warnings or possible dismissal.

The investigators should decide whether the SAP will be submitted for peer review before the analyses are started. Journals such as the BMC journal *Trials* expedite protocol (and hence SAP) publication provided the trial is registered and the study has peer review funding from agencies such as CIHR or NIH.

Privacy Considerations

Are there any special privacy considerations established by the local research ethics board or provincial/national/international legislation or good practice that need to be recognized within the reporting functions? If so, they should be documented.

Appendices

1. Define all short forms and abbreviations used in the write-up of the analysis.
2. Define all common symbols used in the study.

What Is in the Literature about SAP?

In *Statistics in Medicine* on pages 202–204 there are some suggestions to check your SAP.[14] This includes a list of ideas that go into making up an SAP:
- Start with objectives.
- Develop the background and relevance.
- Plan your materials.
- Plan your methods and data.
- Define the subject population.
- Ensure your sample size will satisfy your objectives.
- Anticipate what statistical analysis will yield results.
- Plan the bridge from results to conclusions.
- Anticipate the form in which your conclusions will be expressed.

Once these are listed, to improve the SAP: (1) work backward through the logic process, (2) analyze dummy data, and (3) play the role of the Devil's advocate like a reviewer might.

In *Seeing Through Statistics* there is a list of ten questions that one can ask of each graph to make it easier to understand:[15]
1. Does the message of interest stand out clearly?
2. Is the purpose or title of the picture evident?
3. Is a source given for the data, either with the picture or in an accompanying article?
4. Did the information in the picture come from a reliable, believable source?
5. Is everything clearly labeled, leaving no ambiguity?
6. Do the axes start at zero or not?
7. Do the axes maintain a constant scale?
8. Are there any breaks in the numbers on the axes that may be easy to miss?
9. For financial data, have the numbers been adjusted for inflation?
10. Is there information cluttering the picture or misleading the eye?

One of the few statistics books that suggests an SAP is *Presenting Medical Statistics from Proposal to Publication* on page 24.[16] Here the authors have a Box 3.12: Information on Plan of Statistical Analysis, with six bullet points:
- Distinguish between primary and secondary analyses.
- State the outcomes to be analyzed and the groups compared.
- State methods of analysis, significance tests, and level of significance to be used.
- State assumptions which need to be verified.
- List confounders to be investigated and possibly adjusted for in a multifactorial model.
- If there are several outcomes, describe the strategy for dealing with the possibility of spurious significant findings (type I errors).

The authors also show an example of an SAP in Box 3.13 in an early pregnancy study. In the present author's opinion this example is too short to qualify as an adequate discussion of all the relevant details in a proper SAP. The present author was unable to identify such statements in other references.[3,6,10,11,12,14,15,17]

A published and transparent SAP might help avoid the errors of mis-reporting of outcomes in health research demonstrated with CIHR RCTs in the article by Chan et al.[1]

Conclusion

Having a properly constructed SAP helps to prevent embarrassing headlines about scientific misconduct, and gives clear direction to staff and all investigators of what the key ideas of the study are, including the primary outcome, design considerations, and details of all planned analyses as well as the future presentations and publications.

Suggested Reading

Chan A-W, Krleza-Jeric K, Schmid I, Altman DG. Outcome reporting bias in randomized trials funded by the Canadian Institutes of Health Research. CMAJ 2004;171:735–740

Lang TA, Secic M. How to Report Statistics in Medicine. Annotated Guidelines for Authors, Editors, and Reviewers. 2nd ed. Philadelphia, PA: American College of Physicians; 2006

Mosteller F, Perkins M, Morrissey S. Writing about numbers. In: Bailar JC III, Hoaglin DC eds. Medical Uses of Statistics. 3rd ed. Toronto: Wiley; 2009:353–367

References

1. Chan A-W, Krleza-Jeric K, Schmid I, Altman DG. Outcome reporting bias in randomized trials funded by the Canadian Institutes of Health Research. CMAJ 2004;171:735–740; letter in CMAJ 2005;172:857
2. Bhandari M, Joensson A. Clinical Research for Surgeons. New York: Thieme; 2009
3. Meinert CL. Clinical Trials: Design, Conduct, and Analysis. Oxford: Oxford University Press; 1986:86
4. Bailar JC III, Mosteller F. Guidelines for statistical reporting in articles for medical journals: amplifications and explanations. In: Bailar JC III, Hoaglin DC, eds. Medical Uses of Statistics. 3rd ed. Toronto: Wiley; 2009:325–342
5. Guyatt G, Rennie D, Meade, MO, Cook DJ. Users' Guides to the Medical Literature: A Manual for Evidence-Based Clinical Practice. 2nd ed. New York: McGraw Hill Medical; 2008
6. Shea BJ, Grimshaw JM, Wells GA, et al. Development of AMSTAR: a measurement tool to assess the methodological quality of systematic reviews. BMC Med Res Methodol 2007;7:10
7. Moher D, Cook DJ, Eastwood S, Olkin I, Rennie D, Stroup DF: Improving the quality of reports of meta-analyses of randomised controlled trials: the QUOROM statement. Quality of Reporting Meta-analyses. Lancet 1999;354:1896–1900
8. Bhandari M, Joensson A, Schemitsch E, Robioneck B, eds. Writing Your Research Paper for Publication. New York: Thieme; 2010
9. Boutron I, Moher D, Tugwell PSL, et al. A checklist to evaluate a report of a nonpharmacological trial (CLEAR NPT) was developed using consensus. J Clin Epidemiol 2005;58:1233–1240
10. van Belle G. Statistical Rules of Thumb. 2nd ed. Toronto: Wiley; 2008
11. Robbins NB. Creating More Effective Graphs. Toronto: Wiley; 2005
12. Lang TA, Secic M. How to Report Statistics in Medicine. Annotated Guidelines for Authors, Editors, and Reviewers. 2nd ed. Philadelphia, PA: American College of Physicians; 2006
13. Library for Health Research Reporting. Available at www.equator-network.org/index.aspx?o=1015. Accessed April, 2010.
14. Riffenburgh RH. Statistics in Medicine. 2nd ed. Burlington, MA: Elsevier Academic; 2006
15. Utts JM: Seeing Through Statistics. 2nd ed. Toronto: Duxbury; 1999
16. Peacock J, Kerry S. Presenting Medical Statistics from Proposal to Publication. New York: Oxford University Press; 2007
17. Wang R, Lagakos SW, Ware JH, Hunter DJ, Drazen JM. Reporting of subgroup analyses in clinical trials. In: Bailar JC III, Hoaglin DC, eds. Medical Uses of Statistics. 3rd ed. Toronto: Wiley; 2009:343–352

23

Regression Analysis

Eleanor M. Pullenayegum

Summary

Regression analysis is a powerful technique, and is particularly useful in observational studies where there are several confounding variables to be adjusted for. This chapter will provide an overview of three types of regression: linear regression for continuous outcomes (e.g., weight), logistic regression for binary outcomes (e.g., mortality), and proportional hazards regression for time-to-event outcomes (e.g., survival time). The focus will be on how to interpret and report the regression coefficients, together with a discussion of how to build a regression model.

Introduction

Regression analyses are widely used in research studies, particularly with observational designs. In this chapter we shall explore why regression analyses are useful, how they are undertaken, and how they should be reported.

Why might one consider doing a regression analysis? There are two main reasons: to make predictions, and to understand associations. The reason for undertaking the regression has important implications for how the regression is done.

Regression analyses can be used to predict outcomes for future patients. For example, we might want to predict the probability of survival after 5 years, or the quality of life of a patient 1 month after surgery. At first glance, this seems like an immediate output of a regression analysis, since regression expresses the outcome as a function of a number of baseline covariates. However, when using a regression equation for prediction, it is important to have a measure of its predictive accuracy. It is here that the difficulty arises: a model will always fit the data on which it was developed better than it will fit any new data, in the same way that a shoe, once worn in, will fit its owner better than it will fit another person with exactly the same shoe size. For this reason, when developing models for prediction one should split the data into a training set, on which the model is fit, and a validation set, on which the predictive ability of the model is evaluated. Clearly, this implies the disadvantage of being unable to use the whole dataset to describe associations.

However, it is relatively rare that a researcher's primary objective in considering a regression model is one of pre-

diction. The primary objective would be prediction if the intention were to take the regression model and create a formula (for example in Microsoft Excel) into which data from future patients could be input in order to provide an estimate of the probability of an event occurring or a prediction of a continuous outcome. In most cases, however, researchers are interested in describing associations between an outcome and a set of covariates. Even though the covariates may at times be referred to as "predictors," the main objective is not to develop a formula for predicting events, but rather to understand what patient factors may dispose toward a favorable or an adverse outcome.

> **Key Concepts: Regression Analysis Is Usually Used to Understand Associations**
> In most examples of regression analyses in the medical literature, the objective of the analysis is not to make predictions, but to understand associations.

By far the most common purpose of a regression analysis, then, is to describe relationships amongst variables. If there are just two variables this can of course be achieved by other methods. Regression becomes most useful when it is used to describe the association between more than two variables, for example when we want to understand the association between two variables after accounting for confounding variables. This is particularly relevant for observational studies, where factors which predispose subjects to having the exposure of interest may also be associated with the outcome.

As an example, consider the following study of the relationship between preoperative anemia and perioperative mortality. Beattie et al.[1] found that in unadjusted analyses the odds ratio for perioperative death amongst anemic as compared to nonanemic patients was 4.74 [95% confidence interval (CI) 3.3–6.7; $P < 0.0001$], and that, after adjusting for known confounding factors, the odds ratio became 2.36 (95% CI 1.57–3.41; $P < 0.0001$). It is not surprising that anemia should be associated with perioperative mortality, since it is also associated with a host of other factors (e.g., advanced age, diabetes, coronary artery disease, renal dysfunction). We know that older patients are at greater risk of death than younger patients, so if anemia is associated with age it is no surprise that it is also associated with death. The question is whether, after accounting for age and any other important covariates, anemia confers any additional risk. Equivalently, we might ask whether, amongst two patients who are the same age,

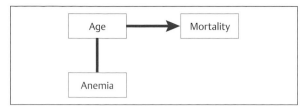

Fig. 23.1 Association between anemia and mortality that is due solely to age.

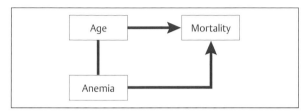

Fig. 23.2 Association between anemia and mortality that is due both to a direct effect and to an effect through age.

one who is anemic has a greater risk than the one who is not.

In the context of regression analyses, *confounding* is an important concept. One variable confounds the relationship between two other variables if it is related to each of the other variables in such a way that, if not accounted for, the true association of interest is distorted. In the above example, age confounds the relationship between anemia and mortality. Thus, in **Fig. 23.1**, we can trace a relationship between anemia and mortality through age, and so if we were to compare mortality rates according to anemia status, we would see a relationship, but it would be conferred only because older patients are both more likely to be anemic and also more likely to die. We are actually interested in the relationship between anemia and mortality *after accounting for age*, as seen in **Fig. 23.2**—namely, is there a direct path from anemia to mortality without going through another covariate?

A classic example of confounding is that the risk of dying from lung cancer is strongly associated with carrying a cigarette lighter. However, after accounting for smoking status, the association would drop dramatically. Similarly, in developed countries we would expect to see a strong relationship between having pierced ears and longevity; however, this relationship would change considerably after accounting for gender.

Key Concepts: Confounding
Confounding occurs when the relationship between two variables is distorted by a third variable. For example, in an observational study, age would confound the relationship between total knee replacement and quality of life if older patients were less likely to get a knee replacement and also more likely to have lower quality of life.

There are three commonly used types of regression: linear, logistic, and proportional hazards regression. These regression methods assume that there is one outcome (sometimes also described as a *dependent variable*) which is to be described in terms of one or more covariates (also sometimes described as *predictors* or *independent variables*). In our anemia example, the outcome was death, and the covariates were anemia, age, and a number of other patient-level variables. Linear regression is used for continuous outcomes, logistic regression is used for binary outcomes, and proportional hazards regression is used for time-to-event outcomes (e.g., survival time). We shall consider each in turn before concluding with some general points on model fitting.

Jargon Simplified: Dependent Variable
The dependent variable is the outcome variable that you wish to describe in terms of baseline covariates. For example, if your question is how anemia is associated with perioperative mortality after noncardiac surgery, your outcome, and hence your dependent variable, is mortality.

Jargon Simplified:
Independent Variable, Predictor, or Covariate
These three terms all mean the same thing, that is, the patient factors whose association with the outcome is modeled in the regression. In the above example mortality is the outcome and anemia is a covariate. Other examples of covariates in this setting might be age and gender.

Linear Regression

In a linear regression, a continuous outcome is regressed onto one or more covariates. These covariates can be either continuous or categorical.

Examples from the Literature: The Effects of Stress and Coping on Surgical Performance During Simulations
Wetzel et al. report on the effects of stress and coping on surgical performance during simulated operations.[2] They state that the quality of the end product was measured using end product assessment (EPA), and participating surgeons included both residents and attending surgeons. Analysis was by linear regression, and the authors report that in the noncrisis simulation "a high coping score and experience significantly enhanced EPA (β_1 0.279, 0.009–0.460, P = 0.04; β_2 0.571, 4.328–12.669, P < 0.001; respectively)." What do β_1 and β_2 mean in this context?

How Is a Linear Regression Model Specified?

In this example, we are interested in the association between coping and performance, and the association between stress and performance; however, since one might expect more experienced surgeons to have better coping, less stress, and better performance, experience is a confounding variable that must be adjusted for. We thus consider a linear model, as follows:

$$EPA_i = \beta_0 + \beta_1\, stress_i + \beta_2\, coping_i + \beta_3\, experience_i \\ + \varepsilon_i \;\; \varepsilon_i \sim iid\; N(0,\, \sigma^2).$$

In this model, EPA_i is the EPA for the i-th surgeon, $stress_i$ is the stress for that same surgeon as captured using the STAI,[3] $coping_i$ is the number of coping strategies that the i-th surgeon has, and $experience_i$ is the number of years of experience for the i-th surgeon. ε_i represents the difference between the actual and the predicted EPA, and is also referred to as the error term or the residual. It is assumed that these error terms are independent of one another and all represent random draws from a common normal distribution.

What Do the Regression Results Mean?

How are the resulting regression coefficients interpreted? It is simplest in the first instance to focus on the case where there is just a single covariate to be included in the model—we shall suppose that we include just years of experience. Then the regression equation is

$$EPA_i = \beta_0 + \beta_1\, experience_i + \varepsilon_i$$

where ε is a mean-zero random error.

For the sake of illustration, we have fitted this model on some hypothetical data and plotted the results in **Fig. 23.3**. Note that when years of experience is zero, the mean EPA score will be β_0, since the error term is on average zero. Thus β_0 is the point at which the regression line hits the y-axis, which in our hypothetical data is about 11. For each additional year of experience, the mean EPA will increase by β_1, and thus β_1 is the slope of the regression line (in our hypothetical data, this is around 0.2).

Thus, in the full regression including stress, coping, and experience, the regression coefficients β_0, β_1, β_2, and β_3 are interpreted as follows. β_0 represents an intercept and is usually not of interest (it represents the mean EPA amongst surgeons with a score of zero on the STAI, no coping strategies, and no years of experience!). β_1 represents the increase in EPA for each unit increase in the STAI amongst surgeons who have the same number of coping strategies and the same number of years of experience. That is, if one cohort of surgeons has a self-assessed stress of 11, two coping strategies and 5 years of experience, and another has a self-assessed stress of 12, two coping strategies, and 5 years of experience, we would expect the difference in mean EPA between the second and the first cohort to be β_1. Note that the numbers 11, two, and five were chosen arbitrarily; the same result would apply if we were to change these choices.

Similarly, β_2 represents the increase in EPA for each additional coping strategy, and β_3 represents the increase in EPA for each additional year of experience.

What Have We Assumed?

There are several assumptions implicit in this model. Firstly, the relationship between the covariates and outcome is assumed to be linear. Thus, in our example, increasing years of experience from two to three leads to the same increase in outcome as increasing them from 10 to 11. Depending on the setting, this assumption may not always be realistic. In fact, for the purposes of illustration we have simplified the actual analysis used by Wetzel et al.: in their analysis they found a nonlinear association between years of experience and the outcome (see Reality Check below). Secondly, the observations are assumed to be independent of one another; an example of nonindependence would be if two surgeons were in the simulation together. Thirdly, the residuals are assumed to follow a normal distribution (that is, if they are plotted on a histogram, it should be bell-shaped). This might fail if, for example, the outcome of interest were measured on a five-point scale. Finally, the variability of the residuals is assumed not to depend on any of the covariates. This assumption might be questionable for certain types of outcome, for example health utilities, where observations tend to cluster close to one.

Reality Check: Reporting Results

In their analysis of the effects of stress and coping on performance in surgical simulations Wetzel et al. report "a high coping score and experience significantly enhanced EPA (β_1 0.279, 0.009–0.460, $P = 0.04$; β_2 0.571, 4.328–12.669, $P < 0.001$; respectively)."[2] What do β_1 and β_2 mean in this context?

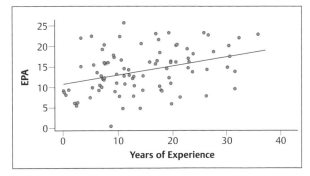

Fig. 23.3 End product assessment (EPA) score as a function of years of experience for a hypothetical set of data.

Performance is measured by the end product assessment (EPA). A regression coefficient of 0.279 for coping means that one additional coping strategy was associated with a mean increase of 0.279 in EPA score.

The regression coefficient for experience is harder to interpret, as in their analysis Wetzel et al. log-transformed (to base 10) years of experience. This means that a 10-fold increase in years of experience is associated with an additive increase of 0.571 in EPA. For example, an increase in years of experience from 1 to 10 would be associated with an increase of 0.571 in EPA.

This illustrates the trade-off between correctly capturing the shape of association between a covariate and the outcome, and having regression coefficients that are easy to interpret. In this example, it was necessary to log-transform experience in order to describe the nature of the association; however, the resulting regression coefficient has a less intuitive interpretation than the coefficient of coping, which was left untransformed.

Is the Model Any Good?

Linear regression will give an estimate of the proportion of the variance in the outcome that is explained by the covariates in the model, often called the R^2. In the case of a single covariate, the R^2 is simply the square of the Pearson correlation coefficient. Thus, if in our example we had seen a Pearson correlation coefficient of 0.3, it would follow that 9% of the variance in EPA is explained by years of experience ($0.3^2 = 0.09 = 9\%$). In the case of several covariates in the same model, the R^2 represents how much of the variability they jointly explain, and hence is not directly related to the correlation coefficient between any two variables. Since the R^2 will always increase as more variables are added to the model, for the purposes of model fit the adjusted R^2 is sometimes used; this is simply the R^2 with a penalty for the number of variables in the model.

Logistic Regression

What Do We Mean by "Logistic"?

Examples from the Literature: Risk Associated With Preoperative Anemia in Noncardiac Surgery
In a study of the relationship between preoperative anemia and perioperative mortality, Beattie et al. found that in unadjusted analyses the odds ratio for perioperative death amongst anemic as compared to nonanemic patients was 4.74 (95% CI 3.3–6.7; P <0.0001), and that, after adjusting for known confounding factors, the odds ratio became 2.36 (95% CI 1.57–3.41; P < 0.0001).[1]

At the beginning of this chapter we introduced a study investigating the association between preoperative anemia and perioperative mortality. Here the outcome of interest is mortality, a binary outcome. Linear regression is not appropriate as the assumptions of the regression, for example normality of the residuals, will not hold. We are interested in the probability of mortality, which is constrained to lie between 0 and 1 and hence is not suited to linear regression models because, for example, if we attempted to fit a model $P = \beta_0 + \beta_1 \times age$, we would likely find that for older patients, the predicted probability P fell below 0, something we know to be impossible. For this reason, we do not model the probability P itself; rather we model the logistic transform (or logit), namely $\log(P/(1-P))$. The reasons behind this are mathematical; however, the main point to note is that whilst P must lie between 0 and 1, logit(P) can take on any value at all. Put another way, if logit(P) = a, then $P = 1/(1 + e^{-a})$, which will always give a probability between 0 and 1 regardless of the value of a. Again for mathematical reasons, all logs are natural logs, that is, to base e.

While the reasons for choosing a logistic transform are relatively unimportant in our context, the consequences of doing regressions on the logit of the probability are vital. The ratio $P/(1-P)$ is the odds of the event—in our example the odds of perioperative mortality. In everyday use, we most commonly use odds in the context of gambling. For example, when we say that the odds of our favorite team's winning a match are 4:1, we mean that amongst many similar matches, we would expect our team to win 4 out of 5 times and lose 1 out of 5 times; thus, the probability of winning is 4/5 or 80%, but the odds are 4/1 = 4.

Jargon Simplified: Odds
The odds of an event is the probability that the event will occur divided by the probability that it will not occur. For example, if the odds of survival after a particular procedure are 7, this could be equivalently expressed by saying that the odds are 7:1 (seven to one), meaning that out of eight procedures, one would expect seven to result in survival.

In previous regression examples we have considered continuous covariates (e.g., stress score), that is, covariates which take on numerical values, so in considering a regression of the log odds of perioperative mortality onto anemia and any potential confounders, we must first consider how to include a categorical covariate, such as anemia, in a regression model. This can be done through the use of a *dummy variable*. That is, we define a new variable which will take on the value 0 or 1 depending on the anemia status of the individual; most typically we would define anemia = 1 if the patient is anemic and 0 otherwise. (Note that although we have introduced dummy variables in the context of logistic regression, they are used in exactly the same way when incorporating categorical covariates into a linear regression).

What Is a Logistic Regression?

A simple regression model, that does not account for any confounders, would then be

Probability of death $= P_i$
$\mathrm{logit}(P_i) = \beta_0 + \beta_1 \times$ anaemia

that is,

$\mathrm{logit}(P_{\text{not anaemic}}) = \beta_0$
$\mathrm{logit}(P_{\text{anaemic}}) = \beta_0 + \beta_1.$

Thus it follows that β_0 is the log odds of death for those who are not anemic, or, equivalently, $1/(1 + \exp(-\beta_0))$ is the odds of death for nonanemic individuals. As with linear regression, the intercept is not of much interest; rather, we are interested in β_1. As can be seen from the above, β_1 is the difference in log odds of death for anemic as compared to nonanemic individuals. Since the difference in logs is the log of the ratio, it follows that *β_1 is the log odds ratio of death for anemic as compared to nonanemic patients.* On fitting this model, the regression coefficient for anemia (β_1 in our model) is 1.56, with standard error 0.18. Since we usually do not think on a log scale, we usually report not β_1 but the odds ratio itself, e^{β_1}, which in our example is $e^{1.56} = 4.74$.

How Should the Results of a Logistic Regression Be Reported?

It is important to report a confidence interval for the odds ratio in addition to the point estimate in order to communicate the degree of uncertainty associated with the estimate. Provided sample sizes are sufficiently large, the distribution of the regression coefficients (i.e., the log odds ratios) will be approximately normal. Most statistical software will report the regression coefficients together with their associated standard errors (SE), and 95% confidence intervals can then be constructed as ($\beta - 1.96 \times$ se, $\beta + 1.96 \times$ se). These can be converted to confidence intervals for the odds ratios themselves by exponentiating: ($\exp[\beta - 1.96 \times$ se], $\exp[\beta + 1.96 \times$ se]). Thus in our example a 95% confidence interval for the regression coefficient β_1 (the log odds ratio) is $1.56 - 1.96 \times 0.18$ to $1.56 + 1.96 \times 0.18$, or 1.2 to 1.9. Rather than reporting on the log scale, however, we transform to the odds ratio scale itself by taking exponentials: $e^{1.2} = 3.3$ and $e^{1.9} = 6.7$, and so we can report that the odds ratio of perioperative

mortality for anemic as compared to nonanemic patients is 4.74 with a 95% confidence interval of 3.3–6.7.

We Need to Adjust for Confounders!

It is not, of course, the unadjusted relationship between anemia and mortality that is of interest, but rather the association after adjusting for potential confounders. Confounders in this case are age, in-hospital status, history of congestive heart failure, preoperative renal dysfunction, preoperative beta-blockers, angiotensin-converting enzyme (ACE) inhibitors, nonsteroidal anti-inflammatory drugs (NSAIDs), and red blood cell (RBC) transfusions (1–2, 3–4, 5–10, >10 units vs. None). This last covariate is ordinal, and is represented not by a single dummy variable, but by four (one minus the number of categories), which we shall denote by RBC1, RBC2, RBC3, and RBC4. There are a number of ways in which this might be coded, but the most natural choice is RBC1 = 1 if 1–2 transfusions and 0 otherwise, RBC2 = 1 if 3–4 transfusions and 0 otherwise, RBC3 = 1 if 5–10 transfusions and 0 otherwise, RBC4 = 1 if >10 transfusions and 0 otherwise. Thus if a patient received any transfusions, one, and only one, of RBC1, RBC2, RBC3, and RBC4 would be equal to 1, and patients who received no transfusions would have all four dummy variables set to zero.

In the adjusted model, β_1 is 0.89 with standard error 0.20, so the adjusted odds ratio is $e^{0.89} = 2.43$ with a 95% confidence interval of 1.65 to 3.60. Note that the drop in the odds ratio on adjusting for confounding factors is typical: as confounding factors are introduced we come closer to measuring the causal association between anemia and mortality, rather than the causal association plus associations arising from confounding. For instance, once adjusted for history of preoperative renal dysfunction, the odds ratio becomes 2.08 with a

95% confidence interval of 1.22 to 3.53; when adjusted for the preoperative beta-blocker metoprolol, the odds ratio becomes 1.67 with a 95% confidence interval of 1.05 to 2.68; and when adjusted for ACE inhibitors, the odds ratio becomes 0.56 with a 95% confidence interval of 0.33 to 0.95.[1]

Proportional Hazards Regression

When Would Proportional Hazards Regression Be Needed?

Binary outcomes such as 1-year mortality or 5-year need for reoperation are perhaps the most common outcomes in surgical research. In many cases, however, we may not have complete follow-up information. This could happen for one of two reasons. Firstly, if recruitment into the study is slow, there may be a need to close the study before everyone has been followed for the entire duration of interest; this is known as *administrative censoring*. Secondly, in studies with longer follow-up, some individuals may leave the study early; this is known as *loss to follow-up*. In such studies, rather than treating the outcome as missing, it is usually preferable to take the time to the event as the outcome of interest, and to treat the time as censored if the event is not observed to occur. For example, in a study where survival time is the outcome of interest, a patient who was recruited into the study and at the end of 4.5 years of follow-up was still alive has what is known as a *censored* survival time. We know that the event occurred after 4.5 years, but we do not know when after that time it occurred.

There are two properties of such time-to-event data that make linear regression an inappropriate analysis. Firstly, time-to-event data tend to be skewed and hence the residuals from a regression model will usually not follow a normal distribution. Secondly, any analysis must account for the censored nature of the data. Treating survival times amongst those who have not been observed to die as missing would seriously bias the analysis since those who survive longer are more likely to have incompletely observed survival times![4]

Examples from the Literature: Social Deprivation and Prognostic Benefits of Cardiac Surgery
Using a large prospective observational cohort of almost 45 000 patients, Pagano et al. describe the association between social deprivation and mid-term mortality amongst patients having had cardiac surgery.[4] They report that "Multivariable analysis identified social deprivation as an independent predictor of mid-term mortality (hazard ratio 1.024, 95% CI 1.015–1.033; $P < 0.001$) … Adjustment for smoking, body mass index, and diabetes reduced but did not eliminate the effects of social deprivation on mid-term mortality (1.017, 95% CI 1.007–1.026, $P < 0.001$)."

In this section we shall explore how multivariable analysis with time-to-event outcomes is undertaken, and how to interpret a hazard ratio.

Although there are other options, regression analysis of time-to-event data is typically done through a Cox proportional hazards model. Here, instead of modeling survival time directly, we model the *hazard* of the event of interest, which can be thought of as an instantaneous incidence of the event (the rate at which the event occurs amongst those who are still at risk, evaluated over a very narrow time interval). This solves the censoring problem because once someone is censored they are simply dropped out of the risk set and so disappear from both the numerator and the denominator of the incidence. Naturally, the incidence will vary over time. One of the attractive features of a proportional hazards model is that the shape of the hazard function is left unspecified. What is modeled, however, is the impact of covariates on the hazard—for example, with two treatment groups it is the ratio of the hazards in the two treatment groups that is modeled. Specifically, the model assumes that the ratio of the hazard in the treatment relative to the control group remains constant over time, that is, the hazards are *proportional*.

Key Concepts: Hazards
The *hazard* of an event is the instantaneous incidence of the event. While the hazard will usually vary over time, in many settings it is reasonable to assume that the ratio of hazards between two patient groups (e.g., treated vs. untreated) is constant over time. Thus the assumption is known as the *proportional hazards* assumption.

How Is a Proportional Hazards Regression Specified?

The model for a proportional hazards regression is

$$hazard_i(t) = hazard_0(t)\exp(\beta_2\chi_2 + \cdots + \beta_p\chi_p).$$

Suppose for now that our regression equation contains just a single covariate; for example, suppose we are modeling survival time after heart surgery and want to investigate the effect of gender without accounting for any potential confounders. If we code gender as a dummy variable, for example gender = 1 for men and gender = 0 for women, then we would have

$$hazard_i(t) = h_0(t)\exp(\beta \times gender_i).$$

That is,

$$hazard_{woman}(t) = h_0(t)$$
$$hazard_{man}(t) = h_0(t)\exp(\beta)$$

and so

$$\frac{\text{hazard}_{man}(t)}{\text{hazard}_{woman}(t)} = \exp(\beta).$$

Thus $\exp(\beta)$ is the ratio of the hazard for men to the hazard for women, that is, it is a hazard ratio. $h_0(t)$ in this equation is known as the baseline hazard, or, the hazard for those whose covariates are all equal to zero. This portion of the regression model is left unspecified and can depend on the time t in any way we wish. In our example, however, we are interested not in gender but in social deprivation. In our example, social deprivation is captured using Carstairs scores,[5] and the regression model used is:

$$\text{hazard}_i(t) = h_0(t)\exp(\beta_1 \text{Carstairs}_i + \text{other covariates}).$$

Other covariates include EuroScore, a measure of cardiac operative risk, and type of cardiac procedure (CABG, CABG + valve(s), CABG + valve(s) + other, CABG + other, Valve(s) only, Valve(s) + other).

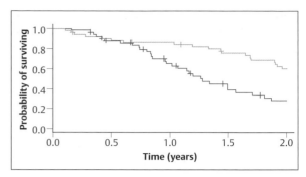

Fig. 23.4 A hypothetical example of nonproportional hazards, for example in comparing a surgical intervention to a nonsurgical intervention. In this example the surgical group, represented by the light blue line, initially experiences worse mortality. However, after the initial period, mortality in the nonsurgical group, represented by the dark blue line, catches up, and then exceeds, mortality in the surgical group.

Reality Check: Interpreting Regression Coefficients for Continuous Covariates

How might the reported hazard ratio of 1.024 and associated 95% confidence interval of 1.015 to 1.033 be interpreted? It may seem that the size of the effect is very small; however, the Carstairs score is not a binary variable but rather a continuous variable ranging from –5.71 (least deprived) to 21.39 (most deprived). Thus the hazard ratio of 1.024 represents a 2.4% increase in hazard for each additional point on the Carstairs score. The median Carstairs score in this sample was –0.54, with first and third quartiles of –2.19 and 2.27 respectively. What would be the difference in hazard between an individual in the third quartile as compared to the first? This represents an increase in Carstairs score of 2.27 + 2.19 = 4.46. Our model tells us that, all other covariates remaining the same, the ratio of the hazard for someone with a Carstairs score of 2.27 to someone with a score of –2.19 would be $\exp(\beta_1 \times 2.27)/\exp(\beta_1 \times (-2.19)) = \exp(\beta_1 \times 4.46) = 1.024^{4.46} = 1.11$, that is, we would have an 11% increase in hazard. The 95% confidence interval for this increase can be obtained similarly: $1.015^{4.46}$ to $1.033^{4.46}$ or, 1.068 to 1.155, meaning a 7% to 16% increase in hazard.

Notice that unlike linear and logistic regression, our proportional hazards regression does not have an intercept term (no β_0). This is because it would be redundant: any terms that do not vary between individuals can be incorporated in the baseline hazard h_0. Moreover, whilst it is possible to derive estimates of the baseline hazard, in most applications this is not a quantity of interest, in the same way as the intercept from a linear or logistic regression is usually uninteresting.

What Have We Assumed?

It is important to ask whether the assumption of a constant hazard ratio over time is reasonable. This assumption may be particularly questionable when comparing a surgical to a pharmacological intervention, as with the surgical intervention one might expect higher perioperative mortality, but if surgery was successful it might be reasonable to expect the hazards of death to decline. See **Fig. 23.4** for an illustration.

How Should the Results of a Proportional Hazards Regression Be Reported?

As with logistic regression, it will usually be more informative to report not the regression coefficients themselves, but rather the implied hazard ratios and their associated confidence intervals. After calculating the regression coefficients and their confidence intervals, the hazard ratios can be found by taking exponentials.

Note that a hazard ratio is not the same as a relative risk. The hazard ratio is the ratio of two instantaneous incidences, assumed to be constant over time, whereas the relative risk is the ratio of two prevalences at a specific point in time.

Jargon Simplified: *b* or *beta*

b and *beta* are totally unhelpful terminology that should not be used in abstracts or in the text of a results section. Both usually refer to regression coefficients from a regression model. In the case of a linear regression, the regression coefficient for a particular covariate describes the unit increase in the outcome variable that occurs when that covariate increases by one unit. In logistic regression and proportional hazards regression the regression coefficients represent log odds ratios and log hazard ratios respectively, and should usually be exponentiated in order to report the odds ratio or hazards ratio in the text.

Model Building

Many users of regression techniques ask about how to build a model. In addressing this question we shall focus on the case where the purpose of the model is to understand associations, rather than to make predictions. It is usually wise to start with a univariate analysis exploring the relationship between each of the covariates and the outcome in turn, in order to gain an understanding of the associations that are present in the data. How the analysis progresses depends on the situation at hand. If there is a primary association of interest and just a few distinct baseline demographic characteristics to adjust for, then in many cases these can simply be entered into the regression model. In such cases there is usually no need to remove covariates that are not significant in the model; there is no reason why all the covariates in a regression model need to be significant.

> ### Key Concepts: Model Building
> Whilst automatic model fitting strategies are popular and convenient, they do not necessarily address a study's unique question. Often it is preferable to build the regression model based on an understanding of the variables in the model and in such a way as to answer the study's research question(s). There is nothing wrong with including covariates in the model when their regression coefficients are not significant.

If there are a large number of potential confounders to adjust for, it is often helpful to consider only those which show some association with the outcome on univariate analysis. Entering too many covariates into a model can cause model overfitting, where instead of modeling genuine features of the data, we end up modeling data quirks. Results from models with overfitting will tend not to replicate in subsequent studies, and will often not make sense. There is no hard and fast rule, but generally simulation studies have shown that having at least ten observations for each covariate in a linear regression model generally avoids overfitting (so if there were 20 covariates, I would need 200 subjects in the study).[6] For logistic regression, this rule of thumb becomes ten events *and* ten nonevents for each covariate (so if there were 20 covariates, I would need to have at least 200 events and at least 200 nonevents; in other words, the number of subjects is driven by the least common outcome).[7,8] For proportional hazards regression, the rule of thumb is ten events per covariate.[9] It is important to remember that these are rules of thumb to avoid overfitting, and do not guarantee adequate power for detecting any given association.

If the number of potential covariates is large compared with the number of subjects, even after filtering out those not approaching significance on univariate analysis, it can be helpful to refine the regression model by considering only those covariates that approach statistical significance. It can also be helpful to consider the covariates in groups; for example, to ask separately which demographic characteristics are important, which elements of patient history are important, which elements of patient care are important etc., and then to consider only those identified within each cohort in a multivariable analysis. Moreover, in some settings there may be two or more covariates that are collinear, that is, very highly associated with one another. An example would be body mass index and weight. In these cases, it is usually both unwise and unnecessary to include both covariates in the model, even if both are significant when entered into the model together, as the regression coefficients will usually not make sense. Often in such settings one coefficient will be large and positive whilst the other is large and negative. Besides using common sense, this type of collinearity can also be evaluated using variance inflation factors.[10]

Automatic model fitting strategies are implemented in many software packages. These can sometimes be helpful, but should be used with caution. Forward selection begins with a list of candidate covariates and a null model including just an intercept, and at each stage includes the covariate that is not currently in the model that would lead to the best improvement in fit of the model (which usually corresponds to the covariate with the smallest *P* value on inclusion). The process stops when there is no covariate not currently in the model that would have a significant *P* value on inclusion. Backward selection does the opposite: it begins with all the covariates in the model and at each stage excludes the variable that leads to the smallest loss of fit (which usually corresponds to the covariate in the model with the largest *P* value). The process stops when all the covariates in the model are significant. The forward procedure can be refined so as to reconsider variables that have been included but are no longer significant, and similarly the backward procedure can be refined so as to reconsider variables that have been excluded but would at a later point be significant if included.

The major difficulty with these automatic selection procedures is that they are primarily concerned with building a model that predicts outcome well, not with answering the specific question of interest. For example, if the question were, "Is anemia associated with an increased risk of perioperative mortality after other important patient pre-surgery factors have been accounted for," there is nothing in the automatic selection procedures that will by default ensure that anemia is in the model, although many software packages will allow it to be forced into the model. Similarly, in some cases variables such as age and gender might be considered such important factors based on external evidence that the results should be adjusted for them; however, the automatic selection process will not necessarily honor this, particularly if there are other variables strongly associated with them. Backward selection procedures can run into trouble when there is a very large number of covariates, or where two or more covariates are collinear; in these cases the initial models that are fit may be unstable or have regression coefficients that are unreasonable, and since subsequent stages of the selection procedure are built on the initially unstable models, the final results may be questionable. Importantly, automatic selection procedures do not provide either a P value or a measure of effect size for variables excluded from the model.

Jargon Simplified: Univariate Regression
Univariate regression is a regression model with just a single outcome and a single covariate.

Jargon Simplified: Multivariate Regression Analysis
Multivariate regression analysis provides a mathematical model that attempts to explain or predict the dependent variable (or outcome variable or target variable) by simultaneously considering two or more independent variables (or predictor variables).[11]

Jargon Simplified: Multivariable Regression
Multivariable regression is a regression model with more than one covariate (predictor).

Goodness of Fit

Whilst a detailed discussion of goodness of fit is beyond the scope of this chapter, it is an essential component of fitting a regression model. The first component of goodness of fit relates to assessing whether the assumptions of the regression model are met. For a linear regression, this would include assessing normality of the residuals (often by plotting a histogram). For linear, logistic, and proportional hazards regression, linearity of the associations can be assessed by plotting residuals versus the covariates.

Other components of goodness of fit assess how well the values predicted by the model agree with the actual outcomes. This can be done through the R^2 for a linear regression, a Hosmer–Lemeshow test, or the area under the receiver-operating characteristic (ROC) curve for logistic regression,[12] and the pseudo-R^2 for proportional hazard regression.

See Hosmer and Lemeshow, 2000 or Norman and Steiner, 2008 for a fuller treatment of the goodness of fit.[12,13]

Conclusion

Regression analysis is a powerful tool for describing associations between variables, particularly in the context of observational studies subject to confounding. Regression models are best constructed through a careful understanding of relationships between variables rather than through automated procedures.

Suggested Reading

Hosmer DW, Lemeshow S. Applied Survival Analysis: Regression Modeling of Time to Event Data. New York: Wiley; 1999
Hosmer DW, Lemeshow S. Applied Logistic Regression. 2nd ed. New York: Wiley; 2000
Norman GR, Streiner DL. Biostatistics: The Bare Essentials. 3rd ed. New York: McGraw-Hill; 2008

References

1. Beattie WS, Karkouti K, Wijeysundera DN, Tait G. Risk associated with preoperative anemia in noncardiac surgery: a single-center cohort study. Anesthesiology 2009;110: 574–581
2. Wetzel CM, Black SA, Hanna GB, et al. The effects of stress and coping on surgical performance during simulations. Ann Surg 2010;251:171–176
3. Marteau TM, Bekker H. The development of a six-item short-form of the state scale of the Spielberger State-Trait Anxiety Inventory (STAI). Br J Clin Psychol 1992;31:301–306
4. Pagano D, Freemantle N, Bridgewater B, et al. Social deprivation and prognostic benefits of cardiac surgery: observational study of 44 902 patients from five hospitals over 10 years. BMJ 2009;338:b902
5. Morgan O, Baker A. Measuring deprivation in England and Wales using 2001 Carstairs scores. Health Stat Q 2006; 31:28–33
6. Freedman LS, Pee D. Return to a note on screening regression equations. Am Stat 1989;43:279–282
7. Harrel F, Lee KL, Matchar DB, Reichert TA. Regression models for prognostic prediction: advantages, problems and suggested solutions. Cancer Treat Rep 1985;69:1071–1077
8. Peduzzi P, Concato J, Kemper E, Holford TR, Feinstein AR. A simulation study of the number of events per variable in logistic regression analysis. J Clin Epidemiol 1996;49: 1373–1379
9. Peduzzi P, Concato J, Feinstein AR, Holford TR. Importance of events per independent variable in proportional hazards regression analysis. II. Accuracy and precision of regression estimates. J Clin Epidemiol 1995;48:1503–1510
10. Mansfield ER, Helms BP. Detecting multicollinearity. Am Stat 1982;36:158–160
11. Guyatt GH, Rennie D, Meade M, Cook D, eds. Users' Guide to the Medical Literature: A Manual for Evidence-Based Clinical Practice. 2nd ed. New York: McGraw-Hill; 2008
12. Hosmer DW, Lemeshow S. Applied Logistic Regression. 2nd ed. New York: Wiley; 2000
13. Norman GR, Streiner DL. Biostatistics: The Bare Essentials. 3rd ed. New York: McGraw-Hill; 2008

24

Survival Analysis

Laurent Audigé, Monica Daigl

Summary

Survival analysis is the appropriate analytical technique to use to investigate time-to-event (survival) data. Such data are characterized by a clearly defined outcome event that may be experienced during the follow-up period by all or some subjects enrolled in a clinical study. The subjects who do not experience the event during their observation period (including subjects lost to follow-up) are said to be "censored." The strength of survival analysis is that it considers all observed subjects in the study, including those being censored. The analysis aims to describe the probability of survival (traditionally, the event being mortality) or failure (occurrence of the event) for all subjects up to and at any follow-up time. This enables prediction of if and when events are likely to occur. We illustrate this technique using several datasets of trauma patients considering mortality, but also favorable outcomes such as achievement of full weightbearing and return to work. Life tables, Kaplan–Meier estimates of the survival and failure function are presented, as well as the log-rank test to compare groups of patients. We introduce the concept of hazard ratio to quantify differences and the underlying proportional hazard assumption. We encourage using survival analysis in orthopaedic studies as the nature of many outcomes documented following surgery is that of time-to-event data.

Introduction

When choosing the most clinically relevant outcomes to assess the effectiveness of therapeutic interventions, the nature and format of the outcome data, as well as the research hypotheses, determine which methods should be used for the statistical analysis. For instance, in orthopaedics, when we compare two interventions in terms of a continuous outcome such as the functional Constant Score,[1] we might use a t-test. When the outcome of interest is binary, such as the occurrence of a complication, we might use the chi-square test. When time plays a role and we are interested in knowing not only whether an event occurred, but also how long it took for the event to occur, time-to-event analysis is the appropriate analytical approach. Time-to-event analysis is often referred to as "survival" analysis because the outcome of interest has most often been the time until death (i.e., the survival time),

for example in oncological studies. Death is also a commonly used outcome measure in surgical studies. However, the event of interest could be any other clinically relevant outcome, such as the achievement of pain-free full weightbearing, hospital discharge, or return to work. The occurrence of these events is often referred to as a "failure" even though the outcome might be favorable.

Survival analysis methodology is uncommon in orthopaedics.[2] However, some recent examples demonstrate its applicability as they address patient mortality following hip fractures,[3-5] prosthesis loosening, reoperation or poor function following total shoulder replacement,[6] and the development of avascular necrosis after acetabular fracture surgery.[7] In this chapter we discuss some of the specific issues affecting the way time to occurrence of an event is expressed and quantified, as well as how to evaluate the effect of factors (e.g., fracture type or surgical interventions) on the time to occurrence of an event. We guide the reader through simple methodological steps to collect and analyze time-to-event data, as well as the presentation of the results. Throughout this chapter we will use data from two prospective studies: one is a small pilot study assessing the time to achievement of full weightbearing following treatment of a tibia fracture in 31 patients (unpublished data) and the other is a larger prospective cohort study assessing the time to return to work after treatment of a distal radius fracture with locking compression plate (LCP) in 155 patients who were employed before the injury. This last dataset was extracted from a previously reported cohort study.[8-10]

Examples from the Literature: Additional Reading Material Regarding Survival Analysis

An introduction to survival analysis in medical research is available in general statistics textbooks for medical researchers such as Altman,[11] Armitage et al.,[12] and Kirkwood and Sterne.[13] Ohno-Machado presents the technique in the context of medical prognosis.[14] Collett[15] provides a comprehensive account of statistical methods for modeling survival data as well as an introduction to survival analysis using SAS software. Cleves et al.[16] focus on the application of survival analysis with Stata software. Finally, good tutorials are provided by two series of articles published in the *British Medical Journal*[17-19] and the *British Journal of Cancer*[20-23].

Documenting Time-to-Event (Survival) Data

Time-to-event data are characterized by the following features:
- For any subject, a clear starting point of the period of risk can be identified (e.g., the day of trauma or the day of surgical intervention).
- A well-defined and measurable study outcome is available (e.g., death, discharge from hospital, pain-free full weightbearing, return to work).
- Only one event can occur in any subject (or we would consider only the first occurrence for any event that could have remissions, e.g., occurrence of a local complication).

Survival data are collected in the form of two variables: a continuous variable for the time from the start of the period at risk to the time of occurrence of the event or end of the observation period (most often recorded in days, but could be weeks, months, or years, depending on the research setting), and a binary variable for the occurrence of the event (usually coded as 1 = event observed/ 0 = event not observed). When an event is observed, the continuous variable contains the time when the event occurred; when no event is observed, time is that of dropout or end of the study. At this point we would like to underline the importance of documenting the actual date of dropout of subjects (e.g., according to the research settings, the date of last visit or the date of discontinuation or death).

Key Concepts: Censoring

When the event of interest could not be observed for an individual, it is said to be censored. Censoring is defined as the occurrence (or possible occurrence) of the event when the subject is not under observation. This can occur in different ways, as summarized in **Fig. 24.1**.
Right censoring is the most common form of censoring that we need to deal with in the analysis of survival data. It occurs when a subject is no longer under observation and the outcome of interest was not observed in that subject. The subject might be lost to follow-up during a study or the study might end before all subjects could experience the event. The term *right* refers to the

fact that censoring occurs after the subject was recruited in a study, that is, on the *right*-hand side of **Fig. 24.1**.

At this stage, two important assumptions underlying the methods for survival analysis described in this chapter should be considered:
- Losses to follow-up (hence censoring) should be independent of the study outcome. In other words, lost subjects should have the same experience regarding the event as subjects remaining under observation in the study.
- Recruitment in a clinical study can be spread over a fairly long period of time, such as many years or even decades. The methods described assume that the survival experience of the first and last subjects enrolled is similar. This would imply that, for example, the procedures that affect the event of interest remain unchanged over the time of data collection.

Examples from the Literature: Survival Analysis in Orthopaedics and Traumatology

Survival analysis is becoming more popular in the field of orthopaedics and traumatology. Shortt and Robinson reported on mortality after low-energy fractures in patients over 45 years of age.[24] Over 12 years until 1999, 18 019 patients with fractures of the hip, wrist, or humeral neck were documented in a single center, and 6020 (33.4%) died during the study period. The subject survival probabilities were estimated within the 1st year, between 1 and 5 years, and then up to 10 years after the injury. The data were compared to mortality in the general population to show that low-energy trauma was associated with prolonged higher mortality in younger age cohorts, possibly owing to associated medical comorbidities (leading to the injury), and only higher mortality within 1 year after the injury in elderly subjects.

The Rationale for Time-to-Event (Survival) Analysis

Because time-to-event data are recorded on a continuous scale, an investigator might be tempted to use common statistical methods for the analysis of this type of data, such as the t-test and/or linear regression. Nevertheless, these methods are not appropriate for two reasons: the most important one is censoring, since time-to-event remains unknown for those subjects. The other reason is asymmetry, as most time-to-event data have distributions skewed to the right with some subjects experiencing the event very late. Methods that assume normality are therefore inappropriate.

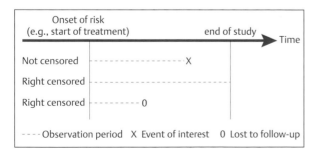

Fig. 24.1 Most common censoring of survival data.

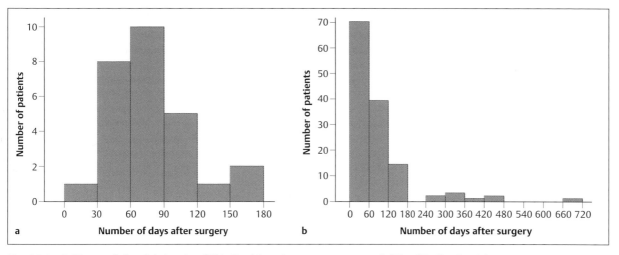

Fig. 24.2a, b Time to full weightbearing (Tibia Study) or time to return to work (Distal Radius Study).
a Tibial Study.
b Distal Radius Study.

Reality Check: Example Datasets

We illustrate these properties here with the data from the Tibia Study (endpoint of interest was time to full weightbearing) and the Distal Radius Study (time to return to work). The distribution of the end points can be found in **Fig. 24.2**.

In the Tibia Study (n = 30 patients) the distribution of the time to full weightbearing is fairly close to a normal distribution, with mean time to full weightbearing at 79 days. However, this average is based on data from 27 instead of 30 subjects. We documented one patient censored on day 6 (lost to follow-up after hospital discharge) and two patients who did not bear their full weight by the last follow-up examination on days 188 and 190, respectively. If we had followed up these two patients until they were eventually able to achieve full weightbearing, we would have obtained a greater average.

In the Distal Radius Study (n = 155 patients), the time to return to work was unknown for 23 patients (15%), 16 of whom were lost before the last follow-up at 2 years. In addition, the distribution of the time to return to work is clearly right-skewed (mean: 86 days, median: 56 days), with some patients again being later to return to work.

Although the mean time-to-event statistic might provide useful information, it intrinsically assumes noncensoring, and thus may be influenced by the length of follow-up. This means that results depend upon the settings and peculiarities of the particular studies, as shown for the Tibia and Distal Radius studies above. In order to enhance the comparability of findings across settings, we should avoid using this statistic for the purpose of describing time-to-event data.

Methods for Survival Analysis

Survival data are usually summarized by means of the *survival curve*. This curve plots the percentage of subjects who did not experience the event of interest up to a particular time, for example, from day of surgery to 1 week.

There are two methods from which to derive the survival curve, namely actuarial life tables and Kaplan–Meier. While both methods aim at the graphical representation of the survival curve, they differ in terms of the mathematics underlying the calculation of the survival probability and therefore produce slightly different plots.

Actuarial Life Tables for Grouped Data

Life tables are the method of choice when grouped data is available, such as when summary rather than individual data are provided. Life tables were developed to summarize long-term subject survival by dividing the life span into intervals during which the probability of dying was reasonably constant. An example of an actuarial life table of simulated survival data (mortality) is presented in **Table 24.1**. We will now examine how the table was prepared.

The number of subjects at risk refers to the beginning of the interval. For each time span we need to count the number of subjects lost to follow-up (censored observations). The life tables method assumes that these patients were lost on average at the midpoint of the corresponding interval (this information is usually not available for grouped data) and calculates the conditional probability of dying during each interval according to the adjusted number of subjects at risk over the time interval. For example, the risk of experiencing the event during the first interval is given by 20/75.5 = 0.265. The probability of surviving the

Table 24.1 Actuarial life table for risk of death following surgery (simulated data)

Time intervals, months	No. of subjects at risk, N	No. of subjects lost to follow-up (censored)	Adjusted no. of subjects at risk	No. of events (death)	Conditional survival probability	Cumulative survival probability
0–3	76	1	75.5	20	0.735	0.735
3–6	55	2	54	5	0.907	0.667
6–9	48	3	46.5	3	0.935	0.624
9–12	42	2	41	1	0.976	0.609

interval is therefore given by one *minus* the risk of experiencing the event (1 – 0.265 = 0.735). It should be noted that this is a *conditional* probability, that is, it is valid on the condition that the event did not occur in the preceding intervals. For instance, the probability of surviving between 3 and 6 months is 0.907, on condition that the subject survived the first 3 months.

The *cumulative* survival probability is calculated as the probability of not experiencing the event from the onset of the observation period (e.g., the start of treatment). From a mathematical point of view it is calculated as the product of the interval-specific survival probability with the previous ones; for instance, in our example table it is 0.735 × 0.907 × 0.935 = 0.624 for the third interval. The cumulative survival probability is used to produce a *survival curve* as shown in **Fig. 24.3**. Depending on the research question we may be more interested in the *failure curve*. This curve starts at zero and goes up as subjects experience events and is given by one *minus* the cumulative survival probabilities (see **Fig. 24.3**). The failure curve is particularly of use in describing rare events.

Jargon Simplified: Survival Function

The survival function $S(t)$ is the probability that a subject's time to event will exceed some specified time. For each time point (t) this function provides a probability that a subject will not experience the event of interest before or on that particular time [$P(T > t)$, meaning that the time T of occurrence of the event is greater than t].

$$S(t) = P(T > t)$$

The survival curve is a representation of the survival function. It goes *down*, starting at 1 (100%) and dropping toward 0 (0%) when subjects have experienced the event.

Jargon Simplified: Failure Function

The failure function is the subject's probability of not surviving—also referred to as experiencing the event within some specified time. The failure curve is a representation of the failure function, starting at 0 (0%) and going *up* to the proportion of subjects who experience the event within the period of observation.

Jargon Simplified: Hazard Function

The hazard function represents a probability divided by time: it represents the probability of experiencing an event in the next time interval, given that it was not experienced previously. The hazard is often simply interpreted as a conditional probability: for example, if return to work was measured on a daily basis, the hazard

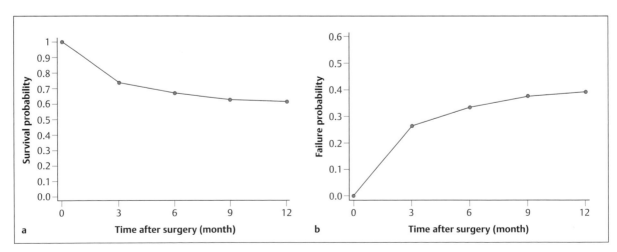

Fig. 24.3a, b Cumulative survival and failure curves derived from an actuarial life table.
a Survival curve.
b Failure curve.

at 2 months can be seen as the probability of a subject returning to work the next day after having been on sick leave for 2 months after surgery. The hazard function is used for *analytical purposes*, such as for comparing subject groups with regard to their survival experience and quantifying the effect of prognostic factors.

Kaplan–Meier Method for Individual Data

Kaplan–Meier (K–M) is the method of choice when individual data are available.[19,25] This method differs from the actuarial life tables by two important points:

- The K–M estimate does not depend on discrete time intervals defined by the investigator. Each table row is determined to be the time at which the next subject (or subjects) experiences the event of interest. Therefore, there is no assumption that the withdrawals occur uniformly during the considered intervals and that the risk of the event is constant across the predefined intervals as each event determines a new interval.
- Censored observations between two events are considered as subjects at risk only up to the time of the first of the two events.

Reality Check: Kaplan–Meier Table

The table that serves for the derivation of the K–M survival curve for the Tibia Study is presented in **Table 24.2**. This table is constructed as follows: the time of event (days) is presented in order of ranking, then at each time of event (full weight bearing), the number of subjects at risk of experiencing the event and still in the study at that time, the number of censored observations (occurring between the time of the event and the time of the next event occurrence), and the number of events are considered. Note that when both censoring and event occur at the same time, the event is assumed to have occurred first. In this example, one subject was lost to follow-up after hospital discharge 6 days after

treatment and therefore is not counted for the following event time at 35 days and risk estimation. The probability of experiencing the event at each time point, conditional upon having not experienced the event up to that time (hazard), is estimated. For example, the probability of experiencing full weightbearing at 35 days is 1/28 = 0.036. The survival and failure functions are calculated as in actuarial life tables.

Presenting the K–M table is best suited to a small sample size, because with large databases and many events such tables could end up being very long. The survival function is usually presented graphically as a step function starting at 1 and decreasing over time, as illustrated in **Fig. 24.4** for the time to full weightbearing data of the Tibia Study. The failure function may be more appropriate for favorable and/or rare outcomes.[26] To ease interpretation of the results, the number of subjects at risk at each planned follow-up examination can be presented in the figure, as can a 95% confidence interval band.

Examples from the Literature: Risk Factors for Revision after Shoulder Arthroplasty

Fevang et al.[27] analyzed survival data from 1825 subjects documented in the Norwegian Arthroplasty Register between 1994 and 2005. Kaplan–Meier failure curves (note that failure curves go upward) for prosthesis revision were drawn over a 12-year period for 1531 hemiprostheses (including resurfacing hemiprostheses), 225 reversed total prostheses, and 69 Neer total prostheses. The author presented the K–M failure curves with a 95% confidence band (**Fig. 24.5**) to demonstrate good results with the use of hemiarthroplasty. The poorer prognosis documented in relation to revision surgery associated with reverse or Neer total prosthesis is somewhat mitigated by the larger confidence band, which is due to the smaller sample size.

Table 24.2 Excerpt of the Kaplan–Meier (K–M) table from the Tibia Study

Time t, days	No. of subjects at risk, N	No. of subjects lost to follow-up (censored)	No. of events	Conditional failure probability	Cumulative survival probability	Cumulative failure probability
1	30	1	1	0.033	0.967	0.033
35	28	0	1	0.036	0.932	0.068
36	27	0	1	0.037	0.898	0.102
41	26	0	1	0.038	0.863	0.137
48	25	0	2	0.080	0.794	0.206
53	23	0	1	0.043	0.760	0.241
56	22	0	1	0.045	0.725	0.275
58	21	0	1	0.048	0.691	0.310
[...]						

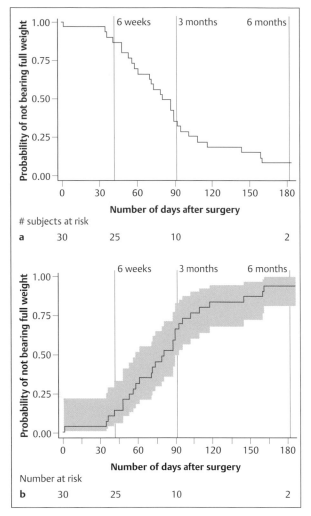

Fig. 24.4a, b Kaplan–Meier survival and failure functions for the Tibia Study.
a Survival function.
b Failure function (with 95% confidence interval band).

Comparing Groups

In this section we introduce the log-rank test to compare survival curves, as well as the concept of hazard ratio (HR) for quantifying the effect of prognostic factors such as treatment. For more details regarding Cox regression, refer to Chapter 23.

Two failure functions representing the probability of returning to work for two separate subgroups of subjects in the Distal Radius Study are presented in **Fig. 24.6**. The patients were grouped according to the severity of their fracture (AO classification type A or B versus type C[28]). The failure (or survival) functions are a powerful means of identifying differences in trends over time. We may note that—depending on the outcome—with a long enough follow-up time, nearly all patients might experience the event in any group. In the example above, the probability of return-

ing to work within 6 months (181 days) after surgery is about 90% in both groups.

Having observed the difference in terms of probability of returning to work for the two groups of patients in the Distal Radius Study, we are interested in knowing whether the difference is genuine or if it may have arisen only by chance. We are interested in testing the null hypothesis that the two curves do not differ.

The *log-rank test* (also known as the *Mantel–Haenszel test*) is the most commonly used approach to test whether the overall survival (or failure) functions in two or more groups are equal. No assumption is made as to the distribution of time-to-event in compared groups. At each time point of occurrence of an event, the observed number of events is compared with the expected number of events under the null hypothesis that there is no difference between the groups (i.e., the survival function is equal) and χ^2 statistic is computed.

It should be noted that the log-rank test gives equal weight to each time point, irrespective of the number of subjects at risk. The *Wilcoxon* (or *Breslow*) *test* is an alternative test that puts more weight on the initial part of the curves where sample size is larger, and thus is more sensitive to differences early in the time period.

For the two curves in **Fig. 24.6**, the *P* value associated with the log-rank test is 0.211, indicating that the observed difference between the two curves is not statistically significant at a 5% level. Interestingly, the *P* value associated with the Wilcoxon test is 0.038, indicating a statistically significant difference between the two curves. It is for this reason that it is critical to specify in advance the test used to compare curves as well as the time point of interest, in order to avoid post hoc decisions. Again interestingly, should we have studied return to work only up to 2 months after surgery (we simulated these data by setting all subjects not returned to work at 2 months as censored), the log-rank test would have shown a statistically significant difference (*P* = 0.037).

The nonparametric tests described have some limitations. For instance, they do not directly provide an effect size. However, we do often want to quantify the effect of surgical intervention (possibly while adjusting for confounding variables), or evaluate the effect of one or more potential prognostic variables. The most commonly used approach for this is the Cox proportional hazards regression model.[29]

We will now consider a simple model for the comparison of two groups. Cox regression makes no assumptions about the form of the hazard curves, but it assumes proportionality among the two curves:

$$\frac{h_{\text{group A}}(t)}{h_{\text{group B}}(t)} = constant$$

where *h* is the hazard and *t* is the time.

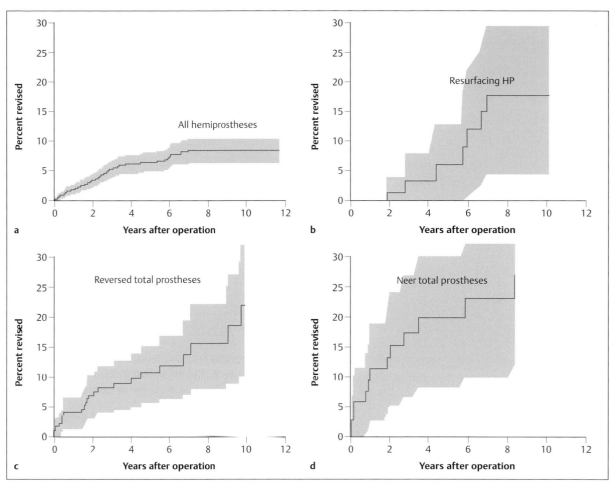

Fig. 24.5 Kaplan–Meier failure curves with 95% confidence interval bands.
Reproduced with permission from Fevang et al.[27]

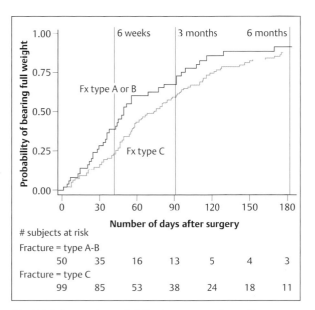

Fig. 24.6 Return to work following surgery for patients experiencing an AO type C vs. a type A or B radius fracture (Fx).

Reality Check: Comparison between Groups
Continuing to use the Distal Radius Study, we explored the effect of several factors on time to return to work by means of Cox regression. In addition to fracture type (AO type A or B vs. type C), we considered the implant type (LCP 2.4 mm vs. 3.5 mm), the surgical approach (volar vs. dorsal), whether the dominant hand was injured (Yes/No), and age. All variables were included in a multivariable Cox regression model. We found a borderline significant HR of 1.48 for fracture type (95% CI 1.0–2.2; $P = 0.050$) and a positive significant effect of the 2.4-mm LCP (HR = 1.7; 95% CI 1.2–2.5; $P = 0.006$), indicating that subjects receiving the thinner plate have higher chances of returning early to work.

Jargon Simplified: Hazard Ratio
The hazard ratio (HR) is the ratio between two hazards: the hazard of experiencing the event in the intervention group at a given point in time over the hazard of experiencing the event in the control group at the same time point. This ratio is interpreted similarly to risk ratios. An HR of one means that there is no effect associated

with the predictor variable under investigation, hence events occur at the same pace in both groups. When the predictor reduces the probability of occurrence of the event, the HR is less than one; when the factor is associated with an increase of risk, the ratio is greater than one.

The Cox model can be used to adjust for confounding variables when assessing the effect of specific factors such as surgical interventions, as well as to build a prognostic model to explain associations between factors and outcome or to make predictions on the survival experience of specific subjects.

Examples from the Literature: Length of Stay, Mortality, Morbidity, and Delay to Surgery in Hip Fractures

Lefaivre et al.[5] investigated the effect of the time from admission to surgery on the time to hospital discharge (acute length of stay) in 607 patients operated on for hip fractures. Forty-eight patients (7.9%) were censored during hospitalization because of death. The Cox proportional hazard model was applied, while the analysis was adjusted for co-morbidity, age, gender, and type of fracture. A delay to surgery of 1 day was found to be associated with a later hospital discharge (HR = 0.91; 95% CI 0.83–0.99).

Examples from the Literature: Factors Determining the 1-Year Survival after Operated Hip Fracture—A Hospital-Based Analysis

Ho et al.[4] reviewed 409 patients operated on for hip fractures between 1998 and 2006 in one hospital. Using multivariable Cox regression they examined the associations between many prognostic factors and the 1-year survival rate, including co-morbidities, age, gender, low preoperative hemoglobin level and high creatinine level, delay to operation, duration of operation, arthroplasty, and length of hospital stay. Among other significant factors, a delay to operation of more than 48 hours was associated with poorer survival compared to surgery within 24 hours of trauma (adjusted HR 2.86; 95% CI 1.08–7.54).

Checking the Proportional Hazards Assumption

The log-rank test and Cox regression methods assume that the ratio of the hazard functions for the two groups is constant over the time period of observation. The first step to verify the proportional hazards assumption is to plot the survival or failure function for each group on the same graph and consider their patterns visually (as in **Fig. 24.6**). When the assumption holds true the two curves should diverge and never cross at any time. More formally, the assumption can be tested by plotting the cumulative hazard function on a log-log scale. The plotted lines for

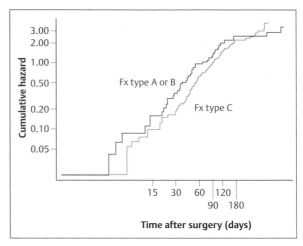

Fig. 24.7 Cumulative hazard plot of the Distal Radius Study data plotted on a log-log scale.

the two groups should run parallel in cases of proportionality, as illustrated in **Fig. 24.7** for the Distal Radius Study.

Key Concepts: Cumulative Hazard Function
The cumulative hazard function is the sum of the hazard experienced up to a given time point. While the hazard function goes up and down with time, the cumulative hazard function can only go up and is therefore easier to interpret and to use for graphical purposes. It can be demonstrated that if the proportional hazard assumption holds true, the cumulative hazard functions plotted on a log-log scale run parallel.

Practical Considerations in the Design of Time-to-Event Studies

We would like to briefly summarize a series of aspects that we deem important when planning a survival analysis. The choice of the outcome as well as its measurement technique should be considered carefully. The event of interest must be clearly defined and be as objective as possible. Moreover, it should be easy to assess, so that time to occurrence may be recorded accurately. In studies of surgical interventions in orthopaedics, patients are under daily observation during hospitalization until discharge; afterward they are only examined at a few follow-up visits. After hospital discharge, patient-assessed outcomes that can be assessed on a daily basis might be more appropriate than radiological parameters that are only assessed at certain time points.

Some events can be directly observed and their time of occurrence can be accurately recorded (e.g., hospital discharge, initiation of full weightbearing, return to employment, revision surgery for joint prosthesis, and death). At each planned visit it might be possible for the subject to recall the time of occurrence of targeted events, or patients might even be required to keep personal records at home between visits.

The length of follow-up in studies of time-to-event outcomes should be defined according to the research question. When planning a study using survival analysis, it is helpful to have a good idea of the shape of the failure function of the primary event within a practical follow-up time. For instance, a 3-month follow-up period of observation might be appropriate to study achievement of full weight-bearing in patients with tibia fractures, but not for patients undergoing arthroplasty.

Survival analysis can be performed using any major statistical software packages (e.g., SAS, SPSS, Stata). As results might be quite susceptible to the techniques used, we recommend making use of a statistical analysis plan that defines the details of the statistical methods before the data is collected, in order to avoid post hoc evaluations.

Conclusion

When studying outcomes related to events that may occur at any time within the follow-up period and beyond, survival analysis is the appropriate analytical technique to use because it examines not only the occurrence of an event of interest, but also the time distribution of occurrence. It accounts for all enrolled and observed persons, whatever their actual follow-up period and whether or not they experienced the event.

Survival analyses are also becoming more popular in the framework of trauma and orthopaedic research. We would like to encourage investigators to consider it in orthopaedic studies, because the nature of many outcomes following surgery is that of time-to-event data.

References

1. Constant CR, Murley AH. A clinical method of functional assessment of the shoulder. Clin Orthop 1987;214:160–164
2. Evans JM. The use of survival analysis for the evaluation of musculoskeletal therapy. J Manipulative Physiol Ther 2005;28:374
3. Söderqvist A, Ekstrom W, Ponzer S, et al. Prediction of mortality in elderly patients with hip fractures: a two-year prospective study of 1,944 patients. Gerontology 2009;55:496–504
4. Ho CA, Li CY, Hsieh KS, Chen HF. Factors determining the 1-year survival after operated hip fracture: a hospital-based analysis. J Orthop Sci 2010;15:30–37
5. Lefaivre KA, Macadam SA, Davidson DJ, Gandhi R, Chan H, Broekhuyse HM. Length of stay, mortality, morbidity and delay to surgery in hip fractures. J Bone Joint Surg Br 2009;91:922–927
6. Kasten P, Pape G, Raiss P, et al. Mid-term survivorship analysis of a shoulder replacement with a keeled glenoid and a modern cementing technique. J Bone Joint Surg Br 2010;92:387–392
7. Reddix RN, Russell G, Woodall J, Jackson B, Dedmond B, Webb LX. Relationship between intraoperative femoral head bleeding and development of avascular necrosis after acetabular fracture surgery. J Surg Orthop Adv 2009;18:129–133
8. Souer JS, Ring D, Matschke S, Audige L, Marent-Huber M, Jupiter JB. Effect of an unrepaired fracture of the ulnar styloid base on outcome after plate-and-screw fixation of a distal radial fracture. J Bone Joint Surg Am 2009;91:830–838
9. Jupiter JB, Marent-Huber M. Operative management of distal radial fractures with 2.4-millimeter locking plates. A multicenter prospective case series. J Bone Joint Surg Am 2009;91:55–65
10. Souer JS, Ring D, Jupiter JB, Matschke S, Audige L, Marent-Huber M. Comparison of AO type-B and type-C volar shearing fractures of the distal part of the radius. J Bone Joint Surg Am 2009;91:2605–2611
11. Altman DG. Practical Statistics for Medical Research. 1st ed. Chapman and Hall/CRC; 1990
12. Armitage P, Berry G, Matthews JNS. Statistical Methods in Medical Research. 4th ed. Oxford: Wiley-Blackwell; 2001
13. Kirkwood BR, Sterne JAC. Essential Medical Statistics. 2nd ed. Oxford: Blackwell Science; 2003
14. Ohno-Machado L. Modeling medical prognosis: survival analysis techniques. J Biomed Inform 2001;34:428–439
15. Collett D. Modelling Survival Data in Medical Research. 2nd ed. Chapman and Hall/CRC Press; 2003
16. Cleves M, Gould W, Gutierrez R, Marchenko Y. An Introduction to Survival Analysis Using Stata. 2nd ed. College Station, Texas: Stata Press; 2008
17. Bland JM, Altman DG. The logrank test. BMJ 2004;328:1073
18. Altman DG, Bland JM. Time to event (survival) data. BMJ 1998;317:468–469
19. Bland JM, Altman DG. Survival probabilities (the Kaplan-Meier method). BMJ 1998;317:1572
20. Bradburn MJ, Clark TG, Love SB, Altman DG. Survival analysis Part III: multivariate data analysis—choosing a model and assessing its adequacy and fit. Br J Cancer 2003;89:605–611
21. Bradburn MJ, Clark TG, Love SB, Altman DG. Survival analysis part II: multivariate data analysis—an introduction to concepts and methods. Br J Cancer 2003; 89:431–436
22. Clark TG, Bradburn MJ, Love SB, Altman DG. Survival analysis part IV: further concepts and methods in survival analysis. Br J Cancer 2003;89:781–786
23. Clark TG, Bradburn MJ, Love SB, Altman DG. Survival analysis part I: basic concepts and first analyses. Br J Cancer 2003;89:232–238
24. Shortt NL, Robinson CM. Mortality after low-energy fractures in patients aged at least 45 years old. J Orthop Trauma 2005;19:396–400
25. Kaplan EL, Meier P. Nonparametric estimation from incomplete observations. J Am Stat Assoc 1958;53:457–481
26. Pocock SJ, Clayton TC, Altman DG. Survival plots of time-to-event outcomes in clinical trials: good practice and pitfalls. Lancet 2002;359:1686–1689
27. Fevang BT, Lie SA, Havelin LI, Skredderstuen A, Furnes O. Risk factors for revision after shoulder arthroplasty: 1,825 shoulder arthroplasties from the Norwegian Arthroplasty Register. Acta Orthop 2009;80:83–91
28. Müller ME, Nazarian S, Koch P, Schatzker J. The Comprehensive Classification of Fractures of Long Bones. Berlin, Heidelberg, New York: Springer-Verlag, 1990
29. Cox DR. Regression models and life-tables. J R Stat Soc 1972;34:187–220

25

Interim Analyses in Randomized Trials

Beate P. Hanson, Ujash Sheth

"Everything that can be counted doesn't necessarily count; everything that counts can't necessarily be counted."
—*Albert Einstein*

Summary

The goal of this chapter is to demonstrate how interim analyses are used to monitor the safety and efficacy of randomized controlled trials. Two classic statistical approaches to interim analyses, the Pocock method and the O'Brien–Fleming method, are presented in addition to the more flexible alpha spending approach. The potential pitfalls associated with stopping randomized controlled trials early for benefit are discussed.

Introduction

In order for clinical research to be ethical, investigators must ensure that a favorable risk–benefit ratio exists.[1] This means that the risks to the patient should be minimized while any potential benefits should be maximized. But what happens when there is an *unexpected* level of harm or benefit seen during a clinical trial? How can we avoid exposing patients to inferior treatments for unnecessarily prolonged periods of time? Should we monitor the data from the treatment arms before the end of the study period? If so, who should be responsible for monitoring the data? What outcomes should be monitored? When should the trial be stopped early? And are there any potential risks associated with stopping the trial prior to its scheduled completion? This chapter will provide answers to these questions in an attempt to present a basic overview of the function of interim analyses in randomized controlled trials.

Interim Analysis Defined

An interim analysis is used to compare the data collected from the treatment and control arms of a randomized controlled trial prior to the scheduled completion of the study to allow for early termination of the trial if unexpected magnitudes of benefit or harm are detected.[2] When a

trial is stopped early for benefit, this means that the accrued information in the trial is sufficient to reject the null hypothesis, whereas if the trial is stopped due to harm the accrued information is sufficient to reject the alternative hypothesis.

> **Jargon Simplified: Null Hypothesis**
> The null hypothesis assumes that there is no significant difference between two groups.

> **Jargon Simplified: Alternative Hypothesis**
> The alternative hypothesis assumes that a significant difference does exist between two groups.

There are a number of compelling reasons to perform an interim analysis. Ethically speaking, we want to ensure that the greatest number of patients receive the most beneficial treatment while minimizing the number of patients exposed to inferior treatments. For cost-efficiency purposes, we want to ensure that we do not waste valuable time and resources prolonging a trial that has already provided convincing evidence. Finally, interim analyses also allow us to determine whether our original assumptions regarding sample size, treatment efficacy, and adverse effects are still valid.[2,3] This is especially important for long-term trials where the study design and sample size calculations are based on preliminary and/or uncertain information from the beginning of the trial.[2]

> **Key Concepts: Interim Analysis**
> Interim analysis is a survey of the data at one or more time points prior to the end of a study to determine whether there is a need to stop the trial early due to efficacy or futility.

Design of an Interim Analysis

An interim analysis may occur at any point in time between trial enrollment and follow-up. However, it should only be conducted when there are enough patients to warrant comparison between groups, otherwise even large treatment effects will be insignificant with smaller sample sizes.[3] In addition, since the number of interim analyses can affect the interpretation of the results of a trial, as we will see later in the chapter, all interim analyses should be planned and described in the study protocol.[2] If an unplanned interim analysis is to be conducted, then before unblinded access is given to treatment comparison data, an amendment to the study protocol must be completed explaining why the need for an interim analysis has arisen.[2]

Most randomized trials compare interventions on a large number of outcome variables. However, when conducting an interim analysis it is optimal if only the major outcome variables are analyzed in order to avoid issues associated with multiple comparisons.[3] In fact, Pocock suggests that investigators should limit the number of major outcome comparisons to one and define formal "stopping rules" for that particular outcome.[4] The remaining treatment outcomes may be used to unofficially evaluate the consistency of the observed difference in the main outcome comparison between treatment groups.[4]

On the surface it may seem as though increasing the number of interim analyses will improve patient safety and potentially be cost-effective; however, conducting an interim analysis comes at a cost. Since interim analysis is a form of multiple testing, the probability of a type I error increases each time an interim analysis is conducted. As a result, Pocock recommends that at least one, but no more than five interim analyses be conducted.[4]

Jargon Simplified: Type I Error

A type I error is also known as an α-error or a false-positive result. Usually, investigators designate how much type I error is acceptable at the beginning of the trial. A nominal significance level, α, of ≤ 0.05 or 5% is commonly used. This means that we accept that there may be a 5% chance that the null hypothesis was falsely rejected.

Reality Check: Sequential Significance Test Method

Suppose we are conducting a randomized controlled trial comparing internal fixation with total hip arthroplasty for displaced femoral neck fractures. Now imagine performing an interim analysis (with a type I error set at $\alpha = 0.05$ for each interim test) every time a new event was recorded for each pair of randomized patients. What would happen to the study-wide false-positive rate? It would increase. Why? Well, the error made in analysis here is that we treated each interim analysis as if it were the only one we performed. Since the data is being analyzed more frequently, the likelihood of a false-positive result increases with each interim analysis.[5] As a result, the combined possibility of falsely rejecting the null hypothesis increases as shown in **Table 25.1**. This hypothetical situation utilizes the *sequential or repeated significance test method* of interim analysis, which is seldom used in practice due to its burdensome nature and penchant for inflating the false-positive rate.[6] So how do we avoid this problem? The next section takes a look at some common statistical methods for preserving the overall type I error at $\alpha = 0.05$.

Table 25.1 False-positive rates in multiple interim tests

Number of tests	False-positive rate
1	0.05
2	0.08
3	0.11
10	0.19
20	0.25

Group Sequential Method

Among all available statistical stopping methods, the group sequential method is arguably the most common and carries out interim analyses at equally spaced intervals.[7] When using the group sequential design, before beginning the trial we must decide how many interim analyses we are going to perform (N) and the number of patients per treatment group that will be assessed between subsequent interim analyses (n).[7] For instance, in a trial where there are two treatment groups, data are analyzed after the results of each consecutive group of 2n patients become available. The two groups are then compared using standard statistical hypothesis testing. If the P value is less than the nominal level of significance, α, then the trial may potentially be stopped, depending on the stopping rules and guidelines established prior to the start of the trial.[7]

In order to perform interim analysis and maintain the overall type I error at a predetermined level (usually 5%), we need to "spend" smaller values of α during earlier tests of significance. Therefore, only very large differences between groups will lead to a significant result. The two classic approaches used to manage α during interim analyses are the Pocock method and the O'Brien–Fleming method. Both methods utilize the number of planned interim analyses to determine the P value at which consideration will be given to stopping the trial. The less commonly used Haybittle–Peto method uses significance levels independent of the number of interim analyses conducted.

The Pocock approach, also known as the fixed nominal level approach, maintains constant significance levels across all interim analyses. This means that in order for a trial with four planned interim analyses to maintain an overall type I error = 0.05, as seen in **Table 25.2**, a P value of 0.018 would be needed to establish significance at each analysis including the final one.[7,8] Critics of this approach point to the fact that if we were to obtain a P value = 0.03 for the previous example it would be deemed not significant. However, if a group sequential approach had not been used, the results from the trial would in fact have been significant.[8] As a result, this approach has fallen out of favor, especially since other methods have been developed to eliminate this important limitation.

Table 25.2 Nominal significance levels according to the number of planned interim analyses conducted by group sequential design

Number of planned interim analyses	Interim analysis	Pocock	Peto	O'Brien–Fleming
2	1	0.029	0.001	0.005
	2 (final)	0.029	0.05	0.048
3	1	0.022	0.001	0.0005
	2	0.022	0.001	0.014
	3 (final)	0.022	0.05	0.045
4	1	0.018	0.001	0.0001
	2	0.018	0.001	0.004
	3	0.018	0.001	0.019
	4 (final)	0.018	0.05	0.043
5	1	0.016	0.001	0.00001
	2	0.016	0.001	0.0013
	3	0.016	0.001	0.008
	4	0.016	0.001	0.023
	5 (final)	0.016	0.05	0.041

Overall α = 0.05. Reproduced with permission from Schulz and Grimes.[8]

The O'Brien–Fleming approach uses very low nominal significance levels during earlier analyses and gradually increases it toward the final analysis.[9] In fact, for a trial with four planned interim analyses, in order to maintain an overall type I error = 0.05, the first analysis would have to yield a P value of 0.0001 to stop the trial (**Table 25.2**), while the second, third, and fourth interim analyses would need P values of 0.004, 0.019, and 0.043 to consider stopping the trial.[9] As you can see, the O'Brien-Fleming approach allows us to preserve most of our intended α level (i. e., 0.05) in addition to our power.[8] Critics of the O'Brien–Fleming approach believe the very low α level used for the first analysis may be too stringent, essentially guaranteeing that the trial is not stopped then.[10]

The Haybittle–Peto approach is yet another group sequential method that is by far the most simple of all the approaches discussed thus far. This approach utilizes extremely cautious stopping criteria by setting nominal levels of significance at a constant 0.001 for all interim analyses regardless of the number conducted (**Table 25.2**). However, during the final analysis the nominal level of significance is set at the standard 0.05.[8,10]

> **Key Concepts: Pocock Method**
> The Pocock method uses the same cutoff for all interim analyses as well as the final analysis.

> **Key Concepts: O'Brien–Fleming Method**
> The O'Brien–Fleming method uses a very strict cutoff early on then relaxes the cutoff as time passes.

> **Key Concepts: Haybittle–Peto Method**
> The Haybittle–Peto method uses a constant cutoff of 0.001 for all interim analyses and a cutoff of 0.05 for the final analysis.

Of the three different group sequential methods reviewed here, there are two limitations that are common to them all. The first is that the number of planned interim analyses must be scheduled prior to the start of the trial. The second is that equal numbers of patients or events are needed between successive analyses.[11] So what happens when we need to conduct an unplanned interim analysis? Or to conduct an interim analysis with an unequal number of patients or events? The next section will take a look at how to address these quite common issues.

Alpha Spending Function

Lan and DeMets developed a more flexible adaptation of the group sequential approach that no longer required the number or time of interim analyses to be planned prior to the beginning of the trial.[11] They proposed a method called the "alpha spending function" which allowed investigators to "spend" the type I error rate, α, a little bit at a time as the trial progressed.[11,12] Use of the alpha spending function assures investigators that the overall type I error at the end of the trial will be the predetermined value of α.[12] All that is needed is the information fraction. The information fraction can be calculated by taking the number of patients randomized at that point of the trial

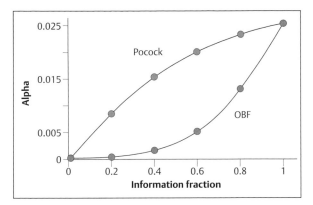

Fig. 25.1 The shape of alpha spending functions for Pocock and O'Brien–Fleming (OBF) type boundaries is depicted here for a one-sided α of 0.025. Reproduced with permission from DeMets and Lan KK.[11]

(i.e., at the time point when the interim analysis is performed), n, and dividing it by the target sample size, N.[11] As a result, the alpha spending function dictates how the predetermined α is spent at each interim analysis as a function of the information fraction.[12] Since Lan–DeMets is a family of alpha-spending curves, the practical applications of the Lan–DeMets family may resemble Pocock, O'Brien–Fleming, and other statistical solutions. However, the dynamic of alpha spending is substantially different between the Pocock and O'Brien–Fleming approaches. The Pocock-type spending function allocates alpha equally and rapidly across the interim analyses. The O'Brien–Fleming-type spending function, on the other hand, allocates little alpha at early stages and saves more alpha spending for the later stages (**Fig. 25.1**).[12]

> **Key Concepts: Alpha Spending Function**
> The "alpha spending function" is a method of describing how the total type I error rate, α, is allocated as a continuous function of the information fraction, which ultimately provides investigators with a corresponding stopping boundary.

Now that we have introduced a number of common statistical methods used during an interim analysis, the question becomes: Who should be responsible for interpreting this information? In the following section we see how data monitoring committees not only assume this role but also play an integral part in the interim analysis.

Data Monitoring Committees

The role of the data monitoring committee is not limited to interpreting the results from the statistical analysis, although that is its primary function. Other activities the committee is involved in include monitoring trial conduct,

assuring patient safety, ensuring ethical conduct of the trial, and assessing the efficacy of the treatment.[13] The data monitoring committee is principally charged with the responsibility for making recommendations regarding whether to continue a trial or terminate it based on the predetermined stopping rules in the study protocol.[2]

The data monitoring committee, or safety data and monitoring board, is composed of clinical scientists who are knowledgeable in the discipline of interest and are familiar with statistical methods. They are an independent group that shares no affiliation with the institutional review board or independent ethics committee.[2] This independence is intended to maintain the confidentiality and integrity of the trial by ensuring that information regarding the efficacy of treatment is not shared with blinded individuals (i.e., patients and investigators).[2] If the investigators and research staff were to learn the results of the interim analysis, that might change their approach to the trial procedures and result in various forms of bias.[12] Investigators and research staff should only be informed about the decision to continue, discontinue, or implement modifications to the trial.[13]

> **Jargon Simplified: Data Monitoring Committee**
> The primary role of the data monitoring committee is to ensure the safety of the study participants by reviewing interim reports for evidence of adverse or beneficial treatment effects. This committee also makes decisions regarding the frequency, timing, and manner in which interim data are analyzed.[14,15]

> **Examples from the Literature: Reporting an Interim Analysis**
> Kirkley et al. conducted a single-center randomized controlled trial to compare arthroscopic débridement in conjunction with physical and medical therapy versus treatment with physical and medical therapy alone in patients with moderate to severe osteoarthritis.[16] The following excerpt from the methods section demonstrates the way in which details of an interim analysis should be reported:
> "A single prespecified interim analysis was performed by an external data monitoring board when one-third of the patients had completed 2 years of follow-up. This analysis was based on an O'Brien–Fleming boundary that specified a P value of 0.0007 to stop the trial because of superiority of treatment and a P value of 0.984 to stop the trial because of futility of treatment."

> **Interpretation**
> Note that the investigators of the trial stated the number of planned interim analyses, the time point at which the analysis was taking place, the statistical method of analysis used, and the P values associated with stopping the trial for efficacy or futility.

Examples from the Literature: Using Interim Analysis to Modify a Randomized Controlled Trial

Camporese et al. performed a randomized controlled trial in adults having arthroscopic knee surgery to evaluate whether low-molecular-weight heparin (LMWH) was superior to graduated compression stockings in preventing deep venous thrombosis and other complications.[17] Patients were randomly assigned to receive graduated compression stockings for 7 days, a daily injection of LMWH (nadroparin) for 7 days, or a daily injection of LMWH (nadroparin) for 14 days. The investigators of the trial utilized the O'Brien–Fleming method for the three planned interim analyses at 40%, 65%, and 80% of the target sample size. Increasing α levels of 0.0006, 0.0045, and 0.0125 were utilized with the final α level set at 0.025. At the time of the second interim analysis, the data monitoring committee discontinued therapy for the 14-day LMWH group. Issues of efficacy and futility were not the reason for their decision; rather, the trial's data monitoring committee had concerns regarding the safety of utilizing a longer LMWH regimen.

Interpretation

This example illustrates how data monitoring committees play an important role during the course of a randomized trial even if they are not making decisions regarding stopping early.

Consequences of Stopping Early for Benefit

Randomized trials that are stopped early for benefit often garner an enormous amount of attention. These are often the trials that the general public hears about on television and the radio. What's more is that a recent systematic review has found that the number of randomized trials stopped early for benefit has nearly doubled since 1990.[18] The general public may interpret this finding as evidence that patient safety has vastly improved over the past two decades. However, in reality trials stopped early for benefit provide interpretational challenges for investigators, clinicians, and even policy makers.[19] The reason for this is inherent to the statistical methods we use to determine our stopping rules, which may in fact systematically overestimate treatment effects.[20] It is believed that this overestimation is a result of large random fluctuations of the estimated treatment effect, especially earlier in the trial.[8] Thus, it is possible that the large beneficial treatment effect used to justify stoppage of the trial may be misleading in some cases. Moreover, in trials where the number of accumulated outcome events is small, the overestimation of treatment effect can be quite large.[21] Serious problems can develop when inflated estimates are used to inform clinical decision making and practice guidelines.[21] As a re-

sult, it has been recommended that investigators of randomized trials ensure that stopping rules in the study protocol demand that a large number of events occur before termination of a trial is considered.[20] There are also a number of other limitations associated with stopping a randomized trial early. One important limitation is that the trial tends to result in a smaller sample size, while incomplete information about side effects and complications of treatment are gathered. The lack of this important information may leave the clinical community unconvinced about the efficacy of the treatment.

Examples from the Literature: Stopping Randomized Trials Early for Benefit and Estimation of Treatment Effects—Systematic Review and Meta-regression Analysis

Source: Bassler D, Briel M, Montori VM, Lane M, Glasziou P, Zhou Q, Heels-Ansdell D, Walter SD, Guyatt GH; STOPIT-2 Study Group.

Context: Theory and simulation suggest that randomized controlled trials (RCTs) stopped early for benefit (truncated RCTs) systematically overestimate treatment effects for the outcome that precipitated early stopping.[20]

Objective: To compare the treatment effect from truncated RCTs with that from meta-analyses of RCTs addressing the same question but not stopped early (nontruncated RCTs) and to explore factors associated with overestimates of effect.

Data sources: Search of MEDLINE, EMBASE, Current Contents, and full-text journal content databases to identify truncated RCTs up to January 2007; search of MEDLINE, Cochrane Database of Systematic Reviews, and Database of Abstracts of Reviews of Effects to identify systematic reviews from which individual RCTs were extracted up to January 2008.

Study selection: Selected studies were RCTs reported as having stopped early for benefit and matching nontruncated RCTs from systematic reviews. Independent reviewers with medical content expertise, working blinded to trial results, judged the eligibility of the nontruncated RCTs based on their similarity to the truncated RCTs.

Data extraction: Reviewers with methodological expertise conducted data extraction independently.

Results: The analysis included 91 truncated RCTs asking 63 different questions and 424 matching nontruncated RCTs. The pooled ratio of relative risks in truncated RCTs versus matching nontruncated RCTs was 0.71 (95% confidence interval, 0.65–0.77). This difference was independent of the presence of a statistical stopping rule and the methodological quality of the studies as assessed on the basis of allocation concealment and blinding. Large differences in treatment effect size between truncated and nontruncated RCTs (ratio of relative risks <0.75) occurred, with truncated RCTs having fewer than 500 events. In 39 of the 63 questions (62%), the pooled effects of the nontruncated RCTs failed to demonstrate significant benefit.

Conclusions: Truncated RCTs were associated with greater effect sizes than RCTs not stopped early. This difference was independent of the presence of statistical stopping rules and was greatest in smaller studies.

Interpretation

The results of this systematic review suggest that the true treatment effect may in fact be negligible or absent in some instances where a randomized trial had been stopped for benefit. Consequently, clinicians and policy makers should be cautious before acting on the results of randomized trials that have been stopped for benefit.

Conclusion

We have reviewed how interim analyses provide investigators with an opportunity to analyze the accrued data before the end of the trial in order to detect trends that may warrant modification of the study protocol or, possibly, termination of the trial. The group sequential methods discussed in this chapter offer an interesting approach to statistical analysis of interim data; however, the major shortcoming of these methods is that they result in an overestimation of the treatment effect. As a result, trials stopped early for benefit can be quite problematic for trial investigators, clinicians, and policy makers. A possible solution would be to ensure that the stopping rules in the study protocol call for a large number of events.

Suggested Reading

Bassler D, Briel M, Montori VM, et al.; STOPIT-2 Study Group. Stopping randomized trials early for benefit and estimation of treatment effects: systematic review and meta-regression analysis. JAMA. 2010;303:1180–1187

Cleophas TJ, Zwinderman AH, Cleophas TF, Cleophas EP. Interim analyses. In: Cleophas TJ, Zwinderman AH, Cleophas TF, Cleophas EP. Statistics Applied to Clinical Trials. 4th ed. Springer; 2009:99–105

Montori VM, Devereaux PJ, Adhikari NK, et al. Randomized trials stopped early for benefit: a systematic review. JAMA 2005;294:2203–2209

References

1. Emanuel EJ, Wendler D, Grady C. What makes clinical research ethical? JAMA 2000;283:2701–2711
2. International conference on harmonisation; guidance on statistical principles for clinical trials; availability—FDA. Notice Fed Regist 1998;63:49583–49598
3. Cleophas TJ, Zwinderman AH, Cleophas TF, Cleophas EP. Interim analyses. In: Cleophas TJ, Zwinderman AH, Cleophas TF, Cleophas EP. Statistics Applied to Clinical Trials. 4th ed. Springer; 2009:99–105
4. Pocock SJ. Clinical Trials. A Practical Approach. New York: Wiley, 1988
5. Everitt BB. Statistical Methods for Medical Investigations. Oxford University Press, 1994
6. Armitage P, McPherson CK, Rowe BC. Repeated significance tests on accumulating data. J R Statist Soc 1969;132:235–244
7. Pocock SJ. Group sequential methods in the design and analysis of clinical trials. Biometrika 1977;64:191–199
8. Schulz KF, Grimes DA. Multiplicity in randomised trials II: subgroup and interim analyses. Lancet 2005;365:1657–1661
9. O'Brien PC, Fleming TR. A multiple testing procedure for clinical trials. Biometrics 1979;35:549–556
10. Geller NL, Pocock SJ. Interim analyses in randomized clinical trials: ramifications and guidelines for practitioners. Biometrics 1987;43:213–23
11. DeMets DL, Lan KK. Interim analysis: the alpha spending function approach. Stat Med 1994;13:1341–1352
12. Friedman LM, Furberg C, DeMets DL. Flexible group sequential procedures—Alpha-spending functions. In. Friedman LM, Furberg C, DeMets DL. Fundamentals of Clinical Trials. 3rd ed. New York, NY; Springer; 1998:266–276
13. Grant AM, Altman DG, Babiker AB, et al.; The DAMOCLES study group. Issues in data monitoring and interim analysis of trials. Health Technol Assess 2005;9:1–238
14. Isaacsohn JL, Khodadad TA, Soldano-Noble C, Vest JD. The challenges of conducting clinical endpoint studies. Curr Atheroscler Rep 2003;5:11–14
15. Nolen TL, Dimmick BF, Ostrosky-Zeichner L, et al. A web-based endpoint adjudication system for interim analyses in clinical trials. Clin Trials 2009;6:60–66
16. Kirkley A, Birmingham TB, Litchfield RB, et al. A randomized trial of arthroscopic surgery for osteoarthritis of the knee. N Engl J Med 2008;359:1097–1107
17. Camporese G, Bernardi E, Prandoni P, et al. Low-molecular-weight heparin versus compression stockings for thromboprophylaxis after knee arthroscopy: a randomized trial. Ann Intern Med 2008;149:73–82
18. Montori VM, Devereaux PJ, Adhikari NK, et al. Randomized trials stopped early for benefit: a systematic review. JAMA 2005;294:2203–2209
19. Briel M, Lane M, Montori VM, et al. Stopping randomized trials early for benefit: a protocol of the Study Of Trial Policy Of Interim Truncation-2 (STOPIT-2). Trials 2009;10:49
20. Bassler D, Briel M, Montori VM, et al.; STOPIT-2 Study Group. Stopping randomized trials early for benefit and estimation of treatment effects: systematic review and meta-regression analysis. JAMA 2010;303:1180–1187
21. Mueller PS, Montori VM, Bassler D, Koenig BA, Guyatt GH. Ethical issues in stopping randomized trials early because of apparent benefit. Ann Intern Med 2007;146:878–881

26

Conflict of Interest Reporting

Guy Klein, Charles T Mehlman, Michael Stretanski

Summary

Collaboration between industry and academia has become omnipresent, leading to widespread concerns for conflict of interest in biomedical research. Disclosure is the most popular method used to identify and discourage conflicts of interest in research. Researchers, peer reviewers, and editors are increasingly required to disclose potential conflicts of interest to journals and academic health centers. In further efforts to limit industrial influence, there are growing requirements for researchers to announce clinical trials and results on public databases.

> **Jargon Simplified: Conflict of Interest**
> "A conflict of interest is a set of circumstances that creates a *risk* that professional judgment or actions regarding a primary interest will be unduly influenced by a secondary interest."[1]

Introduction

Partnerships between academia and industry have led to a plethora of valuable medical innovations and spawned countless companies and economic successes. For example, graduates and faculty of the Massachusetts Institute of Technology (MIT) alone have founded more than 4000 companies, which employ more than 1.1 million persons and net $232 billion in revenue.[2] However, as academic and industry relationships have grown more entwined, the public and many medical professionals have become concerned that conflicts of interest may influence clinical practice, biomedical research, and medical education.[3]

Ethical misconduct is surprisingly widespread in the scientific community.[4] Martinson et al. found that 15.5% of US scientists funded by the National Institutes of Health (NIH) admitted to changing the design, methodology, or results of a study in response to pressure from a funding source.[4] Industry provides 60% of all funding for biomedical research and 70% of the money for clinical drug trials.[5] Twenty-five percent of all biomedical researchers receive financial support from profit-driven companies.[6] Not only is industry funding a large percentage of research, there is also evidence that it is funding the most influential studies. Eighty-four percent of the most frequently cited randomized controlled trials between 1994 and 2003 were funded at least in part by industry.[7] Patsopoulos

et al. suggest that findings such as this "are in line with the scenario of "Academic Inc.," with academic medicine evolving into an efficient enterprise that is directed by profit and has strong ties to other profit-making corporate structures."[7]

The pervasiveness of funding is not without consequences: studies have demonstrated that industry-funded research is more likely to result in positive (pro-industry) outcomes[6,8–10] and biased study designs.[6] Industry-sponsored research is also less likely to result in negative findings, and more likely to restrict investigator behavior.[6,9] Conflict of interest undermines the integrity of academic medicine and threatens the well-being of clinical research subjects.[11]

Disclosure is currently the most popular method used to identify and discourage conflicts of interest in research. This is reflected by the American Medical Association (AMA), who stated "that the best mechanism available to assuage public (and professional) doubts about the propriety of a research arrangement is full disclosure and that such disclosure should be made to the journals that publish the results of the research."[12] However, prominent researchers have made arguments that full disclosure is not the best mechanism to identify or prevent conflicts of interest in the research setting. Richard Horton, editor of *The Lancet*, has expressed his belief that the arguments in favor of full disclosure are based upon three fallacies: "(1) scientific writing cannot be free from prejudices; (2) financial conflicts of interest are of greater concern than academic, personal, and political rivalries and beliefs; and (3) disclosure can heal the wound inflicted by financial conflict."[13]

Examples from the Literature: The Case of ReGen's Menaflex Collagen Scaffold Product

There have been several prominent examples of controversies involving clinical research and alleged or documented conflicts of interest. Recently, the ReGen company developed the Menaflex Collagen Scaffold product, designed to be implanted during arthroscopic knee surgery to repair a damaged meniscus. The attempts by ReGen to gain approval by the Food and Drug Administration (FDA) for its device have become the center of a public controversy. In 2006, a top ReGen executive served as the vice chairman of a review panel whose role was to provide independent oversight of a clinical trial, violating conflict of interest requirements.[14] The FDA sent a letter to the company notifying them of a violation of conflict of interest requirements. The company replied, saying it would address the problem and "prevent similar conflicts of interest in the future." A year later, FDA reviewers unanimously and repeatedly determined that the device was unsafe. However, after "extreme, unusual, and persistent pressure" from four New Jersey legislators (Senators Robert Menendez and Frank R. Lautenberg and Representatives Frank Pallone Jr. and Steven R. Rothman), the FDA overruled their own scientist reviewers and approved the device. It was later revealed that the legislators who had pressured the FDA had received $26 000 in political contributions from ReGen executives.[15] The subsequent public outcry prompted the Institute of Medicine to review and change the process by which medical devices are evaluated by the FDA, leading to greater emphasis on evaluating the safety and effectiveness of potential new devices.[16] In March, 2010, the Center for Medicare and Medicaid Services (CMS) announced that it would deny reimbursement for the Menaflex product, stating that the "device has never met the FDA's standard for approval, much less CMS's more rigorous one." In their report, the CMS stated that there is "no evidence of improved outcomes" and, pertinent to this topic, "The data reported in the journal article[17] were different from the data submitted to the FDA ... The discrepancy in the adverse events reported in the published article on the RCT and the data provided to the FDA is disconcerting. Discrepancies in reported patient outcomes data also creates concerns about the reliability of study results published in peer reviewed journals and begs the question of what resources can be relied on with confidence to make evidence based-decisions in health care."[18] Notably, the authors of the article whose results are inconsistent with those reported to the FDA disclosed receiving substantial funding from ReGen.[17] Unfortunately, their disclosure did not prevent the publication (in a highly prestigious journal) of an incomplete or biased data set. Recently, the FDA has asked an outside agency to review its decision to approve the Menaflex product.

Legal Implications

At the 2008 annual meeting of the American Academy of Orthopaedic Surgeons (AAOS), only 71% of presenters who received payments from biomedical companies actually disclosed their potential conflict of interest.[19] This finding raises the question of why highly successful and educated surgeons had difficulty complying with the requests for disclosure at the AAOS. If the guidelines for disclosure are unclear, the Physician Payments Sunshine Act will hopefully shed light on this gray area. Signed into law as part of the Patient Protection and Affordable Care Act, this legislation mandates disclosure of gifts and payments greater than $100 to doctors from the pharmaceutical, biologic, and medical device industries.[20] The litmus test for the acceptability of a researcher's relationship with industry may be to pose the rhetorical question, "If the details of the association were described in detail on the front page of the newspaper would the reaction be positive or negative?" If the researcher would want to hide details, this suggests that the relationship may be unacceptable. Hopefully, the Sunshine Law will provide this type of transparency.

Several large drugmakers have already established public databases on the internet in order to disclose payments made to physicians. However, the current versions of these websites have been criticized for being difficult to use.[21] Additionally, in an effort to prevent and identify sponsor influence on clinical trials (including the nonpublication of negative results), the Food and Drug Administration Amendments Act of 2007 mandates that new clinical trials are required to be publicly listed prior to the start of the study at ClinicalTrials.gov and results are required to be published within 12 months of completing the study.[22] **Table 26.1** presents a historical perspective on the increasing demand for conflict of interest disclosure.

Table 26.1 Timeline of important events in conflict of interest disclosure

1970s	Conflict of Interest begins to be used in the codes of ethics for the medical profession.
1980	Bayh–Dole Act is passed, encouraging greater partnership between academia and industry.
1984	The New England Journal of Medicine was one of the first biomedical journals to implement a conflict of interest policy.
1985	The Journal of Bone and Joint Surgery (American) implements a conflict of interest policy.
2004	ICJME makes its initial call for mandatory clinical trial registration.
2007	Food and Drug Administration Act Amendment of 2007 is passed, making it federal law to register most interventional clinical trials at outset and to disclose trial results (for marketed products) by 12 months after study completion on www.clinicaltrials.gov.
2008	The ReGen Menaflex product is approved by the FDA after a controversial process and the publication of incomplete data in a premier journal. Its future status remains in question.
2009	The Institute of Medicine publishes the report "Conflict of Interest in Medical Research, Education, and Practice."
2010	Physician Payments Sunshine Act takes effect requiring disclosure of gifts and payments to physicians over $100.

Types of Conflict of Interest

Financial conflict of interest is the most widely discussed. However, it is far from the only conflict of interest that may influence researchers. It has been suggested that "financial conflicts are only the most visible and perhaps the least scientifically dangerous."[23] Academic, personal, and political rivalries and beliefs may create stronger conflicts of interest than financial pressures and should be included in disclosures. Patients in clinical trials have been found to be equally, if not more, concerned with intrinsic conflicts of interest compared with financial conflicts.[24]

Who Should Disclose Conflicts of Interest?

It is widely and strongly suggested that principal investigators and staff members who share responsibility for the design, conduct, or reporting of results of a sponsored project should disclose potential conflicts of interest. While not often the focus of many conflict of interest studies or debates, peer reviewers and journal editors hold highly influential positions and should also report potential conflicts of interest. A recent survey of journals found that while 93% have conflict of interest policies for authors, only 46% and 40% have conflict of interest policies for peer reviewers and editors respectively.[25]

Industry funding is also pervasive and influential in continuing medical education, where commercial sponsors supply approximately half of the $2 billion in annual income that continuing medical education providers receive.[26] Given the prevalence of industry in medical education, it is reasonable to expect instructors involved in medical education to disclose potential conflicts of interest.

When Must Conflicts of Interest Be Disclosed?

Conflicts of interest may be required to be disclosed to journals, academic medical centers, health care institutions, and funding agencies.

The requirement for disclosure in medical journals has recently increased dramatically. In 1995, 75% of journals required authors to disclose conflicts of interest. Today, it has been estimated that 89–94% of journals require author disclosure. However, the nature and breadth of these disclosures varies between journals. The International Committee of Medical Journal Editors (ICMJE) is a consortium of hundreds of medical journals who agree upon a uniform set of standards for the reporting of manuscripts. The ICMJE has published a consensus statement regarding their preferred conflict of interest disclosure protocol for authors. An example of their conflict of interest disclosure form is available at: http://www.icmje.org/coi_disclosure. pdf. The importance of the work of the ICMJE to standardize disclosure among different journals was highlighted by the work of Weinfurt who studied financial disclosures in the area of coronary stents. Weinfurt found that investigators who authored more than one article often had conflicting financial disclosures in other published articles. Most often, one article contained a statement denying financial interests, while another article by the same author contained no disclosure statement. However, in rare instances, one article disclosed an author's financial interests, while another article declared the author had nothing to disclose.[27]

Researchers at academic health centers (such as medical schools or teaching hospitals) may be required to disclose potential financial conflicts of interest to their employer. A survey of conflict of interest policies at the ten US medical schools that receive the largest amount of research money from the NIH found that, while all ten schools required faculty to disclose financial interests, the depth and detail of those disclosures varied greatly. A comparison of the missions of academic health centers and medical companies illustrated how the goals of these two types of organizations differ and have the potential to create conflicts of interest among employees affiliated with both types of organizations.[28] In addition to public universities, private health care organizations have started to limit compensation employees may receive from industry.[28]

Guidelines and Recommendations for Disclosure

The Institute of Medicine in the USA recently appointed a Committee on Conflict of Interest in Medical Research, Education, and Practice, which published a comprehensive report, "Conflict of Interest in Medical Research, Education, and Practice."

In addition to the Institute of Medicine, the Association of American Medical Colleges (AAMC) and the AMA have published guidelines for disclosure of conflicts of interest. The AMA requires disclosure and prohibits remuneration not commensurate with the efforts of the researcher as well as the purchase or sale of stock belonging to the company for whom the investigator is performing research.[29] The AAMC have published a valuable set of guidelines on conflict of interest in biomedical research[30] that are summarized in **Table 26.2**.

Why Must Personal Financial Interests Be Disclosed?

Financial conflicts of interest have the potential to undermine the work of many well-intentioned researchers and

Table 26.2 Main principles of the Association of American Medical Colleges policy on oversight of individual financial interests in human subjects research

1. With regard to research done on human subjects, all significant financial interests are potentially problematic and require close scrutiny.
2. Researchers with significant financial interests may be permitted to conduct research on human subjects under "compelling circumstances," subject to conditions imposed by a conflict-of-interest committee.
3. Significant financial interests should be fully disclosed to the institutional conflict-of-interest committee and updated regularly.
4. Institutional policies should be "comprehensive, unambiguous, well-publicized, consistently applied, and enforced through effective sanctions."
5. When compelling circumstances permit a researcher with financial interests to conduct clinical research, "rigorous, effective and disinterested monitoring" is crucial.
6. Individuals conducting research on human subjects must know the conflict-of-interest guidelines of their institution and must "act diligently" to fulfill the requirements.

Reproduced with permission from Association of American Medical Colleges, Task Force on Financial Conflicts of Interest in Clinical Research.[30]

disrupt the continued progress of evidence-based medicine. For example, guidelines that direct major clinical decisions are among the most influential of clinical publications. However, conflict of interest reporting has been largely disregarded in many published guidelines.[31]

Failure to disclose potential conflicts invites a number of unpleasant possibilities. If undisclosed conflicts are later discovered by a third party, researchers may have to suffer the appearance of guilt (of influencing a study outcome even if this is not the case), public embarrassment, damage to their career, and/or the devaluation of a valid study.

Glaser and Bero found that most researchers approve of industry collaboration when disclosure is complete and results are freely publicized.[32] However, they expressed concern that "researchers' trust in disclosure as a method to manage conflicts may reveal a lack of awareness of the actual impact of financial incentives on themselves and other researchers." For example, most physicians strongly deny that conflicts of interest could change their judgments; however, they routinely admit that financial incentives could bias the decisions of other researchers.[33] Dana and Loewenstein's review of the topic found that "individuals are often unable to avoid bias, even then it is in their best interest to do so" and "self interest distorts the way that individuals weigh arguments." It is postulated that study participants may also think, *some doctors* may be influenced by conflicts, but not *my doctor*. While some researchers have expressed concern that study participants may react strongly and negatively to learning about poten-

tial conflicts of interest, it has been found that conflict of interest is typically one of the least important topics to study participants.[34] Whether this is indeed the case, researchers should be assured that disclosing potential conflicts is unlikely to affect study recruitment substantially.

> **Reality Check: When What Is Good for the Surgeon Is No Longer Best for the Patient**
> Consider the example of a noble and talented surgeon who, appreciating the need for a new device for his patients, collaborates with a biomedical company to invent a superior piece of equipment. His patients benefit from the device and he becomes highly wealthy from the profits while his patients enjoy better outcomes. However, what happens when a new device comes to the marketplace that is better than his invention. Does the surgeon then stop using his own device? The fiduciary responsibilities and expectations for surgical researchers are on par with those of a rabbi or priest. It is our duty to always do what is best for our patients and not what is best for our pocketbook.

Alternatives to Disclosure Policies

While the calls for disclosure policies have become louder and more widespread, de Melo-Martin and Intemann eloquently argued that disclosure policies largely fail to meet their goals of preventing bias and identifying bias when it occurs. Instead, they suggest that there are numerous alternatives that would be more effective for preventing or identifying bias. De Melo-Martin and Intemann argued that policies such as "rejecting contractual provisions that allow sponsors the right to add their own statistical analyses to manuscripts, prematurely terminate a study for financial or public relations reasons, or suppress results that they find unfavorable would be more effective in reducing bias."[35]

Conclusion

Given the pervasiveness of industry–academic relationships, potential conflicts of interest have become unavoidable and ubiquitous. In response, demands for disclosure have grown louder and more systematic, with dozens of guidelines and reports published on the topic during the past decade. Despite the overwhelming demands for disclosure, there are strong arguments that disclosure of potential conflicts fails to prevent conflicts from actually influencing studies and may give the appearance of foul play where none is present. While it would be foolish (and unnecessary) for researchers to fail to disclose potential conflicts of interest, additional legislation and regulation is required to effectively prevent industrial relationships from distorting the legitimacy of the medical literature.

Suggested Reading

de Melo-Martin I, Intemann K, How do disclosure policies fail? Let us count the ways. FASEB J 2009;23:1638–1642

Hirsch LJ. Conflicts of interest, authorship, and disclosures in industry-related scientific publications: the tort bar and editorial oversight of medical journals. Mayo Clin Proc 2009; 84:811–821

Lo B, Field MJ. Conflict of Interest in Medical Research, Education, and Practice. Washington, DC: The National Academies Press; 2009

Office of Extramural Research. Conflict of Interest Information Resources Available on the Web. Last updated 14 July 2010. Available at http://grants.nih.gov/grants/policy/coi/resources.htm. Accessed August 2010

References

1. Lo B, Field MJ. Conflict of Interest in Medical Research, Education, and Practice. Washington, D. C.: The National Academies Press; 2009
2. Toner M, Tompkins RG. Invention, innovation, entrepreneurship in academic medical centers. Surgery 2008;143:168–171
3. Okike K, Kocher MS. The legal and ethical issues surrounding financial conflict of interest in orthopaedic research. J Bone Joint Surg Am 2007;89:910–913
4. Martinson BC, Anderson MS, de Vries R. Scientists behaving badly. Nature 2005;435:737–738
5. Bodenheimer T. Uneasy alliance—clinical investigators and the pharmaceutical industry. N Engl J Med 2000;342:1539–1544
6. Bekelman JE, Li Y, Gross CP. Scope and impact of financial conflicts of interest in biomedical research: a systematic review. JAMA 2003;289:454–465
7. Patsopoulos NA, Ioannidis JP, Analatos AA. Origin and funding of the most frequently cited papers in medicine: database analysis. BMJ 2006;332:1061–1064
8. Bhandari M, Busse JW, Jackowski D, et al. Association between industry funding and statistically significant pro-industry findings in medical and surgical randomized trials. CMAJ 2004;170:477–480
9. Friedman LS, Richter ED. Relationship between conflicts of interest and research results. J Gen Intern Med 2004;19:51–56
10. Leopold SS, Warme WJ, Fritz Braunlich E, Shott S. Association between funding source and study outcome in orthopaedic research. Clin Orthop Relat Res 2003;415:293–301
11. Blumenthal D. Academic-industrial relationships in the life sciences. N Engl J Med 2003;349:2452–2459
12. Council on Scientific Affairs and Council on Ethical and Judicial Affairs. Conflicts of interest in medical center/industry research relationships. JAMA 1990;263:2790–2793
13. Horton R. Conflicts of interest in clinical research: opprobrium or obsession? Lancet 1997;349:1112–1113
14. Mundy A. Political lobbying drove FDA process. Wall Street Journal; 6 March 2009
15. Harris G, Halbfinger DM. FDA reveals it fell to a push by lawmakers. The New York Times; 24 September 2009
16. US Food and Drug Administration. (2010). FDA Changes Process for Medical Device Advisory Committees. Press release dated 26 April 2010. Available at http://www.fda.gov/NewsEvents/Newsroom/PressAnnouncements/ucm209791.htm. Accessed August 2010
17. Rodkey WG, DeHaven KE, Montgomery WH 3rd, et al. Comparison of the collagen meniscus implant with partial meniscectomy. A prospective randomized trial. J Bone Joint Surg Am 2008;90:1413–1426
18. Center for Medicare and Medicaid Services. Decision Memo for Collagen Meniscus Implant (CAG-00414N), 25 May 2010. Available at http://www.cms.gov/mcd/viewdecisionmemo.asp?from2=viewdecisionmemo.asp&id=235&. Accessed August 2010
19. Okike K, Kocher MS, Wei EX, Mehlman CT, Bhandari M. Accuracy of conflict-of-interest disclosures reported by physicians. N Engl J Med 2009;361:1466–1474
20. Policy and Medicine. Physician payment sunshine provisions: patient protection affordable care act passed the House. Dated 22 March 2010. Available at http://www.policymed.com/2010/03/physician-payment-sunshine-provisions-patient-protection-affordable-care-act.html. Accessed July 2010
21. Wilson D. Data on fees to doctors is called hard to parse. New York Times; 12 April 2010
22. US Food and Drug Administration. Food and Drug Administration Amendments Act (FDAAA) of 2007. Available at http://www.fda.gov/RegulatoryInformation/Legislation/FederalFoodDrugandCosmeticActFDCAct/SignificantAmendmentstotheFDCAct/FoodandDrugAdministrationAmendmentsActof2007/default.htm. Accessed July 2010
23. Donaldson S, Capron AM. Patient Outcomes Research Teams (PORTS): Managing Conflict of Interest. Washington, DC: The National Academies Press; 1991
24. Gray SW, Hlubocky FJ, Ratain MJ, Daugherty CK. Attitudes toward research participation and investigator conflicts of interest among advanced cancer patients participating in early phase clinical trials. J Clin Oncol 2007;25:3488–3494
25. Cooper RJ, Gupta M, Wilkes MS, Hoffman JR. Conflict of interest disclosure policies and practices in peer-reviewed biomedical journals. J Gen Intern Med. 2006;21:1248–1252
26. Accreditation Council for Continuing Medical Education (ACCME). ACCME Annual Report Data 2009. Available at http://www.accme.org/dir_docs/doc_upload/f2e89864-b4c1-428f-8ebe-1ba197a31928_uploaddocument.pdf. Accessed August 2010
27. Weinfurt KP, Seils DM, Tzeng JP, Lin L, Schulman KA, Califf RM. Consistency of financial interest disclosures in the biomedical literature: the case of coronary stents. PLoS One 2008;3:e2128
28. Lo B. Serving two masters—conflicts of interest in academic medicine. N Engl J Med 2010;362:669–671
29. American Medical Association. Opinion 8.031—Conflicts of interest: biomedical research. Available at http://www.ama-assn.org/ama/pub/physician-resources/medical-ethics/code-medical-ethics/opinion8031.shtml. Accessed August 2010
30. Association of American Medical Colleges, Task Force on Financial Conflicts of Interest in Clinical Research. Protecting subjects, preserving trust, promoting progress—policy and guidelines for the oversight of individual financial interests in human subjects research. Available at http://www.aamc.org/download/75302/data/firstreport.pdf. Accessed July 2010
31. Papanikolaou GN, Baltogianni MS, Contopoulos-Ioannidis DG, Haidich AB, Giannakakis IA, Ioannidis JP. Reporting of conflicts of interest in guidelines of preventive and therapeutic interventions. BMC Med Res Methodol 2001;1:3
32. Glaser BE, Bero LA. Attitudes of academic and clinical researchers toward financial ties in research: a systematic review. Sci Eng Ethics 2005;11:553–573
33. Dana J, Loewenstein G. A social science perspective on gifts to physicians from industry. JAMA 2003;290:252–255
34. Weinfurt KP, Hall MA, Dinan MA, et al. Effects of disclosing financial interests on attitudes toward clinical research. J Gen Intern Med 2008;23:860–866
35. de Melo-Martin I, Intemann K. How do disclosure policies fail? Let us count the ways. FASEB J 2009;23:1638–1642

27

Authorship—Modern Approaches and Reporting

Rad Zdero, Emil H. Schemitsch

Summary

As authors, both surgeons and research engineers in the orthopaedics field can influence the thinking of other experts, students, young researchers, and orthopaedic manufacturers. Authorship can also lead to the development of new products, services, and techniques that benefit humanity. The aim of this chapter is to encourage researchers to take their findings out of the ivory tower of academia and into society at large.

Introduction

What is authorship? Let us first understand the word "author." It comes from the Latin word *auctor*, which means "origin" or "source." The dictionary defines an author as the beginner, originator, or creator of something, but particularly of a written work. Yet, in the scientific arena, authors do more than just write with a pen or type on a keyboard. They may be involved in generating an original idea, developing a novel application of an old idea, promoting the idea to an audience in nonwritten ways, and, of course, making a record of these ideas in written form. So, we could define an author as the creator, developer, or promoter of an idea, product, or service.

As authors, therefore, clinicians and engineers involved in orthopaedics research are in a unique position to shape and contribute to the scientific community. Their discoveries can lead to improvement of surgical techni-

ques, optimization of orthopaedic implants, and enhanced training of the next generation of specialists. If asked how they plan on spreading the word about their research results, most researchers would probably say they wanted to submit an article to a recognized academic journal for potential publication. While this may directly benefit other specialists in the field or related fields, there are other options for broadcasting one's results to reach a far wider audience.

Imagine the "River of Research" on whose mighty waves the researcher sails and from which flow "The Four Streams of Authorship," namely, the academic stream, the educational stream, the industrial stream, and the popular media stream (**Fig. 27.1**). This chapter will address each of the streams from a practical standpoint regarding audience, style, format, content, dos and don'ts, and pros and cons, as well as providing a real-world example of a published piece.

> **Jargon Simplified: Author**
> The creator, developer, or promoter of an idea, product, or service.

Academic Stream

What Is It?

The academic stream offers researchers the opportunity to get the word out about their findings to other specialists in the field or related fields. The most familiar option in this stream is the traditional academic peer-reviewed journal which produces paper copies for paid subscribers like individuals, university libraries, and research institutes. These journals also offer paid subscriptions which permit access to electronic versions of individual articles on the World Wide Web, either through their own website or through other institutional websites. Moreover, researchers can publish abstracts or short articles in the so-called proceedings or transactions of conferences, which are based on the posters or podium talks they have given during these same meetings. Slowly, but surely, "open access" peer-reviewed journals are also gaining acceptance and popularity because they offer research articles exclusively in electronic format online for free.

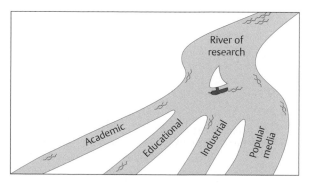

Fig. 27.1 The "Four Streams of Authorship": researchers have the option to make their findings known as authors to various audiences in the academic, educational, industrial, and popular media streams.

Who Is the Audience?

Readers of the academic article or abstract will typically be specialists in the field or a related field. They are the author's own peers. They might be clinicians, engineers, professors, or students active in hospitals, universities, research institutes, and industry. They are highly skilled inquirers seeking information about a specific research question. Consequently, the publication must be suited to their needs and wants. Simply put, journal articles are written by experts for other experts.

What about Style?

The style should have a formal and professional tone. Authors will generally be expected to write in the third person (e.g. "The present authors conducted experiments ..."), but some journals and proceedings permit the use of personal pronouns ("We conducted experiments ..."). Word contractions ("didn't," "weren't," etc.) should never be used. Idioms and jargon ("gold standard," "benchmark tests," "sawbones," etc.) should be employed only if they are well-known terms in that field of research. Otherwise, they should be clearly defined at their initial appearance in the manuscript.

What about Format?

Almost all journals and transactions expect authors to follow a universal structure when reporting their findings. In order of appearance, this includes a title, abstract (or summary), introduction (or background, or objectives), methods (or methodology, or materials and methods), results, discussion, conclusions, and references (or bibliography). In addition, there are usually limitations on the permitted number of accompanying figures, tables, and appendices, as well as word count limits for each section and/or the entire written piece. Shorter pieces such as abstracts, posters, and podium talks at conferences follow a similar pattern.

What about Content?

The content is meant to provide other specialists with new cutting-edge information. As such, the content should be *focused* on answering one or two specific research questions, for example, how changes in one parameter affect the behavior of another parameter. The content should be *relevant* to current challenges being faced in the field or assist in uncovering new knowledge, for example, how a new surgical technique improves the clinical performance of a hip prosthesis. The content should be *systematic* by reporting the chronological steps taken to execute the research project, for example, how scapholunate bone–ligament–bone specimens were obtained from a donor bank, examined for pathology, and mounted into a test apparatus for biomechanical testing. The content should be *comprehensive* by covering a range of salient aspects of the research question(s), for example, how the full range of cortical bone thicknesses from osteoporotic to normal affects the biomechanical properties of the tibia. The content should be *self-critical* by explicitly acknowledging limitations and the need for future work, for example, acknowledging how only a small number of samples per test group were available, causing low statistical power of the study.

What about Authorship?

For academic articles or abstracts, there are some general rules to apply to determine who should be included in the list of authors.[1] Only those who have contributed substantially to a project should be included, although they may have had different roles with respect to general project leadership, study concept and design, literature review, gathering or providing physical resources, performing experiments, building theoretical computer models, executing data analysis, creating figures and tables, and actually writing the article or abstract. Others who made some minor contribution should be recognized in the acknowledgments section.

Special mention should be made of projects to which a large number of people have contributed significantly. This might occur, for instance, when a prospective, large-scale, multicenter randomized controlled trial is undertaken.[2–5] Such a sizable team effort may be broken down into dedicated work groups, such as a project steering committee, a patient recruitment committee, a writing committee, a statistical analysis committee, etc., as well as the individual clinical personnel "on the front lines" who actually carried out patient care and recorded outcomes at their respective centers. When it comes to publishing a journal article, authorship will be credited using the team name or project name, though the names of a few key individuals leading the project may also be listed in addition to the team or project name. Typically in the appendix, however, an explicit list will be provided of all the names of individuals who comprised the various committees and/or who were the principal investigators coordinating the research activities at their particular clinical center, thereby acknowledging their contribution. In this way, everyone who has been formally recognized as a contributor to the study will be able to cite the article in their curriculum vitae (resumé). The details of all of this, of course, will depend on the format and style of the journal in which the paper will be published.

Dos and Don'ts

First, do become familiar with the publication's readership. The article or abstract may be published in various journals or proceedings, which will (or could) have different readerships. For instance, the same biomechanics project on fracture fixation could be published in the *Journal of Orthopaedic Trauma*, whose readers are mostly orthopaedic surgeons, or in the *Journal of Biomechanical Engineering*, whose readers are mostly engineers.

Second, do be aware of the journal's impact factor, which is a numerical score indicating the influence of the journal on the field. This score is based, among other things, on the number of times an article from that journal is cited by other publications.

Third, do choose a journal that is indexed by a well-recognized and widely used online journal directory, such as PubMed (www.pubmed.com), PubMed Central (www.pubmedcentral.com), or Science Direct (www.sciencedirect.com). For "open access" journals, the Directory of Open Access Journals (DOAJ; www.doaj.org) is the most popular online directory. Although Google Scholar (http://scholar.google.com/) is becoming increasingly popular, it has not yet been established as a rigorous and academically recognized resource.

Fourth, do attend strategic conferences where your research can be shared widely with other specialists in the field face to face through posters or podium presentations. Although these events only last for several days, the networking opportunities with scientific peers and industrial contacts may be worth the time and cost.

Fifth, don't delay publication, since other researchers may be working on similar projects and begin publishing before you. As more publications become available on the same topic, your work will become less publishable as time goes on.

Sixth, don't have unrealistic expectations about your publication's impact on the field, since probably only a small portion of fellow researchers or clinicians interested in the specific topic will actually read your article. It will take time for your findings to permeate the scientific community. Research is like Rome—it wasn't built in a day.

Pros and Cons

The main advantage in publishing research findings in academic journals and proceedings is that it may have some influence on the thinking and practice of other specialists in the field. This eventually may translate into substantially improved techniques and devices that are developed in the laboratory or clinic, since scientific colleagues are better positioned to take the next logical steps in future studies. Moreover, adding to the number of your academic publications improves your resumé, thereby increasing the chances for tenure or promotion and improving the prospects for obtaining more research funding when applying for financial grants to the government, private foundations, and industry. The main disadvantage, however, is that your discoveries are being made known only to a relatively small and elite caste of specialists, rather than to wider society, such as government and industry, who also may have an interest in financially supporting your research and commercializing it for societal use.

Real-World Example: Biomechanical Evaluation of Periprosthetic Femoral Fracture Fixation

The following abstract is taken from a research study entitled "Biomechanical Evaluation of Periprosthetic Femoral Fracture Fixation," which was conducted by Zdero and coworkers[6] and published in the *Journal of Bone and Joint Surgery* (American volume). Although the full article is not reproduced here, the abstract is typical of what is written by specialists for other specialists in the academic stream. Note the lack of word contractions, the systematic manner in which the study is described, the use of jargon only understood by other experts in the field, and the emphasis on addressing an ongoing challenge in the field.

*"**Background:** A variety of methods are available for the fixation of femoral shaft fractures after total hip arthroplasty. However, few studies in the literature have quantified the performance of such repair constructs. The aim of this study was to evaluate biomechanically four different constructs for the fixation of periprosthetic femoral shaft fractures following total hip arthroplasty.*

*"**Methods:** Twenty synthetic femora were tested in axial compression, lateral bending, and torsion to determine initial stiffness, as well as stiffness following fixation of a simulated femoral midshaft fracture with and without a bone gap. Four fracture fixation constructs (five specimens per group) were assessed: construct A was a Synthes locked plate (a twelve-hole broad dynamic compression plate) with locked screws; construct B, a Synthes locked plate (a twelve-hole broad dynamic compression plate) with cables and locked screws; construct C, a Zimmer nonlocking (eight-hole) cable plate with cables and nonlocked screws; and construct D, a Zimmer nonlocking (eight-hole) cable plate with allograft strut, cables, and nonlocked screws. Axial stiffness, lateral bending stiffness, and torsional stiffness were assessed with respect to baseline intact specimen values. Axial load to failure was also measured for the specimens.*

*"**Results:** Construct D demonstrated either equivalent or superior stiffness in all testing modes compared with the other constructs in femora with both a midshaft fracture and a bone gap. A comparison of constructs A, B, and C demonstrated equivalent stiffness in all test modes (with one exception) in femora with a midshaft fracture and a bone gap.*

*"**Conclusions:** A combination of a nonlocking plate with an allograft strut (construct D) resulted in the highest stiffness of the constructs examined for treating a peri-*

prosthetic fracture around a stable femoral component of a total hip replacement.
"Clinical Relevance: A locked plate (constructs A and B) should be used with caution as a stand-alone treatment for the fixation of a periprosthetic femoral shaft fracture following total hip arthroplasty, particularly with good bone stock."[6]

Jargon Simplified: Academic Stream
The academic stream is the authorship context in which journal articles and abstracts are written by experts for other experts in the field.

Key Concepts: Authorship in the Academic Stream
• Research is like Rome—it wasn't built in a day!
• Journal articles are written by experts for other experts.

Educational Stream

What Is It?

The educational stream offers the researcher the opportunity to get the word out about their findings to students and up-and-coming researchers. The most familiar option in this stream is the textbook. The researcher can write an entire textbook alone or as part of a small team, write a chapter for a textbook, or edit a textbook by soliciting chapter contributions from other experts in the field. Of course, textbooks are made available by publishers to readers through university libraries, research institutes, bookstores, and website sales. Moreover, researchers who are also university or medical school course instructors can collate their lecture notes, including their latest research findings, into a course notebook for their students.

Who Is the Audience?

Readers of the textbook or course notebook will typically be medical students, graduate students, and undergraduate students. They are generally novices in the field who aspire to improve their skills and enhance their knowledge for their own careers in industry or academia. However, if the material is sophisticated enough and provides some of the latest research findings, the author's own peers may find the publication of personal benefit, such as fellow clinicians, engineers, or professors active in hospitals, universities, research institutes, and industrial settings. Consequently, the textbook or course notebook should be written with their needs and wants in mind.

What about Style?

The style should maintain a formal and professional tone by being written in the third person, avoiding word contractions, and clearly explaining jargon that is commonly used by specialists in the field. However, because the material is often meant to be available to students or young researchers, publishers often want to make the style more "accessible," (i.e., less boring), in order to increase book sales. Moreover, instructors will want to make their course notes academically rigorous, but clear and concise for their students. Consequently, some creativity and humor are sometimes incorporated into figures, tables, and the body of the text itself. After all, the worst thing educators can do is bore their students.

What about Format?

Textbooks and course notebooks almost universally adopt the same logical progressive structure. They usually start with a brief introductory chapter which gives an overview of the field of study and the motivation for writing the book. Subsequent chapters dealing with various topics usually move from defining terms to explaining principles to examining practical case studies or problems. Either at the end of the chapter, or in a separate appendix, additional homework problems or sample tests are given with full worked solutions and/or final answers. There is also usually a glossary at the end of the book which explains frequently used or important terms.

What about Content?

The content is meant to lay the foundations for the education of students and novice researchers, all the while incorporating your own new research findings. As such, the content should be *creative* in order to enhance the enjoyability of the educational process; for example, figures can be made visually appealing by the use of color, cartoons, and design, rather than just informational. The content should be *relevant* to the current challenges that may be faced by the reader once they enter academia or industry; practical examples can be liberally employed to illustrate theories and principles. The content should be *systematic* by moving progressively from the simple to the complex; initial worked examples should be basic in order to illustrate principles, while later worked examples should be more representative of real-world situations. The content should be *holistic* by engaging readers on cognitive, emotive, and tactile levels because of the unique learning style each individual possesses; for example, it should give data and information, it should describe philanthropic benefits, and it should provide practical real-world examples.

What about Authorship?

For academic textbooks or course notes, similar rules for authorship credit apply as for journal articles and abstracts, already discussed above.[1] Only those who contributed substantially to the work should be included as authors, from those who generated the initial concept of the book to those who gathered all the information to be included and those who did substantial editing and finalization of the manuscript. If a textbook or course notebook is really the brainchild of one or two people, their names will appear as the sole authors. If the manuscript is the idea of, and being facilitated by, an editor or team of editors, their names should rightly appear as the main people associated with the work. In this case, individual chapters written by other contributing authors are often explicitly acknowledged somewhere in the book, either in the table of contents, on a "contributing authors" page, or on the first page of each chapter. Lastly, any practical assistance or philosophical feedback from others should be acknowledged in the preface, acknowledgments, or introduction.

Dos and Don'ts

Do take every opportunity, through figures, tables, case studies, practical examples, and references, to inject your own research findings into the textbook or course notebook. Do choose a publisher who has past experience in marketing work in your field of specialty, since they will know which trade shows, book expositions, and online websites to approach. Do be aware that larger publishers tend to keep books in print for a shorter period of time since they market books to have a higher volume of sales at the start, whereas smaller specialty publishers tend to keep books in print for a longer period of time and rely on sales through book longevity. Do recognize that a long-time instructor of a particular university or clinical course will be able to pass on his or her research findings to a steady stream of students from year to year over the long term. Do market your book strategically to other university instructors and clinicians in your field, since they might find it beneficial for their own students. Do take opportunities to have your work translated into other languages, thereby widening your audience.

Don't publish in a textbook any research details that you wish to have published eventually as a journal article, since many journals will not accept previously published work. Don't have unrealistic expectations about your book's immediate impact on the field, since it may take some time to infiltrate scientific circles, clinical practices, and industrial product development.

Pros and Cons

The main advantage in publishing research findings in textbooks and course notebooks is that it could inspire the best and the brightest students to pursue careers in the field. Moreover, authors have the ability to influence the next generation of leaders in the field with their own research discoveries, some of whom may become future colleagues. The best thing educators can do is inspire their students. Additionally, being credited with authorship and/or editorship of a textbook or chapter will greatly enhance your resumé. This can increase the chances of tenure or promotion and may improve the prospects for obtaining future research funding grants from the government, foundations, and industry.

The main disadvantage is that your discoveries are being made known to students and novice researchers, who are not immediately in any position to substantially influence clinical practices, industrial products, or academic knowledge by propagating your ideas. However, in time, some of the readers may become influential researchers themselves who can carry your ideas forward into the future.

> **Real-World Example: Human Factors Engineering**
> The following table of contents gives an overview of a chapter from the book *Human Factors Engineering*.[7] Although a reading of the entire book would be essential to evaluate its educational effectiveness, the table of contents does illustrate how the author's own cutting-edge research findings could potentially have plenty of opportunities to be introduced to students and novice researchers through the numerous practical examples, figures, and further information (e.g., references) being offered.

Chapter 4. Biodynamic Mechanics

4.1 Human Body
  Kinematics
  a. Linear Kinematics
  Example 4.1
  Example 4.2
  Fig. 4.1
  Example 4.3
  Fig. 4.2
  b. Angular Kinematics
  Example 4.4
  Fig. 4.3
  Example 4.5
  Fig. 4.4
4.2 Human Body Kinetics
  a. Mass Systems
  Fig. 4.5
  Example 4.6
  Example 4.7
  b. Elastic Systems

Example 4.8
Fig. 4.6
Fig. 4.7

4.3 Human Body Impact
  and Collision
  a. Human Body
  Impact
  Example 4.9
  Fig. 4.8
  b. Human Body
  Collision
  Example 4.10
  Fig. 4.9
  Fig. 4.10
  Further Information
  Problems (4.1 to 4.12)

> **Jargon Simplified: Educational Stream**
> The educational stream is the authorship context in which textbooks and course notebooks are written by experts for students and young researchers.

> **Key Concepts: Authorship in the Educational Stream**
> The best thing educators can do is inspire their students ... the worst thing educators can do is bore their students.

Industrial Stream

What Is It?

The industrial stream provides the author with an opportunity to make his or her research findings known to organizations and corporations that are creating products for use by society at large. Authors may be under contract with a corporation to do research on a product or technique which the corporation is developing and then give a formal technical report on the results. Alternatively, the authors may have developed a product or technique through their own independent research efforts which they hope eventually to sell to a corporation by providing them with a written report. In cases where these manufactured goods are brought to market, researchers may also be involved in writing and creating user manuals, product catalogs, and brochures.

Who Is the Audience?

Readers of technical reports, in particular, will typically be specialists in the field, because they are either the ones evaluating the potential marketability and technical soundness of a product (e.g., engineers assessing the material properties of a new suture material) or the ones to whom new products or techniques are being marketed (e.g., surgeons being informed about a new hip implant). Moreover, there may be nonspecialists who will read these technical reports, as well as the user manuals, product catalogs, and marketing brochures, because they are interested in other aspects of the product or technique. These interested parties may include lawyers, politicians, purchasing department personnel, business people, patients, hospital trustees, and so forth.

What about Style?

Technical reports, user manuals, and product catalogs should have a formal tone (e.g., written in the third person, no word contractions, and so on) throughout, because their purpose is to inform the reader about the technical aspects of the product or technique, rather than to enter-tain. On the other hand, marketing brochures and other promotional materials targeted toward specialists and nonspecialists do not need to be as formal in tone and allow for some level of creativity in presentation through the use of personal pronouns, word contractions, patient testimonies, colorful illustrations, etc.

What about Format?

Technical reports follow a similar or identical format as an academic journal article, as described earlier, having an abstract (or executive summary), introduction (or background), methods (or methods and materials), results, discussion, conclusions, and references (or bibliography), as well as an array of figures, tables, and appendices. Technical reports are often longer than journal articles because more details of methodology and performance are included for the purposes of ongoing research and development. Also, if you are trying to promote your research idea to a potential corporate buyer, then a section should be devoted to a business plan, marketing opportunities, etc. User manuals focus on practical aspects of using the product and include sections on technical specifications, safety hazards, special features, technical support contact information, and step-by-step instructions. Product catalogs provide brief introductions, numerical data, and assembly diagrams regarding the technical specifications of products with the assumption that readers know how to use the products already. Sometimes, user manuals and product catalogs are combined into one document. Marketing brochures have no standardized structure and are meant to be personal in tone and creative in presentation in order to educate and entertain readers, but they do have key "take home" points about the performance and benefits of the product to persuade the reader to buy it.

What about Content?

The content of technical reports is meant to provide new cutting-edge information about a potential product or technique. Therefore, as with journal articles and abstracts in the academic stream, they should be *focused* on one or two specific research questions, *relevant* to current challenges being faced in the field, *systematic* in reporting the steps to perform the research project, *comprehensive* in covering a range of related aspects of the research question(s), and *self-critical* in recognizing the investigation's or potential product's limitations. The content of user manuals and product catalogs is meant to be purely informational and should only include those technical aspects of the product that will allow the customer or user to easily and safely install, use, troubleshoot, and/or repair the product. The content of marketing brochures should be *holistic*, meaning that it engages readers on intellectual and emotional levels by providing data and information that highlight the philanthropic, practical, and/or financial benefits of the product.

What about Authorship?

Technical reports are similar to academic journal articles and abstracts in purpose, style, format, and content. Therefore, they should include as authors only those people who substantially contributed to the work, as already discussed above.[1] User manuals, product catalogs, and marketing brochures, however, are intended to convey information from a corporate entity to one of their actual or potential customers. As such, these are almost always authored anonymously by individuals or teams inside the corporation. In this way, the customer is left with the impression that the corporation is a unified and professional body, rather than a collection of flawed individuals who are producing these written materials. This may also provide legal protection to individual members of the corporation in case problems with the products or techniques lead to lawsuits. However, authors are explicitly named when a corporation wants to use experts strategically to persuade other experts of the reliability of a product, for example, surgeons writing a marketing brochure to other surgeons about the benefits of a new surgical device or technique. This kind of peer-to-peer persuasion may often be more effective than, say, when sales people try to persuade surgeons to buy a particular product at industrial or professional trade shows.

Dos and Don'ts

Do make sure to have or abide by nondisclosure agreements if, respectively, you are promoting your potential product to a corporation or you are under contract with a corporation to technically assess one of their products. Otherwise, legal repercussions and financial loss could result. Do make sure to be creative when developing marketing brochures, so that the reader will be intrigued by the product and be more likely to purchase it. As the popular proverb states, it's not what you say, but how you say it. Do make sure to appeal to the vested interests of your customer, for example, patient benefits, product performance, financial gain, etc., whether they are a corporation or an individual specialist to whom you wish to sell your product. Do directly compare your product's technical performance to other commercially available products on the market, but only if the performance of your product is superior. Otherwise, there will be no reason to switch to using your product.

Pros and Cons

The main advantage of focusing your research and writing talents in the industrial stream is that you could be involved in seeing a new product come to market that will be of great benefit to patients, surgeons, and design engineers. The real product of a fertile mind is a commercial product that benefits society. Moreover, there may be other spin-off benefits too, such as more industrial partnerships, personal financial benefits, and personal prestige. This could lead to more opportunities for promotions, grants, and tenure.

The main disadvantage is that often only a small group of specialists, like other researchers working in industry, or nonspecialists, like hospital trustees, will ever read about your research, unless it results in a viable commercial product.

Real-World Example: Restoration HA Case Compendium

The following foreword is from a marketing brochure entitled *Restoration HA Case Compendium*.[8] The document is a collection of patient x-rays and brief discussions highlighting the success of the corporation's new restoration hip implant. Note that the document specifically targets orthopaedic surgeons, by focusing on the clinical benefits of the device. This is a strategic approach, since surgeons are the ones from their clinic or hospital who make decisions and/or suggestions about product purchases for patient use. Although written by other experts in the field, the brochure is meant to promote the benefits of the new prosthesis, rather than being an objective critique. Not surprisingly, no patient cases are presented which would be considered failures. "Femoral revision hip surgery has always been a difficult proposition to accomplish when trying to treat the large spectrum of significant and major defects that can occur. Revision surgeons have frequently relied on different manufacturers to cover this wide spectrum of defects.

"The Restoration® HA Revision System has dramatically reduced the number of different components and different styles of components necessary to reconstruct these defects. This system allows correction of a large percentage of typical femoral revision deficiencies without having to resort to multiple systems.

"The stem design, roughened surface, and a nominal thickness of 50μ PureFix™ HA coating demonstrate rapid healing and resolution of pain as well as radiographic demonstration of bone regeneration. The slight taper to the distal aspect of the fully coated stem is designed for easy insertion and may reduce risk of fracture in brittle, deficient femurs. Throughout this compendium, note the abundance of bone regeneration, the lack of proximal stress shielding, the filling in of screw holes, and in general—the restoration of bone stock.

"Overall, this unique revision system has increased the ability of the revision hip surgeon to handle a wide variety of defects, achieve rapid pain relief, and see gratifying radiographic results of bone healing—not only of osteotomies, but filling of bone defects at relatively early time intervals. In my clinical practice, rapid pain relief has been the most dramatic clinical hallmark of use of this stem system. The following 18 case examples illustrate the breadth of cases capably handled by this system."[8]

Jargon Simplified: Industrial Stream

The industrial stream is the authorship context in which technical reports, user manuals, product catalogs, and marketing brochures are written by experts for potential users or customers.

Key Concepts: Authorship in the Industrial Stream

• It's not what you say, but how you say it.
• The real product of a fertile mind is commercial product that benefits society.

Popular Media Stream

What Is It?

The popular media stream offers researchers the opportunity to make their research findings known to an extremely wide audience. Traditional print media such as magazines and newspapers usually have entire sections devoted to news regarding advances in medical science and technology, or at least regularly appearing columns written by consumer advocate reporters. There are also online news magazines exclusively dedicated to reporting the latest medical research to a nonspecialist audience, such as Medical News Today (www.MedicalNewsToday.com) and NewsRX (www.NewsRX.com). Of course, television and radio programs and special interest DVDs are also popular ways of getting news about the latest and greatest in medical science. In our internet age, people all over the world and from every walk of life are also increasingly turning to a variety of websites for the latest in medical and technological information. This includes institutional websites, personal websites, personal blogs, document archives such as Scribd (www.Scribd.com), video archives such as YouTube (www.YouTube.com), social networking sites such as Facebook (www.facebook.com), professional networking sites such as LinkedIn (www.linkedin.com), and online encyclopedias such as Wikipedia (www.wikipedia.com).

Who Is the Audience?

Readers in this stream are usually nonspecialists who have no interest in muddling their way through the insider jargon and technical details often found in journal articles and technical reports. Rather, they want to find out about recent advances in simple ordinary language that they can understand, with a particular interest in what the implications are for patients and the various spheres that make up society at large. This will include patients, patients' family and friends, health watch reporters, consumer advocates, policy makers, lawyers, hospital trustees, business leaders, politicians, and so on.

What about Style?

There is little expectation or desire in the popular media stream for technical complexity in reporting on the latest research findings. Therefore, the style is typically informal. Hence, authors can make use of person pronouns, word contractions, idioms, proverbial sayings, and references to iconic events or personalities, as well as avoiding any and all technical terminology, if they so choose.

What about Format?

There is no standard structure. Structure is based on the preferences of authors or readers, but there is strong tendency toward story telling. Articles usually begin with a catchy phrase, a startling statistic, or a quick summary of a human interest story in order to get the reader's attention. This is often followed by an interview with experts or patients, more factual information in the form of some basic statistics, and some commentary by the authors (reporters) themselves about questions and concerns they have, as representatives of the general public. Articles in magazines and newspapers tend to be short, unless it is a front page or feature article, which gives more in-depth information. Personal blogs, personal websites, interactions on social and professional networking sites, or Wikipedia entries tend to be shorter rather than longer, with perhaps bibliographical references to more technical writings on the subject. Diagrams, photos, and videos can be shaped to suit personal tastes of authors or readers.

What about Content?

The content of popular media is meant to provide reports on the latest cutting-edge research being undertaken. As such, the information must be relatively recent. In fact, when a journalist is the first to report a story it is often called "getting a scoop" or "breaking the story." The information often focuses on the benefits and dangers to society. There will sometimes be a discussion of the legal, ethical, financial, health care policy, and political implications of the research. Sometimes anecdotal information or examples, rather than sheer facts, are preferred because they carry a powerful emotional appeal to the nonspecialist readers that will hold their attention. Personal testimonies and interviews with clinicians, engineers, patients, or other interested parties are also used liberally.

What about Authorship?

In the popular media stream, the researcher has little influence on who should comprise an authorship list. This will be decided by the publisher or editor of the newspaper, magazine, or website, or the producer of the television or radio program. If a researcher is able to arrange an agreement to co-author an article with a print media journalist or an online blogger, or to co-write a television or radio spot or a DVD, they will be in a better position to control authorship credits and distribution of the information. Obviously, researchers are able to substantially shape the authorship credits for information they place on their own personal and institutional websites or in audio and video productions they create themselves.

Dos and Don'ts

Do make sure you have the opportunity to review any material produced by the popular media before it is made public, so that you and your research are not misrepresented. Do make sure the benefits of your research or potential product are highlighted by those who ask permission to report your findings to the public. Do make sure your contact information is accurate and complete, so that readers, viewers, or listeners who are potential funders and collaborators can get in touch with you later. Do make sure that you obtain a patent as soon as possible for your product idea to protect your intellectual property rights.

Don't divulge too many details about your research to reporters or even on your personal or institutional website, especially if it is a product that has not yet been brought to market or for which you are still awaiting patent approval, since there will be no legal barriers to prevent someone from stealing your idea.

Pros and Cons

The great advantage of permitting your discoveries to be made known through the popular media is that information that has reached the public has a chance of becoming "viral" as it wields a vast influence on readership. This can potentially influence the direction of academic research, public health policy, and popular demand for new pro-

ducts and services for the benefit of society at large. As history shows, societal change often happens by educating and empowering people at the grassroots. So, it is important to inform the masses about your research findings.

The main disadvantage is that you no longer have control of your information. Reporters, editors, publishers, bloggers, and webmasters, not to mention the vast array of readers from nearly every walk of life imaginable, are prone to using your information for their own purposes, which may not always be the most noble. There is also the risk that someone might steal your idea before it has become a commercially viable product. Moreover, people may misunderstand the details of your research and accidentally misrepresent it to readers, in a way that makes it difficult to undo the damage to your reputation or product later on. Consequently, the medium chosen to report the information (e.g., newspaper report versus internet blog) will have an influence on how the information is transmitted and understood. After all, as Canadian educator and philosopher Marshall McLuhan wrote, "the medium is the message."[9]

Real-World Example: *Maclean's* Magazine

The following article appeared in the May 15, 2005 edition of *Maclean's*, which is Canada's leading news magazine.[10] It reports on the findings of two research studies regarding the effect of after-hours surgery on patient outcomes. The style, format, and content are typical of written pieces in the popular media, with a de-emphasis on technical details and an emphasis on personal or larger societal implications. Note the use of vernacular sayings such as "A team" and "shin bone," the lack of any bibliographical reference to the titles of the actual studies themselves or the journals in which they were published, the reliance on the personal touch by using interviews with experts, an interest in the behind-the-scenes challenges of hospital bureaucracy, and an emphasis on the effects on patients.

"After-hours fracture surgery leads to complications: broken bones are often fixed at night because of shortages in daytime hospital resources.

"Night-time is definitely not the right time to have routine surgery for a broken bone—it could come with a greater risk for a repeat operation. Two recent studies compared the outcomes of hip, thigh and shin bone fractures surgically repaired during and after regular operating hours. These types of fracture operations are often done at night because of a scarcity of daytime resources rather than medical necessity.

"The results showed that night-time fracture repair was more likely to be associated with complications—particularly an unplanned second operation for removal of painful hardware.

"'Painful hardware is related to surgical technique, which could suffer if the surgeon is tired after already working a full day,' says Dr. William Ricci, co-author of one of the studies and an orthopaedic surgeon at

Washington University and Barnes-Jewish Hospital in St. Louis.

"Ricci and four other orthopedic surgeons—including Dr. Ross Leighton in Halifax—tracked complications among 203 people who had surgery for a thigh or shin bone fracture.

"Patients treated from 3 p. m. to 6 a. m., when the surgeon's 'A team' was likely unavailable, had twice the number of unplanned reoperations compared with those treated from 6 a. m. to 3 p. m., even though the two groups had similar fracture severities. The most common reason for unplanned reoperation was removal of painful hardware.

"In the other study, co-authored by Dr. Timothy Bhattacharyya of Massachusetts General Hospital and Brigham and Women's Hospital in Boston, hip and thigh bone fractures were associated with more complications when repaired at night.

"The same study showed a daytime operating room dedicated to fracture repair can help surgeons get these cases done during regular working hours, but Bhattacharyya says it was 'extremely, extremely, extremely difficult' to convince hospital administration and staff to establish the room.

"Dr. Michael McKee, an orthopedic surgeon at St. Michael's Hospital—the adult trauma center for downtown Toronto—agrees after-hours surgery due to scarcity of daytime resources is a problem in orthopedics. 'That's deleterious from a number of standpoints, both from hospital costs and for probably the quality of care.

"'If you're operating after an 18-hour day ... probably you're not as sharp as you would be during the day, and people who work there at night may not have the knowledge or skills of a lot of the orthopedic equipment we use.'"[10]

Jargon Simplified: Popular Media Stream
The popular media stream is the authorship context in which print and online materials are written by experts and nonexperts to inform society at large.

Key Concepts: Authorship in the Popular Media Stream
- "The medium is the message"—Marshall McLuhan.
- Societal change often happens by educating and empowering people at the grassroots.

Conclusion

Clinicians and engineers involved in orthopaedics research can share their discoveries as authors in academic, educational, industrial, and popular media contexts. This can in-

fluence other experts in the field, students and up-and-coming researchers, corporate leaders, and society at large. Authorship not only adds to the general scientific knowledge available, but also benefits society through the development of new commercially viable products and techniques. Although, for many researchers, the act of scientific discovery is reward enough in itself, the next step of authorship can take their efforts out of the proverbial ivory tower of academia and into society at large for the benefit of others.

Suggested Reading

Biagioli M, Galison P, eds. Scientific Authorship: Credit and Intellectual Property in Science. New York: Routledge; 2002

Zdero R, Schemitsch EH. Authorship: what you should know. In: Bhandari M, Schemitsch EH, Joenssen A, Robioneck B, eds. Getting Your Research Paper Published: A Surgical Perspective. New York and Stuttgart: Georg Thieme Verlag; 2011

References

1. Zdero R, Schemitsch EH. Authorship: what you should know. In: Bhandari M, Schemitsch EH, Joenssen A, Robioneck B, eds. Getting Your Research Paper Published: A Surgical Perspective. New York and Stuttgart: Georg Thieme Verlag; 2011
2. Bhandari M, Guyatt G, Tornetta P 3rd, Schemitsch EH, Swiontkowski M, Sanders D, Walter SD. Randomized trial of reamed and unreamed intramedullary nailing of tibial shaft fractures. J Bone Joint Surg Am 2008;90:2567–2578
3. Leighton RK, Trask K. The Canadian Orthopaedic Trauma Society: a model for success in orthopaedic research. Injury 2009;40:1131–1136
4. Canadian Orthopaedic Trauma Society. Nonoperative treatment compared with plate fixation of displaced midshaft clavicular fractures. A multicenter, randomized clinical trial. J Bone Joint Surg Am 2007;89:1–10
5. Hall JA, Beuerlein MJ, McKee MD; Canadian Orthopaedic Trauma Society. Open reduction and internal fixation compared with circular fixator application for bicondylar tibial plateau fractures. Surgical technique. J Bone Joint Surg Am 2009;91(Suppl 2 Pt 1):74–88
6. Zdero R, Walker R, Waddell JP, Schemitsch EH. Biomechanical evaluation of periprosthetic femoral fracture fixation. J Bone Joint Surg Am 2008;90:1068–1077
7. Phillips CA. Human Factors Engineering. New York: John Wiley and Sons; 2000:87–125
8. Bridle S, Malkani A, Morris H, Sotereanos N. Restoration® HA Case Compendium. Mahwah, NJ: Stryker Corporation; 2005. Available at www.stryker.com
9. McLuhan M. Understanding Media: The Extensions of Man. New York: McGraw Hill; 1964.
10. MacLeans Magazine. After-hours fracture surgery leads to complications: broken bones are often fixed at night because of shortages in daytime hospital resources. Available online at www.macleans.ca/article.jsp?content=20050315_102321_6164. Accessed April 2010.

28
Randomized Trials Reporting Checklists

Ruby Grewal, Joy C. MacDermid

Summary

With an increased emphasis toward evidence-based practice, the results of randomized controlled trials (RCTs) are increasingly being used to guide clinical decisions because they are now regarded as the highest available level of primary research evidence. However, it is overly simplistic to view all RCTs as equal or as high-quality evidence. There is wide variation in the level of quality among RCTs, and the results from a poorly conducted RCT should be regarded with caution.

Introduction

The quality of published randomized clinical trials in the orthopaedic literature has been reviewed in the recent past. Bhandari et al. reviewed the quality of RCTs published in the *Journal of Bone and Joint Surgery* (American volume; JBJS A) between 1988 and 2000.[1] Only 41% of the RCTs in this leading orthopaedic journal reported a concealed method of randomization, suggesting that the remaining 59% of studies were subject to selection bias—a serious threat to internal validity. Other major deficiencies identified included the lack of an a priori sample size calculation (present in only 6% of studies) and power analyses. In fact, only 2% of trials reported a post hoc power calculation when the study results were negative.

A similar review of all RCTs related to the treatment of upper extremity disorders published in the *Journal of Hand Surgery* (American and British volumes) and the JBJS A and JBJS Br (the British volume of *Journal of Bone and Joint Surgery*) from 1992 to 2002 was conducted by Gummesson et al.[2] On the basis of the details provided, they found that only 43% of the reported RCTs were truly randomized studies. Twenty-three percent of published RCTs utilized an inappropriate method of randomization and 34% did not describe the randomization method at all. A quality assessment of the pediatric orthopaedic literature by Dulai et al. found similar results.[3] They reported that 81% of the published RCTs in the journals most commonly used by pediatric orthopaedic surgeons (*Spine, Journal of Pediatric Orthopedics, Journal of Pediatric Orthopedics* Part B, JBJS A, and JBJS Br) failed to meet the standard for acceptability as measured by the Detsky Quality Assessment Scale.[4]

These studies indicate that despite a rigorous editorial process, many well-respected peer-reviewed orthopaedic journals continue to publish trials that appear to be of poor quality. This is a concern, since RCTs with serious underlying methodologic flaws can bias estimates of treatment effects and invalidate their results. During critical appraisal it is necessary to assume that if elements of design are not documented, they were not carried out. However, when the authors of 98 RCTs who had failed to report a variety of bias strategies were contacted, it emerged that in many cases the bias had in fact been addressed: by concealing randomization (96%), blinding participants (20%), blinding health care providers (65%), blinding data collectors (65%), blinding outcome assessors (79%), and blinding data analysts (50%). In cases like these, appraisals can overestimate the potential presence of bias.[5] Thus, poor reporting can also lead to *underestimation* of actual trial quality.

Evidence-based practice requires clinicians to make accurate assessments of study quality so that they can rely on best evidence. A transparent, standardized method of reporting RCTs (both pharmacological and nonpharmacological trials) can reduce errors in estimating study quality and guide authors toward improving either the design or the reporting of trials.

The quality of a study is not ensured by seeing the word *randomized* in the title, nor by seeing it published in a "reputable" journal.

In 1994 two groups of editors, trialists, and methodologists independently published recommendations for a standardized method of reporting clinical trials.[5,6] In 1995, Rennie suggested the two groups combine their efforts and produce a unified statement.[6] The result of this collaboration was the CONSORT statement (*Consolidated Standards Of Reporting Trials*).[7] It was first published in 1996 in *JAMA*, revised in 2001, and most recently revised in 2007. The final iterative process converged to create the CONSORT 2010 "Explanation and Elaboration" document to be found at www.consort-statement.org/.[8,9]

The CONSORT statement is a 25-item checklist and flow diagram that authors are encouraged to use for the purpose of reporting the results of an RCT.[9,10] This checklist can be found at www.consort-statement.org/consort-statement/overview0/. It standardizes reports of the design, analysis, and interpretation of the study, while the flow diagram reports the progress of participants through the trial.[10] This ensures completely transparent reporting, allowing the reader to understand clearly the trial's design, analysis, and interpretation, aiding critical appraisal and interpretation of the results. The CONSORT statement is supported by most leading medical journals and major international editorial groups, and there is evidence to support the contention that the introduction of CONSORT has improved the quality of research reports.[11,12]

While the CONSORT statement works well for most RCTs, there are methodologic issues unique to nonpharmacological trials (NPTs) that also require attention. In NPTs (e.g., surgical trials) it is often impossible to blind participants and care providers or to offer a sham intervention. Because of this, an extension to the CONSORT statement[13] and also the Check List to Evaluate A Report of a NonPharmacological Trial (CLEAR NPT) was developed.[14] This chapter will explore details of the CONSORT statement, the NPT extension to the CONSORT statement, and the CLEAR NPT.

Consort Statement

The requirements for each of the 25 items in the CONSORT checklist are divided into six components: title and abstract, introduction, methods, results, discussion, and other information. Each section will be reviewed below; details of the checklist are given in **Table 28.1**.

Table 28.1 Details of CONSORT statement checklist

Section/topic	Item no.	Checklist item	Reported on page no.
Title and abstract			
	1a	Identification as a randomized trial in the title	
	1b	Structured summary of trial design, methods, results, and conclusions (for specific guidance see CONSORT for abstracts)	
Introduction			
Background and objectives	2a	Scientific background and explanation of rationale	
	2b	Specific objectives or hypotheses	
Methods			
Trial design	3a	Description of trial design (such as parallel, factorial) including allocation ratio	
	3b	Important changes to methods after trial commencement (such as eligibility criteria), with reasons	
Participants	4a	Eligibility criteria for participants	
	4b	Setting and locations where the data were collected	
Interventions	5	The interventions for each group with sufficient details to allow replication, including how and when they were actually administered	
Outcomes	6a	Completely defined prespecified primary and secondary outcome measures, including how and when they were assessed	
	6b	Any changes to trial outcomes after the trial commenced, with reasons	
Sample size	7a	How sample size was determined	
	7b	When applicable, explanation of any interim analyses and stopping guidelines	
Randomization			
Sequence generation	8a	Method used to generate the random allocation sequence	
	8b	Type of randomization; details of any restriction (such as blocking and block size)	
Allocation concealment mechanism	9	Mechanism used to implement the random allocation sequence (such as sequentially numbered containers), describing any steps taken to conceal the sequence until interventions were assigned	
Implementation	10	Who generated the random allocation sequence, who enrolled participants, and who assigned participants to interventions	

Continued ▶

Table 28.1 Continued

Section/topic	Item no.	Checklist item	Reported on page no.
Blinding	11a	If done, who was blinded after assignment to interventions (for example, participants, care providers, those assessing outcomes) and how	
	11b	If relevant, description of the similarity of interventions	
Statistical methods	12a	Statistical methods used to compare groups for primary and secondary outcomes	
	12b	Methods for additional analyses, such as subgroup analyses and adjusted analyses	
Results			
Participant flow (a diagram is strongly recommended)	13a	For each group, the numbers of participants who were randomly assigned, received intended treatment, and were analyzed for the primary outcome	
	13b	For each group, losses and exclusions after randomization, together with reasons	
Recruitment	14a	Dates defining the periods of recruitment and follow-up	
	14b	Why the trial ended or was stopped	
Baseline data	15	A table showing baseline demographic and clinical characteristics for each group	
Numbers analyzed	16	For each group, number of participants (denominator) included in each analysis and whether the analysis was by original assigned groups	
Outcomes and estimation	17a	For each primary and secondary outcome, results for each group, and the estimated effect size and its precision (such as 95% confidence interval)	
	17b	For binary outcomes, presentation of both absolute and relative effect sizes is recommended	
Ancillary analyses	18	Results of any other analyses performed, including subgroup analyses and adjusted analyses, distinguishing prespecified from exploratory	
Harms	19	All important harms or unintended effects in each group	
Discussion			
Limitations	20	Trial limitations, addressing sources of potential bias, imprecision, and, if relevant, multiplicity of analyses	
Generalizability	21	Generalizability (external validity, applicability) of the trial findings	
Interpretation	22	Interpretation consistent with results, balancing benefits and harms, and considering other relevant evidence	
Other information			
Registration	23	Registration number and name of trial registry	
Protocol	24	Where the full trial protocol can be accessed, if available	
Funding	25	Sources of funding and other support (such as supply of drugs), role of funders	

Title and Abstract

The first step in reviewing the applicability, quality, or content of a study is to evaluate the title. Seeing the word "randomized" in the title implies to the reader that this study carries a high level of evidence and is less biased than a nonrandomized trial. For the authors, it is important that the word "randomized" be included in the title as this permits easy identification and recognition of their study when readers are searching online databases. The reader then reads the abstract to review details of methodology and obtain a summary of results. For this reason, the abstract should provide a structured summary of the trial design, methods, results, and conclusions.

Introduction

The introduction provides the reader with pertinent details of the relevant scientific background, helping them to understand the knowledge gaps or treatment controversies that may exist. The introduction should impress upon the reader the rationale for conducting this trial; the research question and the hypotheses to be tested should also be clearly stated.

> **Jargon Simplified: Hypothesis**
> A hypothesis is a tentative explanation for an observation, phenomenon, or scientific problem that can be tested by further investigation. In the case of an RCT, it can be identified by asking: "What question was the trial designed to answer?"

Methods

In order for the reader to understand how the study was conducted, a detailed description of the trial design, along with any important methodologic changes that may have been made to the original study protocol, should be included in the methods. The method of patient recruitment and patient selection should also be explained.

The setting and location where data were collected (e.g., community setting, hospital clinic, in-patient unit, single versus multicenter) should be described, as these may influence the observed results and will also allow readers to judge whether the results are applicable to their own circumstances.

Exact details of both the experimental intervention and the control, including the method of administration (e.g., providers, active ingredients, dosage, adjunctive treatments/health services) should be provided. The *primary* and *secondary outcomes* should be clearly stated, including details on how they were measured. A *sample size calculation* should be provided to assure the reader that the trial was appropriately *powered*.

> **Key Concepts: Primary and Secondary Outcomes**
> The primary outcome is the outcome of greatest importance and the outcome that the trial is powered to answer. Secondary outcomes represent other outcomes of interest, but do not reflect the primary purpose of the trial.

> **Jargon Simplified: Sample Size Calculation**
> A mathematical formula calculates the minimum number of subjects (sample size) necessary to ensure that a difference defined as clinically relevant would be statistically significant with a prespecified level of confidence. This calculation should relate to the primary outcome.

> **Key Concepts: Statistical Power**
> The power of a statistical hypothesis test measures the test's ability to reject the null hypothesis when it is actually false—that is, to make a correct decision about whether groups are different.

The method of randomization should also be clearly reported. Including the word "randomized" in the title does not assure the reader that subjects were truly randomized in an unbiased fashion. Randomization implies that each subject had an equal chance of being assigned to either treatment arm, through a concealed, unbiased process. Many allocation methods such as alternate group assignment, or assignment based on hospital number/date of birth, are subject to bias and are not considered "randomized" because the group allocation cannot be concealed prior to group assignment.

> **Key Concepts: Randomization**
> In order to ensure that the trial is truly randomized, group allocation must occur through a system by which group assignment is concealed so that investigators cannot knowingly or unknowingly influence it.

The process of randomization typically ensures that all known and unknown confounders will be balanced between the two treatment groups. In small trials, certain influential baseline characteristics (e.g., smoking, compensation status) may not be balanced in the final groups, purely as a result of chance. Investigators may use strategies such as stratification or blocking to ensure this does not occur.

> **Jargon Simplified: Stratification**
> Stratification is the process of grouping individuals into "strata" (or layers) on the basis of an important known and measurable characteristic (such as study site, or patient sex or age) to ensure that these characteristics are equally represented across the intervention groups.

> **Jargon Simplified: Block Randomization**
> Blocking randomization is a technique designed to ensure equal distribution of study subjects across treatment groups over time. Blocks of either varying (most common) or equal sizes are created such that each block contains an equal number of treatment and control (or treatment A and treatment B) allocations. The order of treatment allocation within each block is random, and the order of blocks, once they have been created, is also random.

It should be stated whether those administering the interventions and/or those assessing the outcomes were *blinded* to group assignment. If blinding was not possible, this should be clearly explained.

> **Jargon Simplified: Blinding**
> With blinding, patients, clinicians, data collectors, outcome adjudicators, and/or data analysts are unaware of which patients have been assigned to the experimental and which to the control group. In the case of diagnostic tests, those interpreting the test results are unaware of the result of the reference standard, or vice versa.[15]

A detailed description of the methods of statistical analysis used for the primary and secondary outcomes should be given, including any additional analyses that may have been performed. In some trials, it may be ethically necessary to examine interim results before the study is completed (e.g., to evaluate complication rates). Authors should report whether the data was analyzed on multiple occasions and whether this was planned before the trial was started or after.

Results

Outline the flow of participants through each stage of the study (a diagram is recommended), including inclusion, exclusion, randomization, the number receiving the intended treatment, the number successfully completing the study protocol, and the number analyzed for the primary outcome (**Fig. 28.1**). For each group, indicate reasons for any losses or exclusions after randomization.

> **Key Concepts: Flow Diagram**
> The study flow diagram allows the reader to see clearly where and when each subject left the study (due to ineligibility, withdrawal from treatment, being lost to follow-up, exclusion from analysis, etc.) and whether this had any potential to bias the final results.

The results should also include the dates defining the period of recruitment and follow-up, allowing the reader to gain an appreciation of the rate of subject recruitment and place the study in its historical context. The dates also become relevant as medical interventions may evolve over this time, potentially influencing the trial results.

The baseline demographic and clinical characteristics of the enrolled subjects should be provided, allowing the

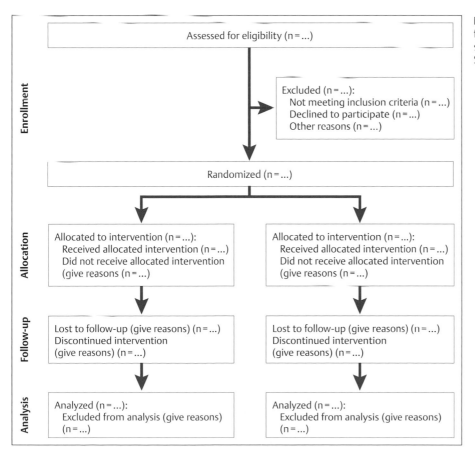

Fig. 28.1 Flow diagram from the 2010 CONSORT statement. Reproduced from Schulz et al.[13]

reader to confirm whether the groups were comparable at baseline. Although the process of randomization is meant to balance both the known and unknown *confounders* between study groups in the trial, there is a chance that the groups may not be equal at baseline. It should be understood that this is the result of chance rather than bias.

> **Jargon Simplified: Confounder**
> A factor that is associated with the outcome of interest and is differentially distributed in patients who are exposed and those who are unexposed to the outcome of interest is referred to as a confounder.[15]

Indicate the number of participants (denominator) in each group included in each analysis. State the results in absolute numbers rather than percentages (e.g., 10 of 20, not 50%). Authors should state clearly which participants are included in each analysis and indicate whether the analysis was by "*intention to treat*". An intention-to-treat analysis is preferred because of the advantage that it avoids bias associated with the nonrandom loss of subjects.

> **Jargon Simplified: Intention-to-Treat Analysis**
> An intention-to-treat analysis is one based on the initial treatment intent (i.e., on initial group assignment) rather than on the treatment eventually administered.

For each primary and secondary outcome, provide a summary of results for each group, the estimated effect size, and its precision (e.g., 95% confidence interval). For binary outcomes, presentation of both absolute and relative effect sizes is recommended.

Report all other analyses performed (subgroup and adjusted analyses) and indicate which were prespecified and which were exploratory.

> **Key Concepts: Exploratory Analysis**
> When multiple analyses are performed (other than those determined prior to data collection) there is an increased risk of false-positive findings. These results should be interpreted with caution in the context of the study in which they are performed, but can be used to generate future hypotheses.

All adverse events or side effects associated with the interventions should be objectively quantified and clearly disclosed. If they resulted in discontinuation of treatment, this should also be clearly stated. This allows the reader to judge the acceptability or usefulness of the intervention being investigated.

Discussion

The discussion allows the authors to discuss and interpret the results of the trial in the context of the current relevant evidence, balancing the advantages and disadvantages of different treatments. The *generalizability* (or *external validity*) of the trial findings can be assessed. The limitations of the trial should also be reviewed, addressing sources of potential bias, imprecision, and, if relevant, multiplicity of analyses.

> **Key Concepts: Generalizability**
> "Generalizability" (or "external validity") refers to the applicability of the trial findings (i.e., can the results be generalized to other settings?)
> If the CONSORT guidelines have been followed, the trial setting, the characteristics of the subjects, the treatments compared, and the outcomes will be clearly evident to the reader. This will allow the reader to determine whether the results of the study can be generalized to other situations (e.g., are these results applicable to patients with different disease severity, or those treated at hospitals which provide a different level of care [primary versus tertiary], or those of a different age?).

Other Information

The authors should also provide the trial registration number and the name of the trial registry, identify where the full trial protocol can be accessed (if available), and report all sources of funding, including all financial support (e.g., supply of drugs), and the role of funders. This allows readers to judge the extent to which the trial may have been modified or influenced.

Nonpharmacological Trials

Nonpharmacological trials (NPTs) account for one in four publications.[16] They evaluate treatment interventions such as surgical procedures, devices, rehabilitation, and/or behavioral interventions and are very common in the orthopaedic literature.

There are many methodologic issues that are unique to NPTs. For example, challenges seen with NPTs in orthopaedic surgery include the feasibility of blinding (it is difficult to blind surgeons and/or subjects as to the treatment being given), difficulty (including ethical problems) in performing sham interventions, and difficulty accounting for the caregiver effect (i.e., treatment success is often dependent on surgeon skill and experience). Small variations in treatment (surgeon experience, nuances of technique, centers' volume of care, rehabilitation protocols, etc.) can influence the overall treatment effect.

To address these and other methodologic issues unique to NPTs, the CONSORT extension to randomized trials of NPTs and the CLEAR NPT were devised. The CONSORT Extension to NPTs was developed in 2006.[13] It consists of extensions to 11 items on the CONSORT checklist, one additional item, and a modification to the flow diagram. The

CONSORT extension to NPTs recommends an additional box to be added for each intervention in the flow diagram, which requires authors to report the median number, together with the interquartile range and maximum and minimum values, of participants treated by each health care provider or center.[13] This information is important to allow others to understand the applicability of the trial's results, which could reveal whether most patients were being treated by only one surgeon or whether all surgeons were treating the same number of patients.[13]

The CLEAR NPT is the Check List to Evaluate A Report of a NonPharmacological Trial (NPT).[14] It was developed in 2005 by a group of epidemiologists, statisticians, members of the Cochrane collaboration, and clinicians involved in planning nonpharmacological clinical trials. While the CLEAR NPT was primarily designed to evaluate the quality of reports, it can also serve as a useful guide to authors planning a nonpharmacological RCT or preparing a manuscript. It consists of a 15-item checklist, with 10 main items and five subitems. Each item is marked as yes, no, or unclear. The 15 items are shown in **Table 28.2**.

Table 28.2 CLEAR NPT checklist

Item	Possible answers
1. Was the generation of allocation sequences adequate?	Yes; No; Unclear
2. Was the treatment allocation concealed?	Yes; No; Unclear
3. Were details of the intervention administered to each group made available?[a]	Yes; No; Unclear
4. Were care providers' experience or skill[b] in each arm appropriate?[c]	Yes; No; Unclear
5. Was participant (i. e., patients') adherence assessed quantitatively?[d]	Yes; No; Unclear
6. Were participants adequately blinded?	Yes; No, because blinding is not feasible; No, although blinding is feasible; Unclear
6.1. If participants were not adequately blinded:	
6.1.1. Were all other treatments and care (i. e., co-interventions) the same in each randomized group?	Yes; No; Unclear
6.1.2. Were withdrawals and lost to follow-up the same in each randomized group?	Yes; No; Unclear
7. Were care providers or persons caring for the participants adequately blinded?	Yes; No, because blinding is not feasible; No, although blinding is feasible; Unclear
7.1. If care providers were not adequately blinded:	
7.1.1. Were all other treatments and care (i. e., co interventions) the same in each randomized group?	Yes; No; Unclear
7.1.2. Were withdrawals and lost to follow-up the same in each randomized group?	Yes; No; Unclear
8. Were outcome assessors adequately blinded to assess the primary outcomes?	Yes; No, because blinding is not feasible; No, although blinding is feasible; Unclear
8.1. If outcome assessors were not adequately blinded, were specific methods used to avoid ascertainment bias (systematic differences in outcome assessment)?[e]	Yes; No; Unclear
9. Was the follow-up schedule the same in each group?[f]	Yes; No; Unclear
10. Were the main outcomes analyzed according to the intention-to-treat principle?	Yes; No; Unclear

[a] The answer should be "yes" for this item if these data were either described in the report or made available for each arm (reference to a preliminary report, online addendum, etc.).

[b] Care provider experience or skill will be assessed only for therapist-dependent interventions (i. e., interventions where the success of the treatment is directly linked to care providers' technical skill). For other treatment, this item is not relevant and should be removed from the checklist or answered "unclear."

[c] Appropriate experience or skill should be determined according to published data, preliminary studies, guidelines, run-in period, or a group of experts, and should be specified in the protocol for each study arm before the beginning of the survey.

[d] Treatment adherence will be assessed only for treatments necessitating iterative interventions (e. g., physiotherapy that supposes several sessions, in contrast to a one-shot treatment such as surgery). For one-shot treatments, this item is not relevant and should be removed from the checklist or answered "unclear."

[e] The answer should be "yes" for this item, if the main outcome is objective or hard, or if outcomes were assessed by a blinded or at least an independent end-point review committee, or if outcomes were assessed by an independent outcome assessor trained to perform the measurements in a standardized manner, or if the outcome assessor was blinded to the study purpose and hypothesis.

[f] This item is not relevant for trials in which follow-up is part of the question. For example, this item is not relevant for a trial assessing frequent versus less frequent follow-up for cancer recurrence. In these situations, this item should be removed from the checklist or answered "unclear."

Table and table footnote reproduced from Boutron et al.[14]

NPT Extension to Consort Statement

The NPT extension to the CONSORT statement utilizes the same format as the CONSORT statement, but adds 11 extensions and one additional item. The following item numbers refer to the NPT extension to the CONSORT statement.[17]

Title and Abstract

The first extension applies to the title and abstract. For NPTs the abstract should also include a description of the experimental treatment, comparator, care providers, centers, and blinding status.

> **Key Concepts: Additional Details Required for Nonpharmacological Trials**
> Providing details as to how the interventions were standardized, what controls were used, the types of centers involved (e.g., high volume, tertiary care), details about the care providers (e.g., community setting, subspecialty trained), and whether blinding was possible allows the reader to make an assessment of the internal and external validity of the trial.

Methods

In addition to item 3 (participants), also elaborate on the participating centers and those performing the interventions. Because experimental interventions can be more difficult to standardize in NPTs, it has been shown that care providers' expertise and centers' volumes of care can influence the treatment effect.[18–22] Therefore, include a description of the qualifications and level of training of care providers, any specific training that may have occurred prior to trial initiation, and the selection criteria for the centers involved. This allows the reader to make an assessment of the risk of bias and the applicability of the results.

The next extension applies to item 4 (interventions). Provide precise details of both the experimental treatment arm and the control group, including a description of the procedure, how the interventions were standardized, and details of how protocol adherence was assessed. Full details of the surgical technique, implants/devices used, and postoperative care must be provided. For rehabilitation, authors should describe the content of each session, delivery (individual or group, whether it was supervised), the number of sessions, and overall duration of the intervention. Describe how each intervention was standardized and how adherence to study protocol was assessed. This facilitates study comparisons, reproducibility, and inclusion in future systematic reviews.

When applicable, in the description of randomization (item 8), explain how care providers were allocated to each trial group. In some NPTs (e.g., surgery), care providers may only be trained to perform one of the two interventions. If so, an *expertise-based RCT* design may be used.

> **Reality Check: Difficulties of Randomization Among Surgeons with Varying Expertise**
> It may be difficult to recruit surgeons to participate in a randomized trial comparing a novel surgical technique with the current standard of care. Many surgeons may only be comfortable with one technique or the other, or they may not have the expertise to perform the novel technique. In an expertise-based RCT, the participating surgeons would be randomized to performing either one technique or the other.

Indicate whether those administering co-interventions were blinded (item 11) to group assignment. If blinding was used, describe the method of blinding, and the similarities of the interventions (e.g., use of sham procedures).

Explain whether clustering by care providers or centers was addressed in the sample size calculation (item 7) and in the statistical methods (item 12).

> **Key Concepts: The Clustering Effect**
> Most RCTs base the statistical analyses on the assumption that observed outcomes in different patients treated by the same physician or in the same center are independent. However, in NPTs, treatment success may be dependent on surgeons' skill or the centers' volume of care. In these trials, observations of subjects treated by the same surgeon or in the same center may be correlated or "clustered." The clustering effect reduces the trial's statistical power and must be accounted for in the sample size calculation and analysis.

Results

In addition to participant flow (item 13), indicate the number of care providers or centers performing the intervention and the number of patients treated by each.

> **Reality Check: Unmasking the Clustering Effect**
> If 10 surgeons are involved in a trial, it is important to know whether the majority of patients were treated by a single surgeon or if all surgeons treated a similar number of patients.

Provide detail of the experimental treatment and comparator as they were implemented (new item). There may have been differences between the intended and the actual administration of the trial. Address any co-interventions or *contaminations* that may have occurred and how they may have influenced the estimates of treatment effect.

Jargon Simplified: Contamination

Contamination is what happens when the control group gets the experimental treatment. For example, in a trial evaluating outcomes seen with and without postoperative physical therapy, some subjects in the "no therapy" group may receive therapy even though this was not intended in the trial design.

In the baseline data (item 15), provide a description of the care providers (case volume, expertise, qualifications) and centers (volume) in both the experimental and the control group.

Discussion

In the interpretation of the results for an NPT (item 20), the choice of the comparator, blinding (feasibility of blinding, risk for bias when blinding is not feasible), balance of expertise of care providers or centers in each group, and any methods used to reduce bias should be discussed (e.g., objective outcomes, independent assessor). Also discuss the generalizability or external validity (item 21) of the trial findings according to the intervention, comparators, patients, care providers, and centers involved in the trial.

CLEAR NPT

The CLEAR NPT addresses many of the same factors (see **Table 28.2** for the complete checklist) as the NPT Extension to the CONSORT statement. The 11 items in the CLEAR NPT include an assessment of the randomization technique, whether treatment allocation was concealed, whether details of the interventions administered to each group were known, care providers' experience, participant adherence to protocol, blinding (of subjects, caregivers, and outcome assessors), standardization of treatment and follow-up, participant flow, and whether outcomes were analyzed according to the intention-to-treat principle.

Conclusion

Both the CONSORT statement and the CLEAR NPT provide readers, researchers, peer reviewers, and editors with tools to objectively assess manuscripts reporting results of randomized trials. While a trial may have been conducted with a reasonable level of rigor, unless these details are clearly communicated to the reader in a high-quality report, critical appraisal is not possible.[3]

Because randomized controlled trials are thought of as providing the highest level of evidence, the reader must be able to judge accurately whether the results justify a change in clinical practice.[2] The CONSORT statement and

CLEAR NPT promote transparency of methodology and if followed would limit opportunities for authors to hide the inadequacies of their study by omitting discussion of key aspects of trial design. Conversely, adherence might also limit the occasions when high-quality studies are assessed in critical appraisals to be of low quality because a lack of reporting is equated with poor design.[5]

As these checklists come to be incorporated throughout the medical literature, they will achieve their goal of improving the quality of RCTs, aiding critical appraisal of the literature and ensuring that only the best evidence is being used to guide future practice decisions.

Suggested Reading

Begg C, Cho M, Eastwood S, et al. Improving the quality of reporting of randomized controlled trials. The CONSORT statement. JAMA 1996;276:637–639

Schulz KF, Altman DG, Moher D; CONSORT Group. CONSORT 2010 statement: updated guidelines for reporting parallel group randomised trials. BMC Med 2010;8:18

References

1. Bhandari M, Richards RR, Sprague S, Schemitsch EH. The quality of reporting of randomized trials in the Journal of Bone and Joint Surgery from 1988 through 2000. J Bone Joint Surg Am 2002;84-A:388–396

2. Gummesson C, Atroshi I, Ekdahl C. The quality of reporting and outcome measures in randomized clinical trials related to upper-extremity disorders. J Hand Surg Am 2004; 29:727–734

3. Dulai SK, Slobogean BL, Beauchamp RD, Mulpuri K. A quality assessment of randomized clinical trials in pediatric orthopaedics. J Pediatr Orthop 2007;27:573–581

4. Detsky AS, Naylor CD, O'Rourke K, McGeer AJ, L'Abbe KA. Incorporating variations in the quality of individual randomized trials into meta-analysis. J Clin Epidemiol 1992;45:255–265

5. Devereaux PJ, Choi PT, El-Dika S, et al. An observational study found that authors of randomized controlled trials frequently use concealment of randomization and blinding, despite the failure to report these methods. J Clin Epidemiol 2004;57:1232–1236

6. Rennie D. Reporting randomized controlled trials. An experiment and a call for responses from readers. JAMA 1995;273:1054–1055

7. Begg C, Cho M, Eastwood S, et al. Improving the quality of reporting of randomized controlled trials. The CONSORT statement. JAMA 1996;276:637–639

8. Moher D, Hopewell S, Schulz KF, et al. CONSORT 2010 explanation and elaboration: updated guidelines for reporting parallel group randomised trials. J Clin Epidemiol 2010;63: e1–37

9. Schulz KF, Altman DG, Moher D; CONSORT Group. CONSORT 2010 statement: updated guidelines for reporting parallel group randomised trials. BMC Med 2010;8:18

10. Moher D, Schulz KF, Altman DG. The CONSORT statement: revised recommendations for improving the quality of reports of parallel-group randomised trials. Lancet 2001;357:1191–1194

11. Moher D, Jones A, Lepage L. Use of the CONSORT statement and quality of reports of randomized trials: a comparative before-and-after evaluation. JAMA 2001;285:1992–1995

12. Egger M, Juni P, Bartlett C. Value of flow diagrams in reports of randomized controlled trials. JAMA 2001;285:1996–1999

13. Schulz KF, Altman DG, Moher D, for the CONSORT Group. CONSORT 2010 statement: updated guidelines for reporting parallel group randomised trials. J Clin Epidemiol 2010;63:834–840

14. Boutron I, Moher D, Tugwell P, et al. A checklist to evaluate a report of a nonpharmacological trial (CLEAR NPT) was developed using consensus. J Clin Epidemiol 2005;58:1233–1240

15. Guyatt GH, Rennie D, Meade M, Cook D, eds. Users' Guide to the Medical Literature: A Manual for Evidence-Based Clinical Practice. 2nd ed. New York: McGraw-Hill; 2008

16. Chan AW, Altman DG. Epidemiology and reporting of randomised trials published in PubMed journals. Lancet 2005;365:1159–1162

17. Boutron I, Moher D, Altman DG, Schulz KF, Ravaud P, for the CONSORT Group. Extending the CONSORT Statement to Randomized Trials of Nonpharmacologic Treatment: Explanation and Elaboration. Ann Intern Med 2008;148:295–309

18. Halm EA, Lee C, Chassin MR. Is volume related to outcome in health care? A systematic review and methodologic critique of the literature. Ann Intern Med 2002;137:511–520

19. Khuri SF, Daley J, Henderson W, et al. Relation of surgical volume to outcome in eight common operations: results from the VA National Surgical Quality Improvement Program. Ann Surg 1999;230:414–429

20. Lavernia CJ, Guzman JF. Relationship of surgical volume to short-term mortality, morbidity, and hospital charges in arthroplasty. J Arthroplasty 1995;10:133–140

21. Birkmeyer JD, Stukel TA, Siewers AE, Goodney PP, Wennberg DE, Lucas FL. Surgeon volume and operative mortality in the United States. N Engl J Med 2003;349:2117–2127

22. Kreder HJ, Deyo RA, Koepsell T, Swiontkowski MF, Kreuter W. Relationship between the volume of total hip replacements performed by providers and the rates of postoperative complications in the state of Washington. J Bone Joint Surg Am 1997;79:485–494

29

Observational Studies Reporting Checklists

Lindsey C. Sheffler, Brett D. Crist, Tania A. Ferguson

Summary

Observational studies are prevalent in the surgical literature but are inherently prone to bias and confounding. The STROBE (*St*rengthening the *R*eporting of *Ob*servational Studies in *E*pidemiology) statement is a checklist of items intended to improve the quality of reporting observational studies.

Introduction

Observational studies differ from experimental "trials" (such as randomized controlled trials, or RCTs). In experimental studies, investigators assign subjects to either a treatment/exposure group or a "control" group. This randomization process allows the creation of two groups that are similar with respect to all variables except the exposure or treatment variable, and thus allows one to determine if an exposure causes an outcome of interest. Observational study designs are used when the assignment of subjects to a treatment or control group is ethically inappropriate or logistically impossible. In observational studies, the investigator identifies a population based on an exposure of interest and draws inferences about the possible effect of the exposure on the outcome. The three most common observational study designs are cohort, case–control, and cross-sectional studies (**Table 29.1**).

Well-designed experimental studies, especially RCTs, represent the highest level of methodology in the hierarchy of research design. Nonrandomized observational studies are an important complement to RCTs and are predominant in the surgical literature in both general surgery (46%) and orthopaedic surgery (88%).[2–4] It is important to understand that observational studies are inherently prone to potential bias and confounding associated with nonrandomization. For this reason, the reporting of observational research is challenging and the author must attempt to unveil any underlying bias or confounding that may have an impact on the observed results.

Table 29.1 Overview of observational study designs

Study design	Description	Outcome measure	Strengths	Weaknesses
Cohort	Subjects are divided into two groups, or cohorts: those with an exposure of interest and those without. The groups are followed prospectively and observed for an outcome of interest.	Relative risk ratio Incidence of disease	Establishes a cause and effect relationship Establishes a sequence of events Can study multiple outcome variables Rare exposures can be studied Regular collection of data reduces recall error	Loss to follow-up Time intensive Expensive Inefficient in studying rare outcomes Potential for confounding variables Potential for sampling bias
Case–control	Subjects who have experienced an outcome (cases) are matched to subjects who have not experienced that outcome (controls). The two groups are then studied retrospectively to determine a causal relationship between unmatched risk factors and the outcome of interest.	Odds ratio	Useful in studying rare outcomes/diseases Relatively quick and inexpensive	Only one outcome variable can be studied Potential for sampling bias in selecting case and control groups Prone to recall bias
Cross-sectional	Each subject in a population is evaluated at a single point in time, often to calculate the prevalence of disease or to establish an association between risk factors and outcome.	Prevalence of disease	Useful in establishing associations Can study multiple outcome variables Relatively quick and inexpensive	Cannot establish a causal relationship between exposure and outcome Cannot efficiently study rare conditions

Information taken from Mann.[1]

Key Concepts: Bias versus Confounding

Bias and confounding can adversely affect the validity and interpretation of an observational study. *Bias* typically occurs early in study design and results in findings or associations that may not reflect truth. Bias thus threatens the validity of the results. *Confounding variables*, on the other hand, are associated with both the exposure and the outcome of interest, so that while the findings may be valid, a cause-and-effect relationship cannot be established between exposure and outcome.[5]

Checklist for Observational Studies: The STROBE Statement

In order to practice evidence-based orthopaedic surgery, a reader must critically appraise the published research, understand the strengths and weaknesses of the study, and determine if the reported results and conclusions are applicable to other clinical situations. For the reader to be able to do this, a research manuscript should clearly describe the research question and study population and further explain how the study was designed to answer the question and if the research methodology/analysis was appropriate to reach the author's conclusions. As stated above, authors of observational studies must examine and disclose potential factors that may threaten the validity and applicability of their findings (please refer to **Table 29.2** for a detailed description of different forms of bias which may impact study findings).

Key Concepts: External Validity

"External validity" refers to the applicability of the results of an investigation to a target population in real world circumstances. It can be threatened by uniqueness of the environment in which the study was performed (a study performed in a level 1 teaching hospital, for exam-

Table 29.2 Bias

Bias	Sampling bias and measurement bias are the most common forms of bias in observational studies. Eight subtypes of biases are explained below.[6]
Sampling bias	A bias that results from the selection of a subject population.
	Prevalence–incidence bias: Enrolling subjects at a later time than the time of exposure may miss fatal or silent cases. *Example:* A study of postoperative deep vein thrombosis (DVT) would be prone to bias if it enrolled subjects who were 10 years out from surgery because it would miss subjects whose DVT was fatal and those who had a DVT that was subclinical.
	Unmasking bias: An exposure that does not cause disease, but causes a symptom that leads the clinician to search for disease. *Example:* A female athlete who presents with secondary amenorrhea receives an intensive diagnostic work-up for osteopenia, whereas a female subject without secondary amenorrhea receives standard screening detection procedures to determine bone health. The investigators claim that the relative risk of osteopenia is higher in women with secondary amenorrhea.
	Nonrespondent bias: A cohort of subjects that respond may differ in exposure and/or outcome from nonrespondents. *Example:* In a survey mailed to subjects recently hospitalized for a traumatic pelvic fracture, subjects are asked about their drug and alcohol use. Only 50% of subjects with documented blood alcohol concentration >80 mg/dL at the time of admission respond whereas 85% of subjects with a blood alcohol concentration <80 mg/dL respond.
	Membership bias: Subjects who are members of a group may have a health status that differs from that of the general population. *Example:* The results of a study exploring the risks of osteoporosis in a group of men recruited from an athletic health club would not be representative of risk factors in the general population.
Measurement bias	A bias that results from the measurement of exposures and outcomes.
	Diagnostic suspicion bias: A subject's medical history may influence the intensity of diagnostic procedures. *Example:* Knowledge of a recent fall in a patient with mild wrist pain may influence a clinician's decision to order a radiograph.
	Exposure suspicion bias: A subject's disease state may influence how vigorously the investigator searches for an exposure. *Example:* An investigator surveys a population of athletes and finds that 5% report anabolic steroid use. A second investigator studying the same population *intensively* questions the male athletes with notable muscle bulk and finds that 35% report use.
	Recall bias: Occurs when patients who experience an adverse outcome have a different likelihood of recalling an exposure than patients who do not experience the adverse outcome, independent of the true extent of exposure.[7] *Example:* When asked about birth history, a parent whose son has brachial plexus birth palsy (BPBP) describes in detail the events surrounding the delivery while a parent whose child does not have BPBP states that her delivery was "normal."
	Family information bias: A subject in a case group with an exposure or outcome of interest may receive family information that differs from that of a subject in a control group. *Example:* A study of subjects with developmental hip dysplasia (DDH) found that 50% of subjects reported a parent with DDH. When the unaffected siblings were asked about their family history, only 30% of subjects reported a parent with DDH.

ple, may not generate results applicable to a small community center). The most common threat to external validity is lack of commonality between the study population and the intended target population. If the study group is not representative of a reader's patients, for example, it may be inappropriate to apply the results to his or her practice.

Key Concepts: Participants

In designing a study, authors hope to make inferences from findings observed in a representative group (sample) which can then be applied to a general (target) population. In order for a reader to determine if it is valid to apply the results of a study to his or her own practice, the study must clearly describe the subjects, how they were selected, what was done to them, and how many of them were available for each point in the study.

The STROBE (*St*rengthening the *R*eporting of *Ob*servational Studies in *E*pidemiology) initiative was established in 2004 in an effort to improve the quality of reporting observational research. A multinational group of methodologists,

researchers, and journal editors met to develop recommendations intended to help investigators write "a clear presentation of what was planned, done, and found in an observational study."[5] This checklist has been adopted by many of the current orthopaedic journals including the *Journal of Bone and Joint Surgery.*[8]

The STROBE statement is an itemized checklist of 22 recommendations considered essential for the reporting of cohort, case–control, and cross-sectional studies (**Table 29.3**). The items provide guidance for transparent reporting of all sections of a research paper: title and abstract, introduction, methods, results, discussion, and funding sources. The recommendations encourage a clear description of study aims, the definition of a testable hypothesis, and guidelines for reporting study limitations and generalizability. Nine of the items are aimed at ensuring a detailed description of the research method including subject selection criteria, variable definitions, identification of potential confounders and biases, sample size calculations, and the use of statistical methods. Five of the checklist items are aimed at improving the transparent description of research results.

Table 29.3 The STROBE statement—checklist of items that should be included in reports of observational studies

	Item no.	Recommendation
Title and abstract	1	(a) Indicate the study's design with a commonly used term in the title or the abstract.
		(b) Provide in the abstract an informative and balanced summary of what was done and what was found.
Introduction		
Background/rationale	2	Explain the scientific background and rationale for the investigation being reported.
Objectives	3	State specific objectives, including any prespecified hypotheses.
Methods		
Study design	4	Present key elements of study design early in the paper.
Setting	5	Describe the setting, locations, and relevant dates, including periods of recruitment, exposure, follow-up, and data collection.
Participants	6	(a) *Cohort study*—Give the eligibility criteria, and the sources and methods of selection of participants. Describe methods of follow-up. *Case–control study*—Give the eligibility criteria, and the sources and methods of case ascertainment and control selection. Give the rationale for the choice of cases and controls. *Cross-sectional study*—Give the eligibility criteria, and the sources and methods of selection of participants.
		(b) *Cohort study*—For matched studies, give matching criteria and number of exposed and unexposed. *Case-control study*—For matched studies, give matching criteria and the number of controls per case.
Variables	7	Clearly define all outcomes, exposures, predictors, potential confounders, and effect modifiers. Give diagnostic criteria, if applicable.
Data sources/ measurement	8*	For each variable of interest, give sources of data and details of methods of assessment (measurement). Describe comparability of assessment methods if there is more than one group.
Bias	9	Describe any efforts to address potential sources of bias.
Study size	10	Explain how the study size was arrived at.

Continued ▶

Table 29.1 Continued

	Item no.	Recommendation
Quantitative variables	11	Explain how quantitative variables were handled in the analyses. If applicable, describe which groupings were chosen and why.
Statistical methods	12	(a) Describe all statistical methods, including those used to control for confounding.
		(b) Describe any methods used to examine subgroups and interactions.
		(c) Explain how missing data were addressed.
		(d) *Cohort study*—If applicable, explain how loss to follow-up was addressed. *Case–control study*—If applicable, explain how matching of cases and controls was addressed. *Cross-sectional study*—If applicable, describe analytical methods taking account of sampling strategy.
		(e) Describe any sensitivity analyses.
Results		
Participants	13*	(a) Report numbers of individuals at each stage of study—e. g., numbers potentially eligible, examined for eligibility, confirmed eligible, included in the study, completing follow-up, and analyzed.
		(b) Give reasons for nonparticipation at each stage.
		(c) Consider use of a flow diagram.
Descriptive data	14*	(a) Give characteristics of study participants (e. g., demographic, clinical, social) and information on exposures and potential confounders.
		(b) Indicate number of participants with missing data for each variable of interest.
		(c) *Cohort study*—Summarize follow-up time (e. g., average and total amount).
Outcome data	15*	*Cohort study*—Report numbers of outcome events or summary measures over time.
		Case–control study—Report numbers in each exposure category, or summary measures of exposure.
		Cross-sectional study—Report numbers of outcome events or summary measures.
Main results	16	(a) Give unadjusted estimates and, if applicable, confounder-adjusted estimates and their precision (e. g., 95% confidence interval). Make clear which confounders were adjusted for and why they were included.
		(b) Report category boundaries when continuous variables were categorized.
		(c) If relevant, consider translating estimates of relative risk into absolute risk for a meaningful time period.
Other analyses	17	Report other analyses done—e. g., analyses of subgroups and interactions, and sensitivity analyses
Discussion		
Key results	18	Summarize key results with reference to study objectives.
Limitations	19	Discuss limitations of the study, taking into account sources of potential bias or imprecision. Discuss both direction and magnitude of any potential bias.
Interpretation	20	Give a cautious overall interpretation of results considering objectives, limitations, multiplicity of analyses, results from similar studies, and other relevant evidence.
Generalizability	21	Discuss the generalizability (external validity) of the study results.
Other information		
Funding	22	Give the source of funding and the role of the funders for the present study and, if applicable, for the original study on which the present article is based.

*Give information separately for cases and controls in case–control studies and, if applicable, for exposed and unexposed groups in cohort and cross-sectional studies.

Note: An Explanation and Elaboration article discusses each checklist item and gives methodological background and published examples of transparent reporting. The STROBE checklist is best used in conjunction with this article (freely available on the Web sites of PLoS Medicine at http://www.plosmedicine.org/, Annals of Internal Medicine at http://www.annals.org/, and Epidemiology at http://www.epidem.com/). Information on the STROBE Initiative is available at www.strobe-statement.org.
Reproduced with permission from von Elm et al.[9]

Key Concepts: Selection Criteria

Inclusion criteria define the main characteristics of the target population that are relevant to the primary research question. Inclusion criteria should be specific and include demographic, clinical, radiographic, and geographic characteristics. The researcher will at times make trade-offs between the scientific goals and the practicalities of performing the research. These compromises should be critically addressed and exposed as they may affect the generalizability of the results.

Exclusion criteria are applied to a subset of patients who generally meet the inclusion criteria of a study but cannot complete the study or possess unique characteristics that may confound the results. Reasons for exclusion may include skeletal immaturity, sex, a history of prior pathology affecting the region of interest, a likelihood of being lost to follow-up, or being unlikely to provide usable data (for example, due to inability on the part of the patient to comply with postoperative precautions or restrictions).

Key Concepts: Reporting of Patient Characteristics

Authors should clearly describe characteristics of study participants (i.e., demographic, clinical, social) and information on exposures and potential confounders. Tables and text boxes are advised (see **Table 29.4**). Authors should report the number of participants at each stage of the study (eligibility, recruitment, enrollment, and follow-up) and include information about subjects who were deemed to be ineligible or who were lost to follow-up. Flow diagrams are very useful for this purpose (see **Fig. 29.1**).

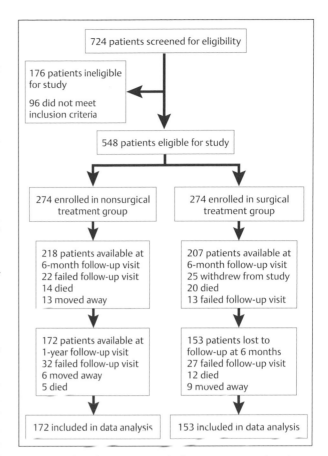

Fig. 29.1 Flow diagram example for a case–control study.

Guide to Investigators: How to Use the STROBE Statement

The STROBE statement is a guideline for authors aimed at improving the quality and clarity of the presentation of their research. Adherence to the STROBE checklist helps an author create a well-written manuscript that exposes potential bias inherent to the study design and alerts the reader to limitations in the generalizability of the results and conclusions. While the STROBE checklist is not intended as a tool for improving study design or research quality, consideration of these items can assist researchers as they define their objectives, hypotheses, study and target populations, variables, research methodology, and statistical methods. We therefore recommend using the checklist during the preparation of the study proposal and/or funding applications.

The following is a user-friendly guide for orthopaedic investigators to help them apply the checklist when preparing manuscripts of observational studies. All item numbers cited refer to checklist items in the STROBE statement (**Table 29.3**).

Table 29.4 Exposures in subjects with (cases) and without (controls) deep vein thrombosis

Variable	Cases, N (%)	Controls, N (%)
All subjects	133 (100)	266 (100)
In-patient surgery	97 (73)	179 (67)
Outpatient surgery	36 (27)	87 (33)
External fixation	20 (15)	53 (20)
Internal fixation	17 (13)	37 (14)
Multisystem trauma	40 (30)	93 (25)
Long-bone fracture	28 (21)	53 (20)
Total joint arthroplasty	42 (32)	69 (26)
Pharmacologic prophylaxis	71 (53)	165 (62)
Smoking	68 (51)	64 (36)
Age >50 years	72 (54)	122 (46)
Body mass index >30	41 (31)	64 (24)
Estrogen use	16 (12)	21 (8)

The STROBE Statement: Explanations of Checklist Items

Title and Abstract

The research title should clearly and concisely inform the reader about the nature of the study and the research method used to investigate the topic. The abstract depicts the key details of the study including why the study was performed, the methods used, the numerical findings, and the study's overall relevance.

Introduction

The introduction explains how the research question was generated and transparently reports the specific aims and hypotheses of the study. By including prespecified hypotheses, the reader can determine if the methods used are appropriate to answering the research question and if the findings support or contradict the hypotheses.

Methods

The methods section should include key study design elements such as the type of observational study and a definition of the exposure(s) and outcome(s) of interest. Authors should also include a description of the population from which subjects are recruited and report when the study takes place (item 4). By including details regarding the research setting, authors provide an important context for the results of the study and allow readers to determine if the findings are generalizable to other settings and populations (item 5).

Transparent reporting of study participants is of high importance given the potential for sampling bias in observational studies (**Table 29.2**). Investigators should define the inclusion and exclusion criteria as well as the sources and methods of recruitment. Matching of case and control groups can reduce the effect of confounding variables, and the rationale behind the selection of matching criteria must be clearly stated (item 6). Furthermore, the investigators should address which confounding variables were accounted for and why these variables were selected (item 7).

Key Concepts: Sampling Strategies
The process of defining a group of study participants representative of a general (target) population is called sampling. The two main categories of sampling strategies are probability and nonprobability sampling.
Probability sampling: The highest standard for ensuring generalizability, probability sampling is a random process used to guarantee that each unit of the general population has a chance of being included in the sample. Three common subtypes of probability sampling are simple random sample, systematic sampling, and stratified sampling.
Nonprobability sampling: Nonprobability sampling does not rely on random assignments or selections. Two modes of nonprobability sampling are convenience sampling and consecutive sampling.

Jargon Simplified: Simple Random Sample
Random numbers are assigned to patients in a population and a subset is selected at random.

Jargon Simplified: Systematic Sampling
Systematic sampling is similar to the above in that all subjects in a population are enumerated, but then a periodic process is used to select the sample (for example, every third patient presenting to the office is included).

Jargon Simplified: Stratified Sampling
Stratified sampling is the process of grouping individuals into strata based on an important known and measurable characteristic (such as study site, patient sex, or age) to ensure that these characteristics are equally represented across the intervention groups.

Jargon Simplified: Convenience Sampling
As the name suggests, in this form of sampling subjects are selected because they are easily accessible to the researcher. This technique is easy, fast, and usually the most logistically feasible method.

Jargon Simplified: Consecutive Sampling
In one of the most common forms of sampling in the orthopaedic literature, consecutive subjects who are eligible for participation in the study are selected. The benefit of using this type of comprehensive sample is that a good representation of the overall population is possible over a reasonable period of time.

Key Concepts: Matching
Matching is a process by which potential confounding variables are identified and cases and controls are "matched" on the basis of these factors such that the groups are the same with respect to them. Matching is associated with important limitations and is fraught with difficulties and therefore not always advised.

In addition to sampling bias, observational studies are prone to measurement bias (**Table 29.2**). A clear description of how data are collected and measured reveals potential biases to the reader that may affect the validity of the study (item 8). For example, radiographic outcome measures (e.g., length, alignment, rotation) will vary with the precision of film acquisition, and small changes in the orientation of the x-ray beam will change the measurement of the outcome variables. Thus, an author using these technologies should describe the steps taken to standardize image acquisition and measurement.

Biased studies are at risk of reporting findings or associations that are invalid (**Table 29.2**). Say, for example, a patient's weight is entered into a total joint registry as 350 lb (159 kg), when in fact the patient weighed only 150 lb (68 kg). This low-risk patient may be inappropriately included in a cohort of morbidly obese patients selected on the basis of weight, and decrease the observed risk of the cohort. While a measurement bias such as the one in this example can be prevented with careful data collection, other biases are more difficult to prevent. In such cases, the authors should report potential sources of sampling and measurement bias (**Table 29.2**) and predict the probable direction and magnitude of the effect on the results (item 9).

In addition to reporting potential biases, the investigator must elucidate the assumptions and calculations used in study design and data analysis. A study must first be appropriately powered so that a difference or association between groups can be detected if it exists. The investigator should inform the reader of how the sample size was calculated or, if it was not calculated, what factors (such as a fixed available sample) determined the sample size (item 10). If a variable is continuous, the author should report linearity or nonlinearity of the data. Furthermore, if a continuous variable is divided into groups, the rationale behind determination of these groups must be addressed (item 11). For example, an investigator interested in studying the incidence of femur fractures in different age groups may divide the continuous age variable into groups of 0–20 years, 21–40 years, and 41–60 years. The investigator should provide the reader with a reason for this grouping (such as a previous publication using similar groupings or an established difference in the risk of traumatic injury between these specific age groups). The reader can thus better understand why the subgroup analysis was performed and analyze what it contributes to the overall findings of the study.

The methods section is also where the investigator should explicitly state all statistical methods used to control for confounding, analyze subgroups, and handle missing data (items 12a–c). The issue of confounding is discussed below.

Key Concepts: Confounding

Confounding can misrepresent the relationship between surgical treatments and outcomes and may result when two pretreatment groups are fundamentally different. Example: An investigator studying the association between type II diabetes and postoperative infection recruits 50 subjects with diabetes (cases) and 50 subjects without diabetes (controls). The subjects undergo the same surgery and postoperatively, the investigator finds that the diabetic group has a higher rate of infection. The investigator, however, did not account for the fact that the subjects with diabetes were significantly more overweight than the control group. Since obesity can increase operative time and thus the risk of

infection, he cannot claim that diabetes alone caused the adverse outcome.

If subgroup analyses are performed, the authors should state if the analysis was planned before or after data collection, since post hoc analyses may be misleading to readers. Missing data points do not preclude subject inclusion in analysis, but authors should report the cause of missing data and employ statistical methods such as weighted estimation to minimize the selection bias associated with missing data. Specific statistical methods may be more appropriate depending on the type of observational study. For example, in a cohort study, loss to follow-up should be addressed, whereas matching and sampling strategy should be described for case–control and cross-sectional studies, respectively. Sensitivity analyses may be used to determine whether the results of the study are consistent when other statistical methods are used and to unmask confounding variables and bias. Investigators should report the type of sensitivity analysis and the rationale behind its use (item 12e).

Results

The results section provides a clear summary of the study participants, outcome data, and secondary analyses that were performed. A flow chart is an effective tool for reporting the number of participants at each stage of the study from eligibility through to follow-up and satisfies items 13 and 14 of the STROBE checklist. **Figure 29.1** is an example of how a flow chart can summarize participant information in a case–control study. In addition to reporting the number of participants who were lost to follow-up, authors should describe the average length of follow-up and the number of participants with missing data (items 14b–c).

Before reporting the results of statistical analyses, descriptive information should be provided about the number of outcomes events (for cross-sectional and cohort studies) or the number of exposures per group (for case–control studies). This can be effectively conveyed in table format, as shown with a hypothetical example in **Table 29.4** (item 15). If the investigators adjusted for potential confounding variables, estimates should include confidence intervals. Unadjusted analyses should also be included so that the reader can compare the results of both analyses (item 16a). If a continuous variable is divided into groups, the range and number of subjects per group should be reported (item 16b), and in studies analyzing the association between exposure and disease, both relative risk and absolute risk should be reported (item 16c). Finally, while the results section should report additional analyses (such as subgroup and sensitivity analyses), the focus of the results section should be on the findings that support or contradict the primary specific aims and hypotheses (item 17).

Discussion

The discussion section provides a context for the main findings of the study and helps the reader understand the validity, generalizability, and relevance of the results. Authors should begin by restating the main results and reporting whether or not the findings support the primary specific aims and hypotheses of the study (item 18). Given the biases to which observational studies are prone, it is imperative that authors report the study limitations, which include potential sources of bias, imprecision of the results, and restrictions to generalizability (item 19). The authors should provide a cautious interpretation of the results to inform the readers of how the study contributes to the existing body of evidence (item 20) and clearly describe whether or not the findings of the study can be applied to other settings and populations (item 21).

Other Information

Funding may introduce a conflict of interest that could influence the overall findings. Authors should report any sources of funding (governmental, nonprofit, industrial/commercial) and elucidate the role of the funding party in study design, data collection, and/or data analysis.

Conclusion

The STROBE statement aims to improve the quality of the written report of observational studies but is limited to the three most common designs (cohort, case–control and cross-sectional). While authors of research utilizing other observational design (case–crossover, case series, etc.) may find the general direction of the checklist useful, the specific design-based items may be more difficult to apply. Moreover, the STROBE contributors warn that the goal of the initiative is not to create a rigid format for the layout of a manuscript.[9] While each item should be clearly addressed in some manner within the body of a manuscript, the format and style of writing should follow the writer's preferences.

The application of the STROBE checklist assists authors in developing a clear, transparent, high-quality manuscript useful to the clinician attempting to practice evidence-based orthopaedic surgery. An author who follows the recommendations of the STROBE checklist should, at the completion of the manuscript, be able to answer yes to the abbreviated list of ten questions outlined in the Reality Check section below.

Reality Check: Application of the STROBE Checklist

If an author has transparently reported an observational study by applying the STROBE checklist, he or she should be able to answer yes to each of the questions in the following abbreviated checklist.

1. Does your *title* describe your study in a manner that would allow a reader to find it with a literature search engine? Does it include the type of study design you used?
2. Is your hypothesis clearly stated within your *introduction*?
3. Based on the study design you chose, is your study prone to *bias*? If so, did you explain how you accounted for potential biases and what residual biases may have affected your results?
4. Is it clear from your manuscript how representative your *participants* are of the general population? Do your results apply to all patients and if not, why?
5. Did you describe the *variables* of interest and potential *confounders* that may have affected your results?
6. Did you report why you chose the *statistical methods* you used? How did you perform the statistical analyses and what assumptions were required? What assumptions were made in calculating your sample size?
7. Are your *results* clearly stated? Is it transparent how many patients were lost to follow-up and why? Did you describe how missing data were handled? Are your graphical representations reader-friendly?
8. Did you clearly state which results were due to *secondary* or *subgroup analyses*? Did you appropriately report both positive and negative findings in your study?
9. Did you clearly analyze the results of your study and provide information regarding the *generalizability* and limitations of your study?
10. Did you state sources of *funding* and/or conflicts of interest?

Observational studies have a prevalent and important role in the orthopaedic literature. However, given the potential biases to which they are prone, it is imperative that authors report the findings of observational studies in a clear and standardized manner. By unveiling the limitations of an observational study and describing potential biases, an author communicates to the reader the context in which the study was performed and allows the reader to judge the applicability of the results to other populations and settings. The STROBE statement can serve as a valuable tool to the orthopaedic surgeon who wishes to improve the quality and clarity of reporting observational studies.

Suggested Reading

Mundi R, Chaudhry H, Singh I, Bhandari M. Checklists to improve the quality of the orthopaedic literature. Indian J Orthop 2008;42:150–164

Vandenbroucke JP, von Elm E, Altman DG, et al. Strengthening the Reporting of Observational Studies in Epidemiology (STROBE): explanation and elaboration. Epidemiology. 2007;18:805–835

von Elm E, Altman DG, Egger M, Pocock SJ, Gotzsche PC, Vandenbroucke JP. The Strengthening the Reporting of Observational Studies in Epidemiology (STROBE) statement: guidelines for reporting observational studies. J Clin Epidemiol 2008; 61:344–349

References

1. Mann CJ. Observational research methods. Research design II: cohort, cross sectional, and case-control studies. Emerg Med J 2003;20:54–60
2. Carr AJ. Evidence-based orthopaedic surgery: what type of research will best improve clinical practice? J Bone Joint Surg Br 2005;87:1593–1594
3. Horton R. Surgical research or comic opera: questions, but few answers. Lancet 1996;347:984–985
4. Mundi R, Chaudhry H, Singh I, Bhandari M. Checklists to improve the quality of the orthopaedic literature. Indian J Orthop 2008;42:150–164
5. Vandenbroucke JP, von Elm E, Altman DG, et al. Strengthening the Reporting of Observational Studies in Epidemiology (STROBE): explanation and elaboration. Epidemiology. 2007;18:805–835
6. Sackett, D.L. Bias in analytical research. J Chron Dis 1979;32:51–63
7. Guyatt GH, Rennie D, Meade M, Cook D, eds. Users' Guide to the Medical Literature: A Manual for Evidence-Based Clinical Practice. 2nd ed. New York: McGraw-Hill; 2008
8. The Journal of Bone and Joint Surgery—Instructions to Authors. Available at: http://www2.ejbjs.org/misc/instrux. dtl. Accessed 2 February 2010
9. von Elm E, Altman DG, Egger M, Pocock SJ, Gotzsche PC, Vandenbroucke JP. The Strengthening the Reporting of Observational Studies in Epidemiology (STROBE) statement: guidelines for reporting observational studies. J Clin Epidemiol 2008;61:344–349

30

Meta-analysis Reporting Checklists

Holly Smith, Nizar Mahomed, Rajiv Gandhi

Summary

In this chapter, the rationale for the creation and use of a meta-analysis reporting checklist is presented. The most widely accepted checklists are introduced for both randomized controlled trials (RCTs) and observational studies, along with their major points of inclusion.

Introduction

A reporting checklist offers guidelines that can be used by an author to increase the methodological soundness and consistency of reporting when preparing a meta-analysis. The checklist items help the author improve clarity and transparency, and ensure completeness of reporting.

The meta-analysis is an increasingly popular source of information among medical professionals who are too busy to read all of the literature available to them. Meta-analyses synthesize data from multiple primary studies to reach a conclusion about the intervention being investigated. They are frequently used to resolve the results of conflicting studies by pooling all available data. Since the results of primary studies are combined, the sample size for each outcome measure is larger, thereby increasing the power of the conclusions that can be made. Although meta-analyses are generally considered to provide the highest level of evidence, they are not immune to bias. Meta-analyses can potentially produce incorrect estimates of treatment effect that can have serious implications for medical practice, patient care, and future clinical research.[1,2]

Several authors have documented that published meta-analyses are frequently of poor quality, throwing the validity of the results into question.[1,3] A recent review of orthopaedic meta-analyses published between 1969 and 2008 found that, despite recent improvements, a large quantity of recently published meta-analyses contain major methodological flaws.[1] The authors assessed the quality of the studies using the Oxman and Guyatt index for meta-analyses.[4,5] The items on this index include reporting, criteria for inclusion of primary studies, comprehensiveness of the search, avoidance of bias in primary studies, inclusions of appropriate validity criteria for primary studies, reporting of statistical methods, and whether the conclusions were supported by the analysis. These items all relate to the methodology and reporting of the meta-analysis, which is just as important to the overall quality of the primary studies.[6] Meta-analysis reporting checklists address all of these criteria. Even if performed with stringent methodology, poor reporting diminishes the value of the conclusions of a meta-analysis. Meta-analysis reporting checklists provide guidelines that enable authors to ensure that their protocol is conducted in a manner that maximizes transparency and clarity. Use of these checklists ensures that the essential components of a well-conducted meta-analysis are included.

Meta-analysis Reporting Checklists

Several different checklists can be used as guidelines for writing a meta-analysis. The choice of checklist depends entirely on the type of primary articles being used. The EQUATOR network (Enhancing the Quality and Transparency of Health Research) is a resource for reporting of health research studies that recognizes reporting guidance for three classes of meta-analyses: those using data from RCTs, those using data from observational studies, and those using individual participant data.[7] The PRISMA (Preferred Reporting Items for Systematic Reviews and Meta-analyses) checklist[8] is recommended for use with meta-analyses of RCTs and can also be used as a guideline for proper reporting of systematic reviews. Meta-analyses performed using data from observational studies are advised to use the MOOSE (Meta-analysis of Observational Studies in Epidemiology) checklist.[9] Meta-analyses of individual participant data can make use of either checklist as applicable.[10]

Meta-analysis reporting checklists are designed to provide a set of guidelines for authors, and should be referred to for a basic framework when writing meta-analyses.

Key Concepts: Sources of Data for Meta-analyses
- Randomized controlled trials
- Observational studies
- Individual patient data

PRISMA (Preferred Reporting Items for Systematic Reviews and Meta-analyses)

The PRISMA checklist consists of 27 items divided on the basis of where they are found in the paper.[11] PRISMA is an update on the QUOROM (*Qu*ality *o*f *R*eporting *o*f *M*eta-analyses) statement that was developed in 1996 with the intention of becoming the "gold standard" of meta-analysis reporting checklists.[12,13] Though effective for many years, the QUOROM statement was revised in 2005 to act as a guideline for writing systematic reviews in addition to meta-analyses.[8] The goal of this transition was to create a more effective, detailed, and comprehensive checklist that would be applicable to both types of papers.

The PRISMA checklist provides recommendations for the structure and content of the abstract and introduction of a systematic review or meta-analysis. The checklist particularly recommends the use of a structured abstract as it provides a balanced overview of the results of the study.[11]

Examples from the Literature: Example of a Structured Abstract[14]

Source: Kuzyk PRT, Guy P, Kreder HJ, Zdero R, KcKee MD, Schemitsch EH. Minimally invasive hip fracture surgery: are outcomes better? J Orthop Trauma 2009;23:447–453

"Objectives: Intertrochanteric hip fractures have high morbidity and mortality rates. The purpose of this study was to determine if minimally invasive plating, nailing, or external fixation operations lead to improved outcomes for intertrochanteric hip fractures compared with standard insertion of a sliding hip screw (SHS).

"Data sources: A systematic search of MEDLINE (1996 to June 2007) and EMBASE (1980 to June 2007) was performed. Results were limited to English language studies. References from eligible studies were reviewed to identify additional studies.

"Study selection: Studies were selected for review based on the following criteria: prospective or retrospective studies comparing minimally invasive plating, nailing, or external fixation to standard insertion of an SHS, exclusion of intracapsular and subtrochanteric hip fractures, and report of outcome data by treatment group to allow for comparison.

"Data extraction: The following outcomes were extracted from eligible studies: operative time, operative blood loss, intraoperative complications, postoperative drop in hemoglobin, postoperative pain, postoperative medical or fracture complications, wound complications, length of hospital stay, and postfracture function.

"Data synthesis: Sufficient data existed among 14 randomized controlled trials to perform a meta-analysis and calculate pooled relative risks for failure of fixation, blood transfusion, and mortality. Relative risks were calculated with 95% confidence intervals using a random-effects model, and an analysis of heterogeneity between pooled studies was conducted. Other outcome measures that were extracted from 17 comparative studies are reported as a systematic review.

"Conclusions: Although a significant heterogeneity exists between pooled studies, minimally invasive hip fracture plating, nailing, or external fixation was associated with a decrease in transfusion rate [relative risk of 0.63 as compared to standard SHS (95% confidence interval 0.41 to 0.96; $I^2 = 83.6\%$)]. There was no significant difference for the other comparisons, including mortality, between minimally invasive plating, nailing, or external fixation and standard insertion of an SHS."

PRISMA provides a list of items to be included in the methods section, such as a description of information sources, search strategy, study selection and data collection process, an evaluation of bias within individual studies and across studies, and a description of summary measures and synthesis of the results.

Examples from the Literature: Example of Study Criteria Reporting[15]

Source: Mason JB, Fehring TK, Estok R, Banel D, Fahrbach K. Meta-analysis of alignment outcomes in computer assisted total knee arthroplasty surgery. J Arthroplasty 2007;22:1097–1106

"A study had to satisfy the following criteria for inclusion: (1) CAS navigated primary TKA; (2) reporting of postoperative implant and limb alignment outcomes; and (3) at least 10 patients in the treatment group. Any rejection of a study had the agreement of two reviewers."

Inclusion of these items greatly increases transparency, and provides readers with crucial information regarding the methodology that is frequently omitted. The checklist further indicates that the results section should include data assessing the risk of bias in the included primary studies. Recommendations for the discussion include the strength of the evidence for each individual outcome investigated, limitations of the study, and final conclusions. For the full checklist refer to **Table 30.1**.

The authors of the PRISMA statement also prepared a flow diagram to be included in the meta-analysis that enables the reader to follow the progression of the literature search (**Fig. 30.1**). When information from the flow diagram and checklist are combined, the original search performed by the authors can be replicated. The reader is thus able to evaluate the thoroughness of the literature search, the likelihood that relevant articles were missed, and any implications that this has for the results of the meta-analysis.

Table 30.1 The PRISMA Checklist

Section/topic	Item no.	Checklist item	Reported on page no.
Title			
Title	1	Identify the report as a systematic review, meta-analysis, or both.	
Abstract			
Structured summary	2	Provide a structured summary including, as applicable: background; objectives; data sources; study eligibility criteria, participants, and interventions; study appraisal and synthesis methods; results; limitations; conclusions and implications of key findings; systematic review registration number.	
Introduction			
Rationale	3	Describe the rationale for the review in the context of what is already known.	
Objectives	4	Provide an explicit statement of questions being addressed with reference to participants, interventions, comparisons, outcomes, and study design (PICOS).	
Methods			
Protocol and registration	5	Indicate if a review protocol exists, if and where it can be accessed (e. g., web address), and, if available, provide registration information including registration number.	
Eligibility criteria	6	Specify study characteristics (e. g., PICOS, length of follow-up) and report characteristics (e. g., years considered, language, publication status) used as criteria for eligibility, giving rationale.	
Information sources	7	Describe all information sources (e. g., databases with dates of coverage, contact with study authors to identify additional studies) in the search and date last searched.	
Search	8	Present full electronic search strategy for at least one database, including any limits used, such that it could be repeated.	
Study selection	9	State the process for selecting studies (i. e., screening, eligibility, included in systematic review, and, if applicable, included in the meta-analysis).	
Data collection process	10	Describe method of data extraction from reports (e. g., piloted forms, independently, in duplicate) and any processes for obtaining and confirming data from investigators.	
Data items	11	List and define all variables for which data were sought (e. g., PICOS, funding sources) and any assumptions and simplifications made.	
Risk of bias in individual studies	12	Describe methods used for assessing risk of bias of individual studies (including specification of whether this was done at the study or outcome level), and how this information is to be used in any data synthesis.	
Summary measures	13	State the principal summary measures (e. g., risk ratio, difference in means).	
Synthesis of results	14	Describe the methods of handling data and combining results of studies, if done, including measures of consistency (e. g., I^2) for each meta-analysis.	
Risk of bias across studies	15	Specify any assessment of risk of bias that may affect the cumulative evidence (e. g., publication bias, selective reporting within studies).	
Additional analyses	16	Describe methods of additional analyses (e. g., sensitivity or subgroup analyses, meta-regression), if done, indicating which were prespecified.	
Results			
Study selection	17	Give numbers of studies screened, assessed for eligibility, and included in the review, with reasons for exclusions at each stage, ideally with a flow diagram.	
Study characteristics	18	For each study, present characteristics for which data were extracted (e. g., study size, PICOS, follow-up period) and provide the citations.	
Risk of bias within studies	19	Present data on risk of bias of each study and, if available, any outcome-level assessment (see item 12).	
Results of individual studies	20	For all outcomes considered (benefits or harms), present, for each study: (a) simple summary data for each intervention group and (b) effect estimates and confidence intervals, ideally with a forest plot.	

Continued ▶

Table 30.1 Continued

Section/topic	Item no.	Checklist item	Reported on page no.
Synthesis of results	21	Present results of each meta-analysis done, including confidence intervals and measures of consistency.	
Risk of bias across studies	22	Present results of any assessment of risk of bias across studies (see item 15).	
Additional analysis	23	Give results of additional analyses, if done [e. g., sensitivity or subgroup analyses, meta-regression (see item 16)].	
Discussion			
Summary of evidence	24	Summarize the main findings including the strength of evidence for each main outcome; consider their relevance to key groups (e. g., health care providers, users, and policy makers).	
Limitations	25	Discuss limitations at study and outcome level (e. g., risk of bias), and at review level (e. g., incomplete retrieval of identified research, reporting bias).	
Conclusions	26	Provide a general interpretation of the results in the context of other evidence, and implications for future research.	
Funding			
Funding	27	Describe sources of funding for the systematic review and other support (e. g., supply of data); role of funders for the systematic review.	

Reproduced with permission from Liberati et al.[11]

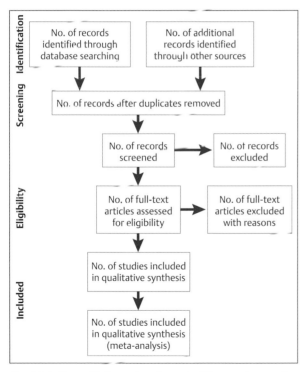

Fig. 30.1 Flow of information through different phases of a meta-analysis. Reproduced with permission from Liberati et al.[11]

MOOSE (Meta-analysis of Observational Studies in Epidemiology)

The MOOSE checklist was created as a reference for authors of meta-analyses using data obtained from observational studies.[9] Although RCTs provide the best evidence regarding an intervention or treatment, they are not always feasible or ethical.[1] In these cases meta-analyses of observational studies can be performed, but the author must take some important factors into consideration in order to optimize the reliability of the results. Observational studies often vary widely in terms of study design, causing a greater amount of heterogeneity than is encountered with RCTs. Increased heterogeneity also occurs between observational studies with respect to populations and outcomes.[9] It has also been reported that observational studies are more prone to confounding and selection bias than RCTs.[16] Thus, as a result of bias and heterogeneity, meta-analyses of observational studies are more challenging to design and interpret.[9]

Key Concepts: Observational Studies
Observational studies that can be used in meta-analyses include cross-sectional studies, case series, case–control design, cohort studies, and studies with historical controls.[9]

Key Concepts: Bias
Bias within a study may take on many forms including selection bias, performance bias, detection bias, and attrition bias.[17] Bias across studies includes publication bias and selective reporting within studies.[8]

Jargon Simplified: Heterogeneity

Heterogeneity means differences among the individual studies that are included in a systematic review; it may refer to study results or to the study characteristics.[18]

Key Concepts: Heterogeneity

Clinical heterogeneity results from differences between individual studies: location, age, sex, severity of disease, dose/intensity of intervention, definition of outcomes.
Methodological heterogeneity results from differences in how individual studies were conducted: study type, methods of analysis, study quality.

The MOOSE checklist includes 35 items, organized in a similar way to the PRISMA checklist, that simplify and improve meta-analysis design. The MOOSE and PRISMA checklists contain many items that are identical or similar, along with a few that are unique to each (**Table 30.2**). The MOOSE checklist provides in-depth guidelines for reporting of search strategy, reflecting the importance of a full description of this step of a meta-analysis.

Examples from the Literature:
Example of Search Strategy Reporting[19]
Source: Hu S, Zhang ZY, Hua YQ, Li J, Cai ZD. A comparison of regional and general anaesthesia for total replacement of the hip or knee: a meta-analysis. J Bone Joint Surg 2009;91-B:935–942
"A search of the literature was undertaken using PubMed (1966 to April 2008), EMBASE (1969 to April 2008), and the Cochrane Library databases using the following keywords: hip replacement, hip arthroplasty, knee replacement, knee arthroplasty, regional anaesthesia, epidural anaesthesia, spinal anaesthesia and general anaesthesia. The terms regional, epidural, spinal, and general anaesthesia were linked with 'or' and combined using 'and' with each subsequent term."

The Methods section of the checklist includes items relevant to data coding, assessment of confounding and heterogeneity, and a description of all statistical methods. Assessment of heterogeneity is particularly important as the degree of heterogeneity will determine whether statistical pooling of data should be attempted, and what types of summary measures are appropriate.[9] The checklist contains several items that emphasize the importance of eval-

Table 30.2 Items included in the PRISMA and MOOSE checklists

Checklist items	PRISMA	MOOSE
Title and abstract		
Title identifies the report as a meta-analysis	√	
Structured abstract	√	
Introduction		
Reference to participants, interventions, study outcomes, and design	√	√
Rationale for the review	√	
Problem definition and hypothesis statement		√
Methods and search strategy		
Description of all information sources and presentation of the search strategy	√	√
Method of study selection and data extraction and coding	√	√
Qualifications of searchers		√
Use of hand searching reported		√
Method of addressing foreign-language articles and unpublished studies		√
Assessment of bias, confounding, study quality, and heterogeneity	√	√
Description of statistical methods and analyses (e. g., sensitivity testing)	√	√
Indication of where a review protocol can be accessed	√	
Statement of summary measures (e. g., risk ratio)	√	
Provision of appropriate graphs and tables		√
Results, discussion, and conclusions		
Description of study selection and characteristics for which data were extracted	√	
Justification for exclusion of studies		
Quantitative assessment of bias within and across studies	√	√
Results of individual studies included	√	√
Synthesis of results	√	√
Discussion of study limitations	√	√
Generalization of conclusions and guidelines for future research	√	
Consideration of alternate explanations for study results		√
Sources of funding	√	√

Table 30.3 The MOOSE checklist

Reporting of background should include:	• Problem definition • Hypothesis statement • Description of study outcome(s) • Type of exposure or intervention used • Type of study designs used • Study population
Reporting of search strategy should include:	• Qualifications of searchers (e. g., librarians and investigators) • Search strategy, including time period included in the synthesis and keywords • Effort to include all available studies, including contact with authors • Databases and registries searched • Search software used, name and version, including special features used (e. g., explosion) • Use of hand searching (e. g., reference lists of obtained articles) • List of citations located and those excluded, including justification • Method of addressing articles published in languages other than English • Method of handling abstracts and unpublished studies • Description of any contact with authors
Reporting of methods should include:	• Description of relevance or appropriateness of studies assembled for assessing the hypothesis to be tested • Rationale for the selection and coding of data (e. g., sound clinical principles or convenience) • Documentation of how data were classified and coded (e. g., multiple raters, blinding, and inter-rater reliability) • Assessment of confounding (e. g., comparability of cases and controls in studies where appropriate) • Assessment of study quality, including blinding or quality assessors; stratification or regression on possible predictors of study results • Assessment of heterogeneity • Description of statistical methods (e. g., complete description of fixed- or random-effects models, justification of whether the chosen models account for predictors of study results, dose–response models, or cumulative meta-analysis) in sufficient detail to be replicated • Provision of appropriate tables and graphics
Reporting of results should include:	• Graphic summarizing individual study estimates and overall estimate • Table giving descriptive information for each study included • Results of sensitivity testing (e. g., subgroup analysis) • Indication of statistical uncertainty of findings
Reporting of discussion should include:	• Quantitative assessment of bias (e. q., publication bias) • Justification for exclusion (e. g., exclusion of non-English-language citations) • Assessment of quality of included studies
Reporting of conclusions should include:	• Consideration of alternative explanations for observed results • Generalization of the conclusions (i. e., appropriate for the data presented and within the domain of the literature review) • Guidelines for future research • Disclosure of funding source

uating the quality of the primary article. Also included is a quantitative assessment and discussion of potential sources of bias using recommended methods such as funnel plots (publication bias). Finally, the MOOSE checklist recommends a discussion of possible alternative explanations for the results, and appropriate generalizations of the conclusions. For the full checklist refer to **Table 30.3**.

Conclusion

Meta-analysis reporting checklists improve the quality of the methodology and reporting of meta-analyses. The PRISMA checklist for systematic reviews and meta-analyses of RCTs and the MOOSE checklist for meta-analyses of observational studies are important reference tools both for authors of meta-analyses and for readers evaluating their quality.

Suggested Reading

Liberati A, Altman DG, Tetzlaff J, et al. The PRISMA statement for reporting systematic reviews and meta-analyses of studies that evaluate health care interventions: explanation and elaboration. Ann Intern Med 2009;151:W65–W94

Riley RD, Lambert PC, Abo-Zaid G. Meta-analysis of individual participant data: rationale, conduct, and reporting. BMJ 2010;340:521–525

Stroup DF, Berlin JA, Morton SC, et al. Meta-analysis of observational studies in epidemiology: a proposal for reporting. JAMA 2000;283:2008–2012

References

1. Bhandari M, Morrow F, Kulkarni AV, Tornetta P 3rd. Meta-analyses in orthopaedic surgery: a systematic review of their methodologies. J Bone Joint Surg 2001;83:15–24
2. Bhandari M, Devereaux PJ, Montori V, Cinà C, Tandan V, Guyatt GH. User's guide to the surgical literature: how to use a systematic literature review and meta-analysis. Can J Surg 2004;47;60–67
3. Gerber S, Tallon D, Trelle S, Schneider M, Jüni P, Egger M. Bibliographic study showed improving methodology of meta-analyses published in leading journals 1993–2002. J Clin Epidemiol 2007;60:773–780
4. Oxman AD, Guyatt GH. Validation of an index of the quality of review articles. J Clin Epidemiol 1991;44:1271–1278
5. Oxman AD, Guyatt GH, Singer J, et al. Agreement among reviewers of review articles. J Clin Epidemiol 1991;44:91–98
6. Dijkman BG, Abouali JAK, Kooistra BW, et al. Twenty years of meta-analyses in orthopaedic surgery: has quality kept up with quantity? J Bone Joint Surg Am 2010;92:48–57
7. Equator network. Guidelines for reporting systematic reviews and meta-analyses. 2010. Available at: http://www.equator-network.org. Retrieved 19 May 2010
8. Moher D, Liberati A, Tetzlaff J, Altman DG; The PRISMA Group. Preferred reporting items for systematic reviews and meta-analyses: the PRISMA statement. PLoS Medicine 2009;6:1–6
9. Stroup DF, Berlin JA, Morton SC et al. Meta-analysis of observational studies in epidemiology: a proposal for reporting. JAMA 2000;283:2008–2012
10. Riley RD, Lambert PC, Abo-Zaid G. Meta-analysis of individual participant data: rationale, conduct, and reporting. BMJ 2010;340:521–525
11. Liberati A, Altman DG, Tetzlaff J, et al. The PRISMA statement for reporting systematic reviews and meta-analyses of studies that evaluate health care interventions: explanation and elaboration. PLoS Medicine 2009; 6(7): e1000100
12. Moher D, Cook DJ, Eastwood S, Olkin I, Rennie D, Stroup DF. Improving the quality of reports of meta-analyses of randomised controlled trails: the QUOROM statement. Lancet 1999;354:1896–1900
13. Egger M, Davey Smith G, Altman DG. Systematic Reviews in Health Care: Meta-Analysis in Context. 2nd ed. London: BMJ Publishing Group; 2001:88,468
14. Kuzyk PRT, Guy P, Kreder HJ, Zdero R, KcKee MD, Schemitsch EH. Minimally invasive hip fracture surgery: are outcomes better? J Orthop Trauma 2009;23:447–453
15. Mason JB, Fehring TK, Estok R, Banel D, Fahrbach K. Meta-analysis of alignment outcomes in computer assisted total knee arthroplasty surgery. J Arthroplasty 2007;22:1097–1106
16. Egger M, Schneider M, Davey Smith G. Spurious precision? meta-analysis of observational studies. BMJ 1998;316:140–144
17. Egger M, Davey Smith G, Altman DG. Systematic Reviews in Health Care: Meta-Analysis in Context. 2nd ed. London: BMJ Publishing Group; 2001:46
18. Guyatt GH, Rennie D, Meade M, Cook D, eds. Users' Guide to the Medical Literature: A Manual for Evidence-Based Clinical Practice. 2nd ed. New York: McGraw-Hill; 2008
19. Hu S, Zhang ZY, Hua YQ, Li J, Cai ZD. A comparison of regional and general anaesthesia for total replacement of the hip or knee: a meta-analysis. J Bone Joint Surg 2009;91-B:935–942

Resources and Contacts for Surgical Research

Meaghan Zehr, Sheila Sprague, Christopher Vannabouathong

Summary

There are multiple educational and supportive resources available for surgical researchers. These resources include mentorship, graduate studies, online course work, textbooks, journal articles, and contract research organizations. This chapter discusses the role of each of these resources, as well as their respective merits and disadvantages.

Introduction

Health care practitioners interested in conducting clinical research may be unaware of what educational and supportive resources are available to them and whether such resources will suit their research needs. Having formal training and adequate support can enhance any research initiative. Educational and supportive opportunities in clinical research exist in the form of mentorships, academia, online courses, literature, workshops, and contract research organizations.

Mentorship

In the health care field, practitioners can take responsibility for teaching, supporting, and assessing the performance of students through mentoring.[1] A mentorship is a valuable resource for individuals pursuing their own research endeavors. Steiner et al. found that students who participated in an ongoing mentorship program reported that they were better prepared for future careers, devoted more time to research, and enjoyed greater research productivity.[2] Selecting an ideal mentor can be a challenging process and some students have reported that their mentors were not easily accessible, that their research ideas were stolen by their mentor, and that they perceived competition with their mentor.[3] In most situations, however, good mentors can provide valuable guidance concerning issues that may not be intuitively understandable to new researchers, and they may also be able to provide guidance on how to find a balance between work and leisure.[3]

When searching for a mentor, some character traits in particular should be regarded as desirable. These include seniority, approachability, accessibility, altruism, understanding, patience, honesty, respect, and open communi-cation.[3] When selecting a mentor, it is helpful to vocalize expectations and ask what expectations the potential mentor may have.[4] If those expectations are in harmony with those of the student, the student should consider devising a research plan, which can represent a written commitment from both the student and mentor.[4]

Key Concepts: Selecting a Mentor
The ideal mentor will exhibit:
- Seniority
- Approachability
- Accessibility
- Altruism
- Understanding
- Patience
- Honesty
- Respect
- Open communication
- Mentors and mentees should have similar expectations for the relationship.

Key Concepts: Pros and Cons of Mentorship
Advantages:
- Better prepared for future career
- Devote more time to research
- Enjoy greater research productivity

Disadvantages:
- May be inaccessible
- Claims of stolen research
- Claims of competition

Graduate Programs

Many academic institutions have graduate programs that focus on teaching the principles of clinical research methodology and epidemiology. Graduate programs teach specific skills from experts in the field of health science, such as research design, research ethics, measurement techniques, statistical methods, and observational and analytical techniques. Graduate study programs are very in-depth and specialized. They provide students with an extensive knowledge base of current health and research trends and prepare students for careers in research by providing opportunities to practice these concepts.

Advantages of graduate studies include the ability to interact with peers and field experts, to practice and apply concepts, and to widen career opportunities. Possible limitations include the obligation of relocating to a university campus, rigid schedule and time demands, and enrollment costs.

An example of a graduate program offered to students interested in research is the multidisciplinary Health Research Methodology program at McMaster University, with topics of study that include research synthesis and design, selection and development of measurement tools, data gathering analysis and interpretation, communication of research results, and knowledge translation.[5] The Medical Sciences program featured at Harvard University is another option for students wishing to pursue careers in research or teaching.[6] This program covers a broad array of subjects in the biomedical science field.[6] Some of the subjects include biostatistics, health economics, health policy analysis, health services research, geography, psychology, sociology, anthropology, and political science.[5]

Key Concepts: Pros and Cons of Graduate Programs
Advantages:
- Specialized, in-depth knowledge base
- Interaction with peers and field experts
- Opportunities for the practice and application of concepts
- Increased career opportunities

Disadvantages:
- Rigid schedule
- Enrollment costs

Online Courses

Online courses or distance education are excellent choices for aspiring researchers with a busy schedule, limited budget, and who are strongly self-motivated. Unlike traditional face-to-face lectures, communication through online courses occurs through various media such as email, bulletin boards, chat rooms, and instant messengers.[7] Lectures can be available through web conferences, word files, teleconferences, bulletin boards, text chat, streaming audio, and film lectures.[7] Because online course work can be completed at the student's discretion and is not confined to a rigid schedule, students can maintain regular full-time work, thereby maintaining a steady income. Students can also avoid relocating, which can incur a significant financial burden. However, because users are not able to communicate face to face, communication may be misinterpreted or infrequent. Also, not every subject of interest is available through distance education. Students may need to be proactive in finding an accredited and relevant program. In addition to possessing basic computer skills, students must also have working access to a high-speed internet connection and computer.

Reality Check: Available Online Courses
The National Institutes of Health offer online training to the general population as well as health care professionals. This training provides a broad overview to define clinical trials and explore their role in the health care community. To register, visit
http://www.nihtraining.com/crtpub_508/index.html.
The National Cancer Institute provides online training to healthcare professionals who are interested in becoming clinical trials investigators, including topics such as patient enrollment, funding, ethics approval, and quality assurance procedures. To register, visit
http://www.cancer.gov/clinicaltrialscourse.
The Medical Research Management organization offers almost 20 online courses designed to expand upon basic principles of good clinical practice and conducting clinical research. To register, visit
http://www.cra-training.com/e-learnings/course-library/default.asp.
The Norton Training Institute offers expert training on good clinical practice to prepare clinical investigative teams to meet requirements and recommendations. To register, visit
http://nortoninstitute.coursehost.com/engine/Academic/Tools/CoursePublicize.asp?
pk=27542&LID=2&ky=d_BPDiQVRgHzDiPRUmf_DgHzJ47OL3vz.

Key Concepts: Pros and Cons of Online Courses
Advantages:
- Flexible schedule
- Can maintain regular full-time work

Disadvantages:
- Potential for communication problems
- Limited topic selection

Textbooks and Journals

Textbooks and journals are excellent resources to better understand the concepts behind health research methodology and statistical methods. While textbooks can provide in-depth knowledge on a topic, readers are cautioned that during the time since the textbook was published, the material may have become outdated.[8] Journal articles are often easily accessible and current, and provide recent information on different aspects of research methodology. Examples of journals devoted to research methodology and clinical trials include *Contemporary Clinical Trials, Controlled Clinical Trials, Journal of Clinical Epidemiology, Trials,* and *Statistical Methods in Medical Research.* Medical and surgical journals may also publish articles or even devote an entire supplement to a methodological issue. For example, the *Journal of Bone and Joint Surgery* (American volume) recently published a supplement devoted to observational research in orthopaedics.[9]

Examples from the Literature
Textbooks
- Bhandari M, Joensson A, eds. Clinical Research for Surgeons. Stuttgart: Thieme; 2009
- Emanuel E et al. The Oxford Textbook of Clinical Research Ethics. New York: Oxford University Press; 2008
- Gallin J, Ognibene F, eds. Principles and Practice of Clinical Research. New York: Academic Press; 2002
- Hulley S, et al. Designing Clinical Research. 3rd ed. Philadephia: Lippincott, Williams and Wilkins; 2007

Journals Devoted to Research Methodology
- *Contemporary Clinical Trials*
- *Controlled Clinical Trials*
- *Journal of Clinical Epidemiology*
- *Trials*
- *Statistical Methods in Medical Research*

Journal Articles on Research Methodology
- Bhandari M, Giannoudis PV. Evidence-based medicine: what it is and what it is not. Injury, International Journal of the Care of the Injured. 2006;37:302–306
- Bhandari M, Pape HC, Giannoudis PV. Issues in the planning and conduct of randomised trials. Injury 2006;37:349–354
- Farrokhyar F, Karanicolas PJ, Thoma A, et al. Randomized controlled trials of surgical interventions. Ann Surg 2010;251:40
- Cook JA. The challenges faced in the design, conduct and analysis of surgical randomised controlled trials. Trials 2009;10:9
- Devereaux PJ, McKee MD, Yusuf S. Methodologic issues in randomized controlled trials of surgical interventions. Clin Orthop Relat Res 2003;413:25–32
- Chung KC, Burns PB. A guide to planning and executing a surgical randomized controlled trial. J Hand Surg Am 2008;33:407–412

Textbooks and journal articles provide information on current clinical research methodologies at a relatively low cost. The journal subscription fee may even be covered by a researcher's university affiliation. Readers must avoid misinterpreting the author's findings and conclusions. Another potential limitation of textbooks and journals is the lack of opportunity to pose questions to experts. Although an author's contact information (mailing or email address) may be provided, communication is often very limited (author may not respond or respond infrequently).

Key Concepts: Pros and Cons of Textbooks and Journal Articles
Advantages:
- Provide current information on clinical research methodologies
- Subscription fees may be covered by university affiliations

Disadvantages:
- No interaction opportunities
- Quality of data may be variable

Courses and Workshops

There are numerous courses and workshops offered to surgical researchers. It is important to consider different options before committing to a course to ensure that it meets your current needs. Workshops are ideal for researchers with time or budget constraints and who prefer face-to-face communication.

It is important to consider the costs of attending courses, including registration fees, travel costs, and the cost of being away from a busy clinical practice. Registration fees tend to reflect the length of time of the course and may include costs such as meals, lecture hall, coordinator fees, lecturer time, parking, and hotel room. Researchers must also consider travel costs, which can be considerable depending on the location of the workshop.

As workshops and courses often offer a large volume of information in a very short time, attendees may feel overwhelmed. Workshops and courses can be fast-paced, not allowing time for participants to take notes and discuss their questions with the instructors. Also, some workshop and course presentations show movie clips, audio, pictures, charts, and graphs. These can be difficult to analyze and interpret during the limited time constraints.

Another important aspect to consider is whether the course or workshop has received continuing medical education (CME) accreditation; this can be confirmed by contacting the course's coordinator.

Key Concepts: Pros and Cons of Workshops
Advantages:
- Short duration
- Low cost
- Opportunities to interact with experts and colleagues
- Receive continuing medical education (CME) credit

Disadvantages:
- Potential to be overwhelmed

Some examples of such courses include the "Principles and Practice of Clinical Research" course and the "How to Teach Evidence-Based Medicine" workshop. The "Principles and Practice of Clinical Research" course is a 2-day, intensive course focusing on surgical research methodology.[10] This course is designed to educate surgeons, surgical trainees, and allied health care professionals on the principles of evidence-based medicine and research methodology. The course's co-founders (Dr. Mohit Bhandari and Dr. Emil Schemitsch) are world-renowned orthopaedic surgeons and researchers, and the course's faculty is comprised of other surgical and clinical experts. The "Principles and Practice of Clinical Research" course was designed to provide participants with a solid foundation in the principles of health research methodology specific to the field of surgery. In order to evaluate the transfer of knowledge, the participants completed a preconference and a postconference test. The results showed a significant improvement in overall participant knowledge about evidence-based medicine and clinical research methods.[11]

The "Evidence-Based Clinical Practice" workshop, chaired by Dr. Gordon Guyatt at McMaster University, focuses on the principles of teaching evidence-based medicine.[12] This course is designed for researchers who are interested in communicating the concepts of evidence-based clinical decision-making to their students. Learning objectives include how to help your quality teams, local policymakers, clinicians, and students interpret the results of comparative effectiveness research and how this understanding can help them translate these results into practice.

Examples from the Literature
Courses and Workshops
- "Principles and Practice of Clinical Research" (www.cmecourses.ca)
- "How to Teach Evidence-Based Medicine" (http://ebm.mcmaster.ca/)
- "Teaching and Leading EBM" (http://www.mclibrary.duke.edu/training/courses/ebmworkshop)
- Global Educator (http://grsolutions.ca)

Contract Research Organizations

Contract research organizations (CROs) are companies who are contracted to help coordinate clinical trials. They are typically contracted by pharmaceutical companies; however, they may also be contracted by individual researchers to help plan, manage, and conduct clinical trials. CROs will ensure the study meets the ethical regulatory requirements of local health care communities. The primary advantage of employing a CRO is the quality assurance, and the primary limitation is often the high start-up cost.[13] The responsibilities of a CRO can vary depending on the needs of the researcher. The CRO can be contracted as a full service provider, where it assumes responsibility for all aspects of a trial.[14] Another role the CRO can assume is a functional provider, where the CRO takes responsibility for only one area of the trial, such as randomization or adjudication

of outcomes.[14] Another possibility is for the investigator to manage one area of the trial, leaving the remainder of the trial to the CRO's direction; this arrangement is referred to as single area outsourcing.[14]

Global Research Solutions (GRS)(http://grsolutions.ca) is an example of a full service CRO, which provides practical research and education support to the medical community. GRS specializes in orthopaedic surgical trials with an expertise in outcomes adjudication using a web-based adjudication system, the Global Adjudicator. GRS also offers clinical trial management, committee management, and image management services. In addition to acting as a CRO, GRS is responsible for developing the Global Educator platform, which offers courses and seminars in the fields of clinical research methodology and techniques in surgery.[15] It is in this capacity that CROs are capable of providing an educational service to young researchers.

Key Concepts:
Contract Research Organization Responsibilities
- Protocol development[16]
- Randomization[16]
- Patient enrollment and follow-up[16]
- Monitoring[16]
- Laboratory services[16]
- Data management[16]
- Outcomes adjudication
- Biostatistics[16]
- Consulting services associated with Government agencies (ethics approval)[16]

Key Concepts: Questions to Ask When Evaluating a Contract Research Organization
- Is it likely I can form a solid partnership with this CRO?[14]
- Is it in the financial interest of this CRO to expend more labor rather than less to complete this project?[14]
- Does it cost more to do a study through this particular CRO?[14]
- What has been the source of communication breakdowns in projects conducted by this CRO in the past?[14]
- Is this CRO more concerned with obtaining the next contract or with performing well on the current project?[14]
- Does this CRO have expertise in my field of study?[17]
- Does this CRO have comprehensive standard operating procedures in place?[17]
- Does this CRO maintain and calibrate its laboratory equipment appropriately?[17]
- How much time does this CRO typically require to implement a study from the time the protocol is approved?[17]
- How much time does this CRO typically require to finalize reports from the time of study completion?[17]
- Does this CRO have good customer service?[17]
- Does this CRO have a reputation for quality?[17]

- Does this CRO have the capacity to address global projects?[14]

Key Concepts: Pros and Cons of Contract Research Organizations
Advantages:
- High-quality results[11,12]
- Experience in patient enrollment and follow-up[12]
- Commercialization insight[12]

Disadvantages:
- High start-up cost

Conclusion

In conclusion, there are many resources available for researchers that can help prepare them for conducting clinical trials by expanding their knowledge base and teaching them the specific skills suited to the field. It is important for researchers to carefully consider the advantages and disadvantages of each available resource and ensure that they select the resources that are most beneficial to their learning objectives and their career aspirations.

Suggested Reading

Bhandari M, Sancheti P, eds. Clinical research made easy: a guide to publishing in medical literature. New Delhi, India: Jaypee Brothers Medical Publishers; 2010

Straus SF, Chatur F, Taylor M. Issues in the mentor-mentee relationship in academic medicine: a qualitative study. Acad Med 2009;84:135–139

Principles and Practice of Clinical Research. Available at http://www.cmecourses.ca/. Accessed on April 16, 2010.

References

1. Marshall M, Gordon F. Exploring the role of the interprofessional mentor. J Interprofessional Care 2010; 24(4):362–374
2. Steiner JF, Curtis P, Lanphear BP, Vu KO, Main DS. Assessing the role of influential mentors in the research development of primary care fellows. Acad Med 2004;79:865–872
3. Straus SE, Chatur F, Taylor M. Issues in the mentor–mentee relationship in academic medicine: a qualitative study. Acad Med 2009;84:135–139
4. K Kjeldsen. A proficient mentor is a must when starting up with research. Exp Clin Cardiol 2006;11:243–245
5. McMaster University. Available at http://www.fhs.mcmaster.ca/hrm/phd_program.html. Accessed online on April 12, 2010
6. Harvard University. Available at http://www.gsas.harvard.edu/programs_of_study/division_of_medical_sciences_at_harvard_medical_school_dms.php . Accessed on April 13, 2010
7. Kuther T. What is an online graduate class like? Available at http://gradschool.about.com/od/distanceeducation/f/OnlineGradPrgrm.htm. Accessed on April 14, 2010
8. Bhandari M, Sancheti P, eds. Clinical research made easy: a guide to publishing in medical literature. New Delhi, India: Jaypee Brothers Medical Publishers; 2010
9. Bhandari M, Morshed S, Tornetta P, Schemitsch E. Design, conduct, and interpretation of nonrandomized orthopaedic studies—a practical approach. J Bone Joint Surg Am 2009;91(Suppl 3):1
10. Principles and Practice of Clinical Research 2010. Available at http://www.cmecourses.ca/. Accessed on April 16, 2010
11. Sprague S, Pozdniakova P, Kaempffer E, et al. The Principles and Practice of Clinical Research Course for Surgeons: An Evaluation of Knowledge Transfer and Perceptions. Can J Surg 2012; 55(1):46–52
12. McMaster University. How to teach evidence-based clinical practice workshop. Available at http://ebm.mcmaster.ca/. Accessed on April 14, 2010
13. Barnes K. Bigger is better, reveals CRO survey. Available at http://www.drugresearcher.com/Research-management/Bigger-is-better-reveals-CRO-survey. Accessed on April 26, 2010
14. Glass HE, Beaudry DP. Study reveals how sponsors rate their own outsourcing abilities compared to other companies. Available at http://appliedclinicaltrialsonline.findpharma.com/appliedclinicaltrials/Project+Management/CRO-Selection-amp-Management/ArticleStandard/Article/detail/591994. Accessed on April 26, 2010
15. Global Research Solutions [cited 2010 May 24]. Available from: http://grsolutions.ca
16. The line between CRO and sponsor responsibilities. Available at http://www.pharmaceutical-int.com/article/the-line-between-cro-and-sponsor-responsibilities.html. Accessed on April 26, 2010
17. A guideline to outsourcing. Available at http://www.mdbiosciences.com/outsourcing/. Accessed on January 28, 2012

Glossary of Terms

Academic stream
The authorship context in which journal articles and abstracts are written by experts for other experts in the field.

Adjudication
Determination of an outcome by an independent person or group of individuals who are not otherwise involved in the study.

Adjudication committee
A group of clinical experts who determine endpoint assessment in a standardized and unbiased manner.[2]

Adverse event
An adverse event is "any untoward medical occurrence in a research participant which does not necessarily have a causal relationship with the treatment."[3] Serious adverse events result in death, are life threatening, require inpatient hospitalization, or result in persistent or significant disability or incapacity, or birth defect. Adverse events which are nonserious do not meet any of these criteria.[3]

Alternative hypothesis
The alternative hypothesis assumes that a significant difference does exist between two groups.

Applicability
Usefulness in clinical practice.

Author
The creator, developer, or promoter of an idea, product, or service.

b or beta (*β*)
Both *b* and beta (*β*) usually refer to regression coefficients from a regression model. In the case of a linear regression, the regression coefficient for a particular covariate describes the unit increase in the outcome variable that occurs when that covariate increases by one unit. In logistic regression and proportional hazards regression the regression coefficients represent log odds ratios and log hazard ratios respectively, and should usually be exponentiated in order to report the odds ratio or hazards ratio in the text.

Bias
Any trend in the collection, analysis, or interpretation of data that can lead to conclusions that are systematically different from the truth.

Binary outcome
An outcome for which there are two mutually exclusive possibilities.

Blind (or blinded or masked)
Patients, clinicians, data collectors, outcome adjudicators, or data analysts unaware of which patients have been assigned to the experimental and which to the control group. In the case of diagnostic tests, those interpreting the test results are unaware of the result of the reference standard or vice versa.[4]

Block randomization
A technique to ensure equal distribution of study subjects across treatment groups over time. Blocks of either varying (most common) or equal sizes are created such that each block contains an equal number of treatment and control (or treatment A and treatment B) allocations. The order of treatment allocation within each block is random, and the order of blocks, once they have been created, is also random.

Central methods center
A central methods center can be a private contract research organization or it can be under the direction of the nominated principal investigator. It is responsible for the day-to-day activities of managing a clinical trial, which includes protocol development, maintaining a centralized randomization system, data management, organization of trial committees, and communication with the clinical centers participating in the study.[5]

Clinical bias
Clinical bias can occur when the decision about when an outcome has occurred is left to the clinician's discretion (e.g., deciding when to readmit patients to hospital or perform additional surgical procedures). Reported study outcomes may then be biased, as clinical decisions by clinicians may not directly relate to the intervention, but rather to clinical preferences instead.

Closed-ended questions
Questions that offer fixed answers that cannot be altered by the respondent.[6]

Coding
The process of assigning labels, called "codes," to data (such as interview phrases or passages) as a means of categorizing concepts and themes that emerge through the qualitative analysis.[7,8]

Composite outcome (or end point)

A composite outcome (or end point) consists of a combination of multiple selected outcomes that are counted and reported as a single "composite" outcome.

Conditional logistic regression

Conditional logistic regression is a type of logistic regression used when there is one or more matched control for each case.

Conflict of interest

"A conflict of interest is a set of circumstances that creates a *risk* that professional judgment or actions regarding a primary interest will be unduly influenced by a secondary interest."[9]

Confounder
(or confounding variable or confounding)

A factor that is associated with the outcome of interest and is differentially distributed in patients exposed and unexposed to the outcome of interest.[4]

Consecutive sample

One of the most common forms of sampling in the orthopaedic literature, a consecutive group including evenly available subjects is selected such that the entire accessible population is studied. The benefit of using this type of a comprehensive sample is that a good representation of the overall population is possible over a reasonable period of time.

CONSORT
(Consolidated Standards of Reporting Trials)

The CONSORT group has articulated various widely accepted standards for the reporting of clinical trials. The CONSORT statement can be found at http://www.consort-statement.org/.

Construct validity

A construct is a theoretically derived notion of the domain(s) we wish to measure. An understanding of the construct will lead to expectations about how an instrument should behave if it is valid. Construct validity therefore involves comparisons between measures, and examination of the logical relationships which should exist between a measure and characteristics of patients and patient groups.[6]

Contamination

Contamination occurs when the control group gets the experimental treatment.

Content validity

In relation to the health-related measures, validity represents the extent to which an instrument is measuring what it is intended to measure.[6]

Convenience sample

Subjects are selected because they are easily accessible to the researcher. This technique is easy, fast, and usually the most logistically feasible method.

Cost–effectiveness ratio

The cost–effectiveness ratio is the ratio of additional costs required to achieve a defined better medical outcome for the patient, e.g., "additional fracture healed."

Crossover

In a crossover, a patient does not receive the intervention to which he or she was randomized but instead receives the other intervention.

Data management

Data management is the list of things one does for data entry into a database, data cleaning, and file construction in preparation for statistical analysis.

Data monitoring committee / Data and safety monitoring board (DSMB)

The primary role of the DSMB is to ensure the safety of the study participants by reviewing interim reports for evidence of adverse or beneficial treatment effects. The DSMB also makes decisions regarding the frequency, timing, and manner in which interim data are analyzed.[10,11]

Deduction

Using data to make conclusions about a predetermined theory or hypothesis; this is the intent of quantitative research[7]

Dependent variable (or Outcome variable, or Target variable)

The target variable of interest; the variable that is hypothesized to depend on or be caused by another variable, the independent variable.[4]

Diagnostic suspicion bias

A subject's medical history may influence the intensity of diagnostic procedures.[1]

Differential expertise bias

A systematic effect on the results of a study caused by an imbalance in the proportion of clinicians with expertise in one procedure over the other.

Dummy variables

A categorical variable that has been recoded into one or more numeric variables (taking values 0 or 1) to allow incorporation into a regression equation.

Educational stream

The authorship context in which textbooks and course notebooks are written by experts for students and young researchers.

Effect size

An easily interpretable value specifying the direction and magnitude of a treatment effect.

End point

An event or outcome that can be measured objectively to determine whether the intervention being studied is beneficial.

Equipoise

Equipoise refers to genuinely not knowing if one treatment is better than another; otherwise ethics forces the physician to prescribe the superior treatment.[12]

Ethnography

A qualitative methodology that seeks to understand patterns, beliefs, and behaviors of a group within a social context, such as a culture or team, through observation and interaction.[7]

Evidence-based medicine

Heath care policies and practices that are derived from the systematic, scientific study of the effectiveness of various treatments.

Exposure suspicion bias

A subject's disease state may influence how vigorously the investigator searches for an exposure.[1]

External validity

The degree to which the results of a study can be generalized beyond the sample studied.

Factorial RCT

A randomized controlled trial (RCT) design whereby two or more study questions are answered at the same time within the same group of study subjects without the need for increased sample size (in the absence of interactions between the study question interventions).

Failure function

The probability of not surviving; also used to refer to experiencing the event within some specified time. The failure curve is a representation of the failure function, starting at 0% and going up to the proportion of subjects experiencing the event within the period of observation.

Family information bias

A subject in a case group with an exposure or outcome of interest may receive family information that differs from that of a subject in a control group.[1]

Fixed-effects analysis

A method of pooling or meta-regression that assumes that all the variability in effect sizes among studies has been accounted for.

Fixed-effects regression

Fixed-effects regression assumes that there is one overall true effect and that each individual study is an estimate of that true effect that varies from the true effect by chance alone. The underlying assumption is that all studies are identical replications from the same population of patients, interventions, and outcome measures.

Forest plots

A graphical diagram depicting the relative strength of treatment effects in multiple studies with minimal heterogeneity.[13–15]

Funnel plots

A graphical diagram displaying the treatment effect against a measure of study size that is used to identify publication bias in a meta-analysis.[13–15]

Grounded theory

A qualitative methodology that uses data from interviews and observations to "ground" the development of a theory; this is an iterative process involving the continuous cycle of data collection and analysis.[7,16,17]

Hazard function

Represents a probability divided by the time. It represents the probability of experiencing an event in the next time interval, given that it was not experienced previously. The hazard is often simply interpreted as a conditional probability. The hazard function is used for analytical purposes, such as for comparing subject groups with regard to their survival experience and quantifying the effect of prognostic factors.

Hazard ratio

The ratio of two hazards (i.e., the hazard of experiencing the event in the intervention group at a given point in time over the hazard of experiencing the event in the control group at the same time point). This ratio is interpreted similarly to risk ratios. A hazard ratio (HR) of one means that there is no effect associated with the predictor variable under investigation, hence events occur at the same pace in both groups. When the predictor reduces the probability of occurrence of the event, the HR is less than one; when the factor is associated with an increase of risk, the HR is greater than one.

Heterogeneity

Differences among individual studies included in a systematic review, typically referring to study results; the term can also be applied to other study characteristics.[4]

Hypothesis
A tentative explanation for an observation, phenomenon, or scientific problem that can be tested by further investigation; e.g., what question was the trial designed to answer?

I^2
A measure of heterogeneity. Specifically, the I^2 measures the proportion of variability in the observed effect sizes that is due to variability between studies.

Incident cases
"New occurrences of a condition (or disease) in a population over a period of time. Incidence refers to the number of new cases of disease occurring during a specified period of time; expressed as a percentage of the number of people at risk."[18,19]

Independent variable (or Predictor, or Covariate)
These all mean the same thing, that is, the patient factors whose association with the outcome is modeled in the regression.

Induction
Using data, observations, or interactions to generate a theory or hypothesis; this process is inherent to qualitative research.[7]

Industrial stream
The authorship context in which technical reports, user manuals, product catalogs, and marketing brochures are written by experts for potential users or customers.

Industry-initiated vs. investigator-initiated
An industry-initiated trial is a study that is developed, sponsored, and coordinated by a pharmaceutical or device company.[5] An investigator-initiated trial is a study that is developed and directed by a researcher.[5]

Intention-to-treat analysis
An analysis based on the initial treatment intent (i.e., initial group assignment), not on the treatment eventually administered.

Interaction
A statistical interaction between two variables occurs when the combined effect of two interventions is more than simply additive. If the combined effect augments the outcome, the interaction is synergistic. If the combined effect is weaker, the interaction is antagonistic.

Internal validity
The degree to which the inferences about the observed differences between two treatment groups of representative patients can be attributed only to the effect under investigation.

Intervention
A specific treatment (or placebo) administered to a study subject. A study question usually involves two or more competing interventions.

L'Abbé plot
A plot of study-level effect size versus a continuous study-level covariate, in which the size of the plotting symbol is proportional to the weight received by the study in the analysis.

Logistic regression
Popular regression technique used to model the relationship of several predictor variables to a dichotomous dependent variable. In case–control studies, the dependent variable is the disease state (present or absent); the independent variables include the exposure of interest.

Matching
Matching involves selecting a control or controls that have the same or a similar value as the case for identified confounding variables (e.g., age, gender).

Membership bias
Membership bias occurs when subjects who are members of a group have (or may have) a health status that differs from that of the general population.[1]

Meta-analysis
A quantitative systematic review in which statistical methods are used to combine the results of two or more studies.

Meta-regression analysis
When summarizing patient or design characteristics at the individual trial level, meta-analysts risk failing to detect genuine relationships between these characteristics and the size of the treatment effect. Further, the risk of obtaining a spurious explanation for variable treatment effects is high when the number of trials is small and many patient and design characteristics differ. Meta-regression techniques can be used to explore whether patient characteristics (e.g., younger or older age) or design characteristics (e.g., studies of low or high quality) are related to the size of the treatment effect.[4]

Methods center
The main facility that captures, stores, and manages data pertaining to the trial.

Minimization
Adjusts the probability of allocation depending on the balance of known important prognostic factors.

Multiple testing
Multiple testing occurs when investigators report the statistical significance of multiple outcomes being tested on

the same set of participants. If we test enough outcomes, the chance of seeing a difference increases just due to chance alone. Caution is needed when a single difference among many nonsignificant findings is reported.

Multivariate regression analysis (or Multivariable analysis, or Multivariable regression equation)

A type of regression that provides a mathematical model that attempts to explain or predict the dependent variable (or outcome variable or target variable) by simultaneously considering two or more independent variables (or predictor variables).[4]

Negative studies

Negative studies are those whose findings are not statistically significant.

Nested case–cohort study design

When a case–control study is incorporated or "nested" into a cohort study. The controls are a random sample selected from the entire cohort (cases and controls) and can be selected immediately (do not have to wait until a case occurs).

Nested case–control study design

When a case–control study is incorporated or "nested" into a cohort study. The cases include the persons with the outcome of interest that occurred during a cohort study. Similar to a case–control study, the controls are the individuals who are at risk in the cohort at the time the case develops but who do not develop the outcome.

Nonrespondent bias

A cohort of subjects who respond may differ in exposure and/or outcome from nonrespondents.[1]

Null hypothesis

The null hypothesis assumes that there is no significant difference between two groups.

Odds

The odds of an event is the probability that the event occurs divided by the probability that it does not occur.

Open-ended questions

Open-end questions are those that offer no specific structure for the respondent's answer.[6]

Ordinal scales

Scales, typically with three to nine possible values, that include extremes of attitudes or feelings (such as from "totally disagree" to "totally agree") and that investigators present to respondents to obtain their ratings of their responses.[6] Ordinal scales can be unipolar, where the scale is anchored at one end by the "zero point" (e.g., "none of the time" to "all the time"), or bipolar, where the "zero point" lies somewhere in the middle (e.g., "totally agree" to "neutral" to "totally disagree").

Outcome

The end result or consequence of interest in a clinical trial.

Outcome ascertainment

Outcome ascertainment is determining when or if the outcome has occurred. To standardize ascertainment among investigators and study centers, the definition of what constitutes an "outcome" needs to be defined at study outset.

Outcome variable (or Dependent variable, or Target variable)

The target variable of interest. The variable that is hypothesized to depend on or be caused by another variable (the independent variable).[4]

Overmatching

Overmatching means matching on variables that are not risk factors. This leads to decreased variance in the exposure variables, but does not control for any additional confounding.

Phenomenology

A qualitative theory that seeks to understand how individuals interpret and experience a particular phenomenon from the perspective of their own contextual framework.[7,20,21]

Popular media stream

The authorship context in which print and online materials are written by experts and nonexperts to inform society at large.

Positive studies

Positive studies are those whose findings are statistically significant.

Prevalence–incidence bias

Enrolling subjects at a later time than the time of exposure may miss fatal or silent cases.[1]

Prevalent cases

"Refers to the total number of people with a disease or condition in a certain population at a certain time. This includes both people who are newly diagnosed and those who have had the disease or condition for a long time. Prevalent cases must have been incident cases at some earlier point."[18]

Publication bias

Occurs when the publication of research depends on the direction of the study results and whether they are statistically significant.[4]

Purposive (theoretical) sampling

A method of sampling in qualitative research that seeks to round out concepts and reflect diversity in a population as information is gathered and theory emerges; this process is "responsive to the data"; participants are selected in each round of sampling with the intent of exploring a concept in greater depth.[22-24]

P value

A statistic that quantifies the probability of the results (or those more extreme) obtained in a research study occurring due to chance alone. By convention, *P* values lower than 0.05 are considered to be "statistically significant," meaning that the results are unlikely to be due to chance alone and are therefore assumed to be due to the intervention under study.

Qualitative heterogeneity

Individual components of a composite outcome are substantially different in clinical importance.

Quantitative heterogeneity

Individual components of a composite outcome occur at substantially different rates.

Random-effects analysis

A method of pooling or meta-regression that allows for unexplained variability in effect sizes among studies.

Random-effects regression

Random-effects regression assumes that no true treatment effect exists, but rather that a distribution of effects exists across different populations. Each study represents a sample from a unique population which estimates that population's true effect with some chance error. The difference between an individual study effect and the mean effect for the entire population is the chance difference between the individual study effect and that population's true effect (within-study variation) plus the difference between that population's true effect and the mean effect for all populations (between-study variation).

Randomization (or Random allocation)

Allocation of participants to groups by chance, usually done with the aid of a table of random numbers. Not to be confused with systematic allocation or quasi-randomization (e.g., on even and odd days of the month) or other allocation methods at the discretion of the investigator.[4]

Randomized controlled trial (or Randomized trial)

A randomized controlled trial (RCT) is an experiment in which individuals are randomly allocated to receive or not receive an experimental diagnostic, preventive, therapeutic, or palliative procedure and are then followed to determine the effect of the intervention.[4]

Recall bias

Occurs when patients who experience an adverse outcome have a different likelihood of recalling an exposure than patients who do not experience the adverse outcome, independent of the true extent of exposure.[4]

Receiver-operating characteristic curve

A figure depicting the power of a diagnostic test. The receiver-operating characteristic (ROC) curve presents the test's true-positive rate (i.e., sensitivity) on the horizontal axis and the false-positive rate (i.e., specificity) on the vertical axis for different cut points dividing a positive from a negative test. An ROC curve for a perfect test has an area under the curve equal to 1.0, while a test that performs no better than by chance has an area under the curve of only 0.5.[4]

Redundancy

Occurs when there are no more new themes identified in qualitative research and response coding becomes repetitive; this may be viewed as an appropriate stopping point for some studies.[23]

Reflexivity

The recognition that a researcher's own contextual framework and worldview influences the collection and analysis of data in qualitative research. In reflexivity, the researcher uses introspective techniques, such as journaling, to understand his or her own role in the qualitative process.[20,22]

Regression model

A statistical model that uses predictor or independent variables to build a statistical model that predicts an individual patient's status with respect to a dependent or target variable.[25]

Reliability

Assesses whether an instrument produces reproducible and internally consistent results.[6]

Residual confounding

Residual confounding arises when a confounding factor cannot be measured with sufficient precision to be quantified for the purposes of statistical adjustment.

Response bias

The tendency for a greater response rate to arise from a group of the sample that is bound by a similar characteristic.[6]

Responsiveness

This is the ability of a tool to detect a significant difference between two populations that is clinically relevant.

Sample size calculation

A mathematical formula that calculates the minimum number of subjects necessary to ensure that a difference defined as being clinically relevant would be statistically significant with a prespecified level of confidence. This calculation should be based on the primary outcome.

Saturation

The point at which no new information emerges from the data. It includes the subsequent categorization of meaningful terms, often into domains and subdomains; this often involves development of a conceptual model which illustrates relationships between domains.[7,16,23]

Selection bias

Selection bias is present when the study and control group subjects differ in the distribution of factors that might affect a given outcome of interest. These factors may be unknown or unmeasurable (e.g., motivation). Selection bias can only be controlled by random allocation into treatment groups such that each subject (with known and unknown characteristics) has an equal chance of being in either treatment group.

Sensitivity

The sensitivity of a test measures the proportion of people who truly have a designated disorder who are so identified by the test. The test may consist of, or include, clinical observations.[4]

Sensitivity analysis

Any test of the stability of the conclusions of a health care evaluation over a range of probability estimates, value judgments, and assumptions about the structure of the decisions to be made. This may involve the repeated evaluation of a decision model in which one or more of the parameters of interest are varied.[4]

Simple random sample

Random numbers are assigned to patients in a population and a subset is selected at random.

Specificity

The specificity of a test measures the proportion of people who are truly free of a designated disorder who are so identified by the test. The test may consist of, or include, clinical observations.[4]

Standardized mean difference

An effect size statistic that can be used for continuous data that standardizes based on the degree of variability of the outcomes. The standardized mean difference specifies in standardized units how much greater than the control the experimental group mean is.

Statistical pooling

The process by which abstracted data from individual studies are combined into a summary statistic that is produced in a meta-analysis.[4]

Steering committee

Committee comprised of investigators, physicians, and other experts not actively involved in the conduct of a study. This committee serves to oversee the data collection processes, direct the implementation of changes in procedures, and evaluate study progress.[10]

Stratification

The process of grouping individuals into strata based on an important known and measurable characteristic (such as study site or patient sex or age) to ensure that these characteristics are equally represented across the intervention groups.

Study question

In the context of a clinical trial, this is a question pertaining to the relationship between interventions and an outcome of interest. A study question usually involves two or more interventions (e.g., is intervention A better than intervention B? Is intervention A better than control?).

Subgroup analysis

Separate meta-analyses performed for different subsets of studies. The selection of studies for subgroup analysis is specified a priori.

Survival function

The probability that a subject's time to event will exceed some specified time. For each time point (t) this function provides a probability that a subject does not experience the event of interest before or on that particular time.

Systematic review

Rigorous review of specific clinical questions which summarize the original research following a scientifically based plan that has been decided in advance and made explicit at every step.

Systematic sampling

Random numbers are assigned to patients and a periodic process is used to select the sample.

Traditional review

A review in which a senior expert in the field summarizes evidence and recommendations for a broad research question.

Treatment effect

The impact of a treatment relative to a control; that is, how much better or worse a particular treatment may be relative to the control. Treatment effects are best assessed in randomized controlled clinical trials, although they may also be estimated from well-designed nonrandomized comparative studies.

Triangulation

Includes data triangulation, investigator triangulation, and theory triangulation. Generally speaking, triangulation is the use of multiple techniques, investigators, or theories in a qualitative study. Findings between methods are compared, not with the intention of reliability reporting, but with the purpose of producing a more comprehensive set of data.[16,23]

Type I error

A type I error is also known as an α-error or a false-positive result. Usually, investigators designate how much type I error is acceptable at the beginning of the trial. A nominal significance level, α, of ≤ 0.05 or 5% is commonly used. This means that we accept that there may be a 5% chance that the null hypothesis was falsely rejected.

Univariate regression

A regression model with just a single outcome and a single covariate.

Unmasking bias

An exposure that does not cause disease, but causes a symptom that leads the clinician to search for disease.[1]

Utilities

Utilities help to quantitatively assess the "value" of a certain health state with utilities between 0 (death) and 1 (perfect health). Utilities can then be transformed into quality-adjusted life years.

Validity

The degree to which the data measure what the data were intended to measure (i.e., the results of a measurement correspond to the true state of the phenomenon being measured). Another word for *validity* is *accuracy*.[26]

References

1. Sackett DL. Bias in analytical research. J Chron Dis 1979;32:51–63
2. Bhandari M, Petrisor B, Schemitsch E. Outcome measurements in orthopedics. Indian J Orthop 2007;41:32–36
3. Health Canada. Drugs and Health Products: Definitions. Available at: http://www.hc-sc.gc.ca/dhp-mps/prodpharma/activit/consultation/clini-rev-exam/definition-eng.php. Accessed February 9, 2010
4. Guyatt GH, Rennie D, Meade M, Cook D, eds. Users' Guide to the Medical Literature: A Manual for Evidence-Based Clinical Practice. 2nd ed. New York: McGraw-Hill; 2008
5. Altman R, Brandt K, Hochberg K, et al. Design and conduct of clinical trials in patients with osteoarthritis: recommendations from a task force of the Osteoarthritis Research Society. Osteoarthritis Cartilage 1996;4:217–243
6. Guyatt G, Rennie D, eds. In: Users' Guides to the Medical Literature: A Manual for Evidence-Based Clinical Practice. Chicago, IL: American Medical Association Press; 2002
7. Beaton D. Clark J. Qualitative research: a review of methods with use of examples from the total knee replacement literature. J Bone Joint Surg Am 2009;91(Suppl 3):107–112
8. Clark JP, Hudak PL, Hawker GA, et al. The moving target: a qualitative study of elderly patients' decision-making regarding total joint replacement surgery. J Bone Joint Surg Am 2004;86:1366–1374
9. Lo B, Field, MJ. Conflict of Interest in Medical Research, Education, and Practice. Washington, DC: The National Academies Press; 2009
10. Isaacsohn JL, Khodadad TA, Soldano-Noble C, Vest JD. The challenges of conducting clinical endpoint studies. Curr Atheroscler Rep 2003;5:11–14
11. Walter SD, Cook DJ, Guyatt GH, King D, Troyan S. Outcome assessment for clinical trials: how many adjudicators do we need? Controlled Clinical Trials 1997;18:27–42
12. Hamilton Health Sciences Research Ethics Board. Available at http://www-fhs.mcmaster.ca/healthresearch/reb/forms.html. Accessed February 26, 2010
13. Ionnidis JP, Trikalinos TA. The appropriateness of asymmetry tests for publication bias in meta-analyses: a large survey. CMAJ 2007;176:1091–1096
14. Lau J, Ioannidis JP, Terrin N, Schmid CH, Olkin I. The case of the misleading funnel plot. BMJ 2006;333:597–600
15. Terrin N, Schmid CH, Lau J. In an empirical evaluation of the funnel plot, researchers could not visually identify publication bias. J Clin Epidemiol 2005;58:894–901
16. Kuper A, Reeves S, Levinson W. An introduction to reading and appraising qualitative research. BMJ 2008;337:a288
17. Lingard L, Albert M, Levinson W. Grounded theory, mixed methods, and action research. BMJ 2008;337:a567
18. Bhandari M, Joensson A. Clinical research for surgeons. New York: Thieme; 2009
19. Bhandari M, Tornetta P, III, Guyatt GH. Glossary of evidence-based orthopaedic terminology. Clin Orthop Relat Res 2003;158–163
20. Kuper A, Reeves S, Levinson W. An introduction to reading and appraising qualitative research. BMJ 2008;337:a288
21. Reeves S, Albert M, Kuper A, Hodges BD. Why use theories in qualitative research? BMJ 2008;337:a949
22. Kuper A, Lingard L, Levinson W. Critically appraising qualitative research. BMJ 2008;337:a1035
23. Giacomini M, Cook D. Qualitative research. In: Guyatt G, Rennie D, Meade M, Cook D, eds. Users' Guides to the Medical Literature: A Manual for Evidence-Based Clinical Practice. 2nd ed. New York, NY: McGraw-Hill; 2008:341–360
24. Corbin J, Strauss A. Basics of Qualitative Research. Thousand Oaks, CA: Sage; 2008:vii–381
25. Samartzis D, Perera R. Meta-analysis: statistical methods for binary data pooling. Spine J 2009;9:424–425
26. Fletcher RH, Fletcher SW. Systematic reviews. In: Sun B, Linkins E, eds. Clinical epidemiology: the essentials. 4th ed. Baltimore, MD: Lippincott Williams & Wilkins; 2005: 205–220

Index